Twelfth Edition

Curren's Math FOR Meds

Dosages and Solutions

Gladdi Tomlinson, RN, MSN
HACC, Central Pennsylvania's Community College

Lou Ann Boose, RN, MSN
HACC, Central Pennsylvania's Community College

Anna M. Curren, RN, MA

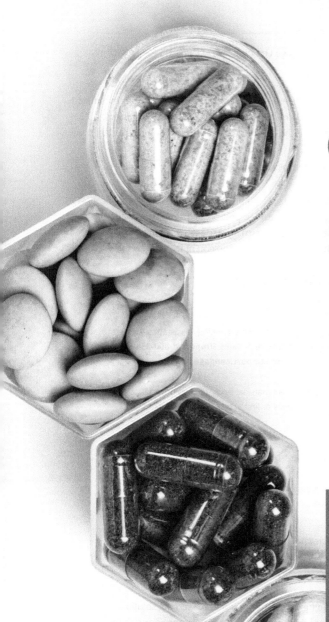

❊ Cengage

Australia • Brazil • Canada • Mexico • Singapore • United Kingdom • United States

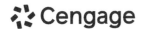

Curren's Math for Meds, **Twelfth Edition**
Gladdi Tomlinson, Lou Ann Boose, and Anna M. Curren

SVP, Product: Cheryl Costantini

VP, Product: Thais Alencar

Product Director: Jason Fremder

Associate Product Director: Laura Stewart

Portfolio Product Manager: Andrea Henderson

Product Assistant: Isaiah Johnson

Learning Designer: Natalie Goforth

Content Manager: Christy Frame

Digital Project Manager: Pradhiba Kannaiyan

VP, Product Marketing: Jason Sakos

Director, Product Marketing: Neena Bali

Product Marketing Manager: Joann Gillingham

Content Acquisition Analyst: Erin McCullough

Production Service: MPS Limited

Designer: Felicia Benett

Cover Image Source: Syringe and vial: ChooChin/Shutterstock.com; Capsules and pills: Natalia Golubnycha/Shutterstock.com.

For product information and technology assistance, contact us at
**Cengage Customer & Sales Support, 1-800-354-9706
or support.cengage.com.**

For permission to use material from this text or product, submit all
requests online at **www.copyright.com.**

Library of Congress Control Number: 2023917267

ISBN: 978-0-357-76807-5

Cengage
5191 Natorp Boulevard
Mason, OH 45040
USA

Cengage is a leading provider of customized learning solutions. Our employees reside in nearly 40 different countries and serve digital learners in 165 countries around the world. Find your local representative at **www.cengage.com.**

To learn more about Cengage platforms and services, register or access your online learning solution, or purchase materials for your course, visit **www.cengage.com.**

Printed at CLDPC, USA, 10-24

Contents

Section 1 Refresher Math

Chapter 1
Relative Value, Addition, and Subtraction of Decimals   2

Chapter 2
Multiplication and Division of Decimals   12

Chapter 3
Solving Common Fraction Equations   23

Section 2 Introduction to Drug Measures

Chapter 4
Metric/International (SI) System   38

Chapter 5
Unit, Percentage, Milliequivalent, Ratio, and Household Measures   50

Section 3 Preparing for Medication Administration

Chapter 6
Safe Medication Administration   60

Chapter 7
Interpreting Drug Labels   72

Chapter 8
Ratio and Proportion   103

Preface

Curren's Math for Meds: Dosages & Solutions, twelfth edition, is your best resource for success in dosage calculations. With a growing record of positive instruction with hundreds of thousands of users, its fully self-instructional approach fosters achievement and confidence as the ideal choice for both learners and instructors.

A large part of the credit for this successful journey lies in the fact that *Curren's Math for Meds,* twelfth edition, has integrated current information, while never losing sight of the students it was designed to teach. Medication labels have been updated to reflect medications currently in use in clinical practice settings. *Curren's Math for Meds* is the only calculations text of its kind that is completely focused to teach from simple to complex. It focuses on dosage calculation and eliminates the unnecessary. Instruction is consistently geared toward clinical realities and offers a solid and seamless learning process from day one until program completion.

Organization

Curren's Math for Meds allows for self-paced study, progressing from basic to more complex information. All learners are encouraged to complete the Refresher Math PreTest on page xviii to determine their competence in basic math skills. Section 1, Refresher Math, is also recommended for all learners, as this information is included in the examples throughout the text. Calculators are used routinely in clinical facilities and on the National Council Licensure Examination (NCLEX) exam, and their use is encouraged in this text. Although calculators are encouraged, students are taught not to rely solely on calculators. They are encouraged to use critical thinking and clinical judgment to evaluate their answers and determine if they are logical. Consistent rounding recommendations are presented throughout the book to prevent inaccuracies in calculations.

Once the fundamental skills are mastered, the learner will move on to the basics needed for calculating dosages and administering medications safely. Metric system units and milliequivalent dosages; reading dosage labels and syringe calibrations; and working with reconstituted drugs and insulin are some of the topics covered, with an emphasis on safety. Hundreds of sample dosage problems will reinforce this information.

With these basic skills solidified, students are prepared to progress to advanced calculations. Calculations based on body weight and body surface area are presented, as well as a chapter on pediatric dosage calculations. Finally, chapters discussing intravenous therapy, intravenous calculations, and intravenous drips are presented.

Features

Curren's Math for Meds, twelfth edition, offers examples and practice problems throughout to enhance comprehension. Answers are provided immediately following the practice problems, allowing the learner to receive immediate feedback on deficits and strengths. Comprehensive summary self-tests are presented at the end of each chapter. The terms *patient* and *client* are used interchangeably throughout the book to identify any recipient of health care. An icon 🔌 is used throughout the chapters to allow learners to easily identify important information and KEY*points.* The most up-to-date equipment and safety devices are depicted in color, and real, full-color drug labels and syringes are included with explanations and dosage problems. Students using *Curren's Math for Meds* will have the tools to safely prepare and administer medications, and to become safe practitioners in a clinical setting.

New to This Edition

▷ Many new medication labels have been added to reflect the most up-to-date information on the market. Additional labels have been added to the practice problems and summary self-tests. A medication label index has been added to this edition.

▷ The order of chapters was revised to present a more orderly flow of information for the students.

▷ A Clinical Relevance consideration is presented in many of the chapters to encourage the student to apply the information in the chapter to the clinical setting.

▷ The three methods of calculation are presented in all the dosage calculation chapters. Students are encouraged to select the method of their choice.

▷ The chapter on IV drips has been enhanced to include additional advanced calculations and medication labels.

▷ Critical Thinking Questions are presented at the end of many of the chapters with answers and rationales.

▷ Appendix A, Equivalents, has been revised to put less emphasis on the apothecary system and instead address equivalents in general. A table with common equivalents used for conversions includes household and metric equivalents. Apothecary equivalents are provided for information only.

▷ Appendix B has been updated with the current ISMP List of Error-Prone Abbreviations, Symbols, and Dose Designations.

▷ Appendix C, Insulin, has been added with information addressing the types of insulin and clinical considerations.

Student Resources

Additional student resources for this product are available online. Sign up or sign in at **www.cengage.com** to search for and access this product and its online resources.

⁂ Cengage WebAssign Prepare for class with confidence using Web Assign from Cengage for *Curren's Math for Meds,* twelfth edition. This online learning platform, which includes an interactive ebook, fuels practice, so you truly absorb what you learn—and are better prepared come test time. Videos and tutorials walk you through concepts and deliver instant feedback and grading, so you always know where you stand in class. Focus your study time and get extra practice where you need it most. Study smarter with WebAssign!

Ask your instructor today how you can get access to WebAssign, or learn about self-study options at www.webassign.com.

Instructor Resources

Additional instructor resources for this product are available online. Instructor assets include an Instructor's Manual, Educator's Guide, PowerPoint® slides, Solution and Answer Guide, and a test bank powered by Cognero®. Sign up or sign in at **www.cengage.com** to search for and access this product and its online resources.

Cengage WebAssign   WebAssign from Cengage for *Curren's Math for Meds*, twelfth edition, is a fully customizable online solution, including an interactive ebook, for STEM disciplines that empowers you to help your students learn, not just do homework. Insightful tools save you time and highlight exactly where your students are struggling. Decide when and what type of help students can access while working on assignments—and incentivize independent work so help features aren't abused. Meanwhile, your students get an engaging experience, instant feedback, and better outcomes. A total win-win!

To try a sample assignment, learn about LMS integration, or connect with our digital course support, visit www.webassign.com/cengage.

Introduction for the Learner

This text will be an important resource throughout your academic studies and career. On completion of your instruction with *Curren's Math for Meds: Dosages & Solutions,* twelfth edition, you will find that you have the calculation skills required to safely practice in your profession. You do not have to be a math expert to be successful in dosage calculations; what you do need is a desire for accuracy and a motivation to learn. If you have not used your math skills for several years, Section 1, Refresher Math, will quickly bring you up to date. *Curren's Math for Meds* is fully self-instructional and lets you move at your own pace through the content. Hundreds of examples and problems will keep your learning on track. Here are some tips to help you get started.

1. Gather a calculator, pencil or pen, and plenty of scratch paper.

2. Start by completing the Refresher Math PreTest on page xviii. This will alert you to those areas in Section 1, Refresher Math, that will need your particular attention. Some of the items in the PreTest and Refresher Math section were designed to be completed without using a calculator, but the choice is entirely yours; when you need a calculator, use one. You must remember, however, that calculator settings vary. Pay careful attention to the rounding recommendations throughout the text.

3. Record the answers to calculations on the scratch paper as well as in your text. This makes checking your answers against those we provide much easier.

4. As you work your way through the chapters, do exactly as you are instructed. The book proceeds from simple to more complex calculations and presents the information in a step-by-step manner. The steps must be followed carefully; jumping ahead may cause confusion. All chapters are designed to let you move at your own speed.

Introduction
for the Instructor

Welcome to the twelfth edition of *Curren's Math for Meds*. Whether you are a seasoned user of this text or are becoming acquainted with it for the first time, we would like to share a few ideas on how to incorporate this bestselling text most effectively into your curriculum. *Curren's Math for Meds* is designed to be used starting early in the students' beginning semester. Many instructors assign the Refresher Math Pre-Test and the entire Section 1, Refresher Math, to be completed before the semester starts, and test on it within the first two weeks. Chapters can also be assigned on a weekly basis at a pace fitting your students' learning needs. In addition, answers found directly after the problem sets in each chapter will provide immediate feedback for the student.

Students have many demands on their schedule, and experience has shown that they learn best when their progress is routinely both encouraged and monitored. A short weekly test of about 10 questions on the content assigned is the ideal way to do this. If a student struggles with the first test, provide a makeup opportunity. If a second test is unsuccessful, you will need to delve more deeply to determine the exact problem and help the student establish a study plan. The content in Section 1 is ideally suited to bring students up to the level of math skills required for success in dosage calculations.

Using the Learning Package

▷ **Clinical Relevance** discussions are presented at the beginning of most chapters in a shaded box to provide applications of the content to the clinical setting. These discussions are useful in providing a context for safe and accurate medication administration.

Clinical Relevance: Two tablets labeled 0.05 mg each are administered to your client. What is the total amount of medication administered? Knowledge of basic information related to calculations involving decimals will provide a foundation for calculation of some basic dosage problems and can be used to determine how much medication is administered to a client. Using critical thinking and application of the principles learned in this chapter, you can determine that the total amount the client has received is 0.1 mg.

▷ An **icon** designates important reminders to help with calculations and to highlight important safety considerations. As you study for your exams, locate these **KEYpoints** and make sure you know and understand them. Consider making flash cards of these considerations.

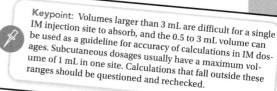 **Key**point: Volumes larger than 3 mL are difficult for a single IM injection site to absorb, and the 0.5 to 3 mL volume can be used as a guideline for accuracy of calculations in IM dosages. Subcutaneous dosages usually have a maximum volume of 1 mL in one site. Calculations that fall outside these ranges should be questioned and rechecked.

▷ **Examples** walk you through each concept in a step-by-step manner, showing the calculation and mathematical processes. Focus on these areas to be sure you understand how to do each different type of calculation.

Example 1 ■

The client weighs 220 pounds and for treatment purposes, we must calculate their weight in kilograms. Recall that 2.2 pounds is equal to 1 kilogram. Recall that, for conversions, D will be the unit of measure we want to convert. In this example, we are given the information of 220 pounds. Use the formula method to set up this conversion.

$$\frac{220\ lb \times 1\ kg}{2.2\ lb} = x\ kg$$

Next, eliminate lb in the numerator and denominator.

$$\frac{220\ \cancel{lb} \times 1\ kg}{2.2\ \cancel{lb}} = x\ kg$$

$$100\ kg = x$$

Answer: After completing the calculation, 220 pounds is equal to 100 kg.

▶ **Problems** for practice are provided throughout each chapter. This is your opportunity to put your skills to the test, to identify your areas of strength, and to also acknowledge those areas where you need additional study. Answers to all problems are printed in the accompanying shaded box. Double-check your calculations if you have difficulty or talk to your instructor for additional help.

Problems 14.3

For each of the following combined R and NPH insulin dosages, indicate the total volume of the combined dosage and the smallest capacity syringe you can use to prepare it; 30, 50, and 100 unit capacity syringes are available.

	Total Volume	Syringe Size
1. 28 units R, 64 units NPH	_____	_____
2. 6 units R, 16 units NPH	_____	_____
3. 33 units R, 41 units NPH	_____	_____
4. 21 units R, 52 units NPH	_____	_____
5. 13 units R, 27 units NPH	_____	_____

▶ Actual **full-color labels** are used to support the problems and examples. Challenge yourself to read the labels carefully and accurately. Are you able to understand the quantity, strength, form, dosing, and administration guidelines for every label you encounter?

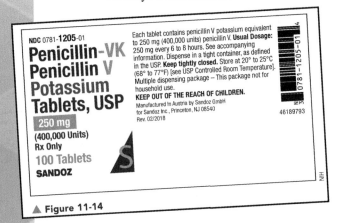

NDC 0781-1205-01

Penicillin-VK
Penicillin V
Potassium
Tablets, USP

250 mg
(400,000 Units)
Rx Only
100 Tablets
SANDOZ

Each tablet contains penicillin V potassium equivalent to 250 mg (400,000 units) penicillin V. **Usual Dosage:** 250 mg every 6 to 8 hours. See accompanying information. Dispense in a tight container, as defined in the USP. **Keep tightly closed.** Store at 20° to 25°C (68° to 77°F) [see USP Controlled Room Temperature]. Multiple dispensing package -- This package not for household use.
KEEP OUT OF THE REACH OF CHILDREN.
Manufactured in Austria by Sandoz GmbH
for Sandoz Inc., Princeton, NJ 08540
Rev. 02/2018

46189793

0781-1205-01

▲ **Figure 11-14**

▶ **Images of syringes** are depicted so that you can gain confidence in perfecting the real-life skill of accurately reading and interpreting syringe calibrations and medication levels.

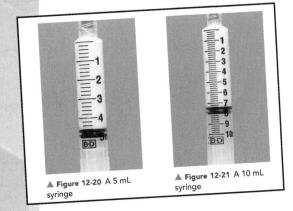

▲ **Figure 12-20** A 5 mL syringe

▲ **Figure 12-21** A 10 mL syringe

▷ **Summary Self-Tests** are located at the end of each chapter. Complete these as you finish studying the material, identify areas where you need to focus, and review the content again until you are confident in your calculating ability. Some of these tests include combined label and syringe questions, where you must calculate a dosage and then measure the dosage on a syringe. This is an excellent tool to test how well you apply your knowledge.

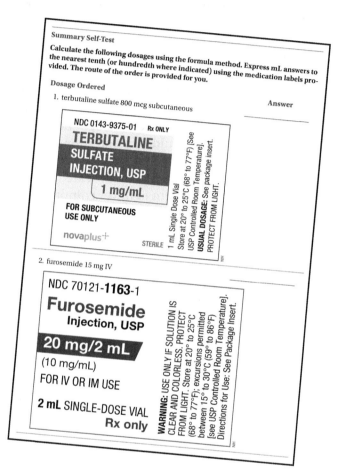

▷ **Critical Thinking Questions** follow the summary self-tests in some chapters. These questions provide challenging situations and encourage practice with exercising clinical judgment and critical thinking.

Critical Thinking Questions

1. Mr. Kline, a 60-year-old male client, has been admitted with a glucose level of 450 mg/dL. The client weighs 120 kg and is scheduled to receive an insulin drip to infuse at 9 units/hr. The IV bag will be prepared by the nurse. The order is to add 35 units to a 250 mL sodium chloride IV bag. Choose the following relevant data as it relates to the preparation and administration of this IV drip. Select all that apply.

   a. Add regular insulin to the IV bag with a 1 mL syringe.
   b. Calculate the flow rate at 7.1 mL/hr.
   c. Use a 50-unit insulin syringe to prepare the IV bag.
   d. Calculate the flow rate at 64.3 mL/hr.
   e. Choose a D_5 NS IV bag for preparation.

Acknowledgments

We offer our thanks to the Cengage team for their belief and confidence in us as new authors to revise a textbook that has been successfully published since the 1990s.

We would like to thank and acknowledge our colleagues at the college and affiliated clinical settings for valuing health care education and modeling safe care.

We offer our thanks to the students who use this book to learn and reinforce safe medication administration, and believe that mastering dosage calculations is imperative for competency and proficiency in practice.

Finally, we would like to acknowledge the late Ron Rebuck, our former Nursing Program Director, for his guidance and support of nursing faculty and his respect for our ideas and our autonomy. He truly believed in the importance of competency in dosage calculation. He was a true advocate for our students and conveyed his love of nursing by educating them to never compromise safe patient care.

Dedications

Lou Ann Boose

I am truly grateful to Gladdi for having the confidence in me to help revise this book dedicated to safe medication administration. I have cherished our years of friendship. A special and loving thank you to my husband, Paul, who supported me unconditionally every day through this journey. To my son Kyle, who makes me so proud and gave me encouragement in my efforts to write this book. To my mom, who at this writing is 91 years old, for her love, encouragement, and her belief in me from infancy on. My dad, who passed away, is always in my heart and is my guiding force. To my siblings Anna May, "Bud," Joyce, and Jennifer, who have always been a great influence in my life. Finally, my work on this book is in loving memory of my son, Justin, who passed away in 2020 from complications related to a car accident in 2007. Justin, you remain forever in my heart. Your journey through the health care system inspires me to teach my students to aim to provide consistently safe, compassionate, and quality care. I love you.

Gladdi Tomlinson

My deepest appreciation and gratitude to my colleague and dear friend, Lou Ann, for taking on this journey with me. Without her creativity and vision, this book would not be possible. To my love, Jeff, a heartfelt thank you for your unending support, love and encouragement to me throughout this endeavor. To my daughter, Jessica, and grandson, Grayson, who always bring me joy and happiness. For my siblings, Tom, Mollie, and Todd, and their everlasting inspiration. To my friend, Barb, who always cared enough to make sure I wasn't overworking. Finally, a special thank you to my parents who gave me love, and guidance throughout the years. I know they would be proud.

Refresher Math PreTest

If you can complete the PreTest with 100% accuracy, you are off to an exceptional start. However, don't be alarmed if you make some errors because the Refresher Math section that follows is designed to bring your math skills up to date. **Regardless of your proficiency, it's important that you complete the entire Refresher Math section of the book.** It includes memory cues and shortcuts for simplifying and solving many of the clinical calculations that are included in the entire text, and you will need to be familiar with these.

Identify the decimal fraction with the greatest value in each set.

1. a) 4.4   b) 2.85   c) 5.3   _____
2. a) 6.3   b) 5.73   c) 4.4   _____
3. a) 0.18   b) 0.62   c) 0.35   _____
4. a) 0.2   b) 0.125   c) 0.3   _____
5. a) 0.15   b) 0.11   c) 0.14   _____
6. a) 4.27   b) 4.31   c) 4.09   _____

Add these decimals.

7. $0.2 + 2.23 =$ _____
8. $1.5 + 0.07 =$ _____
9. $6.45 + 12.1 + 9.54 =$ _____
10. $0.35 + 8.37 + 5.15 =$ _____

Subtract these decimals.

11. $3.1 - 0.67 =$ _____
12. $12.41 - 2.11 =$ _____
13. $2.235 - 0.094 =$ _____
14. $4.65 - 0.7 =$ _____

Perform the following calculations.

15. If tablets with a strength of 0.2 mg are available and 0.6 mg is ordered, how many tablets must you give? _____
16. If tablets are labeled 0.8 mg and 0.4 mg is ordered, how many tablets must you give? _____
17. If the available tablets have a strength of 1.25 mg and 2.5 mg is ordered, how many tablets must you give? _____
18. If 0.125 mg is ordered and the tablets available are labeled 0.25 mg, how many tablets must you give? _____

Round these to the nearest tenth.

19. $2.17 =$ _____
20. $0.15 =$ _____
21. $3.77 =$ _____
22. $4.62 =$ _____
23. $11.74 =$ _____
24. $5.26 =$ _____

Round these to the nearest hundredth.

25. $1.357 =$ _____
26. $7.413 =$ _____
27. $10.105 =$ _____

28. $3.775 =$ _____
29. $0.176 =$ _____

Multiply these decimals. Round your answers to the nearest tenth.

30. $0.7 \times 1.2 =$ _____
31. $1.8 \times 2.6 =$ _____
32. $5.1 \times 0.25 \times 1.1 =$ _____
33. $3.3 \times 3.75 =$ _____

Divide these fractions. Round your answers to the nearest hundredth.

34. $16.3 \div 3.2 =$ _____
35. $15.1 \div 1.1 =$ _____
36. $2 \div 0.75 =$ _____
37. $4.17 \div 2.7 =$ _____

Provide the definitions for the following terms.

38. Numerator

_____

_____

39. Denominator

_____

_____

40. Highest common denominator

_____

_____

41. Product

_____

_____

Solve these equations. Express your answers to the nearest tenth.

42. $\dfrac{1}{4} \times \dfrac{2}{3} =$ _____

43. $\dfrac{240}{170} \times \dfrac{135}{300} =$ _____

44. $\dfrac{0.2}{1.75} \times \dfrac{1.5}{0.2} =$ _____

45. $\dfrac{2.1}{3.6} \times \dfrac{1.7}{1.3} =$ _____

46. $\dfrac{0.26}{0.2} \times \dfrac{3.3}{1.2} =$ _____

47. $\dfrac{750}{1} \times \dfrac{300}{50} \times \dfrac{7}{2} =$ _____

48. $\dfrac{50}{1} \times \dfrac{60}{240} \times \dfrac{1}{900} \times \dfrac{400}{1} =$ _____

49. $\dfrac{35,000}{750} \times \dfrac{35}{1} =$ _____

50. $\dfrac{50}{40} \times \dfrac{450}{40} \times \dfrac{1}{900} \times \dfrac{114}{1} =$ _____

Refresher Math

Relative Value, Addition, and Subtraction of Decimals

Objectives

The learner will:

1. identify the relative value of decimals.
2. add decimals.
3. subtract decimals.

Prerequisites

Recognize the abbreviations mg for milligram, and g for gram, as drug measures.

In the course of administering medications, you will be dealing with decimal fraction dosages on a daily basis. The first two chapters of this text provide a complete refresher on everything you need to know about decimals, including safety measures when you do calculations both manually and with a calculator. We'll start with a review of the range of decimal values you will see in dosages. This will enable you to recognize which of two or more numbers has the greater (or lesser) value—a skill you will use constantly in your professional career.

Clinical Relevance: Two tablets labeled 0.05 mg each are administered to your client. What is the total amount of medication administered? Knowledge of basic information related to calculations involving decimals will provide a foundation for calculation of some basic dosage problems and can be used to determine how much medication is administered to a client. Using critical thinking and application of the principles learned in this chapter, you can determine that the total amount the client has received is 0.1 mg.

Relative Value of Decimals

The most helpful fact to remember about decimals is that our monetary system of dollars and cents is a decimal system. The whole numbers in dosages have the same relative value as dollars, and decimal fractions have the same value as cents: The greater the number, the greater the value. If you keep this in mind, you will have already learned the most important safety measure of dealing with decimals in dosages.

The range of drug dosages, which includes decimal fractions, stretches from millions on the whole number side, to thousandths on the decimal side. Refer to the decimal scale in Figure 1-1, and locate the decimal point, which is slightly to the right on this scale. Notice the whole numbers on the left of the scale, which rise increasingly in value from ones (units) to millions, which is the largest whole-number drug dosage in current use.

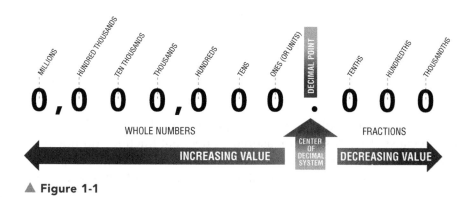

▲ Figure 1-1

 Keypoint: The first determiner of the relative value of decimals is the presence of whole numbers. The greater the whole number, the greater the value.

Example 1 ▪   10.1 is greater than 9.15

Example 2 ▪   3.2 is greater than 2.99

Example 3 ▪   7.01 is greater than 6.99

Problems 1.1

Choose the greatest value in each set.

1. a) 3.5	b) 2.7	c) 4.2	_____
2. a) 6.15	b) 5.95	c) 4.54	_____
3. a) 12.02	b) 10.19	c) 11.04	_____
4. a) 2.5	b) 1.75	c) 0.75	_____
5. a) 4.3	b) 2.75	c) 5.1	_____
6. a) 6.15	b) 7.4	c) 5.95	_____
7. a) 7.25	b) 8.1	c) 9.37	_____
8. a) 4.25	b) 5.1	c) 3.75	_____
9. a) 9.4	b) 8.75	c) 7.4	_____
10. a) 5.1	b) 6.33	c) 4.2	_____

Answers **1.** c **2.** a **3.** a **4.** a **5.** c **6.** b **7.** c **8.** b **9.** a **10.** b

If, however, the whole numbers are the same—for example, **10**.2 and **10**.7—or there are no whole numbers—for example, **0**.25 and **0**.35—then the fraction will determine the relative value. Let's review the fractional side of the scale (refer to Figure 1-2).

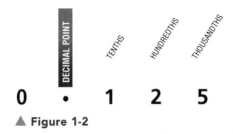

▲ **Figure 1-2**

It is necessary to consider only three figures after the decimal point on the fractional side because drug dosages measured as decimal fractions do not contain more than three digits; for example, 0.125 mg. Notice that a zero is used to replace the whole number in this decimal fraction and in all dosages that do not contain a whole number.

 Keypoint: If a decimal fraction is not preceded by a whole number, a zero is used in front of the decimal point to emphasize the decimal point and identify the number as a fraction. This is known as a leading zero.

Example 4 ▪   0.125   0.1   0.45

Review Figure 1-2 again. The numbers to the right of the decimal point represent tenths, hundredths, and thousandths, in that order. When you see a decimal fraction in which the whole numbers are the same, or there are no whole numbers, stop and look first at the number representing tenths.

 Keypoint: The fraction with the greater number representing tenths has the greater value.

Example 5 ▪   0.3 is greater than 0.27

Example 6 ▪   0.4 is greater than 0.29

Example 7 ▪   1.2 is greater than 1.19

Example 8 ▪   3.5 is greater than 3.2

Problems 1.2

Choose the greatest value in each set.

1. a) 0.4	b) 0.2	c) 0.5	_____
2. a) 2.73	b) 2.61	c) 2.87	_____
3. a) 0.19	b) 0.61	c) 0.34	_____
4. a) 3.5	b) 3.75	c) 3.25	_____

5. a) 0.3   b) 0.25   c) 0.4   _____
6. a) 1.35   b) 1.29   c) 1.4   _____
7. a) 2.5   b) 2.7   c) 2.35   _____
8. a) 4.51   b) 4.75   c) 4.8   _____
9. a) 0.8   b) 0.3   c) 0.4   _____
10. a) 2.1   b) 2.05   c) 2.25   _____

Answers   1. c. **2.** c **3.** b **4.** b **5.** c **6.** c **7.** b **8.** c **9.** a **10.** c

If in decimal fractions the numbers representing the tenths are identical—for example, 0.25 and 0.27—then the number representing the hundredths will determine the relative value.

 Keypoint: When the tenths are identical, the fraction with the greater number representing hundredths will have the greater value.

Example 9 ▦   0.27 is greater than 0.2**5**

Example 10 ▦   0.1**5** is greater than 0.1 (0.1 is the same as 0.1**0**)

 Keypoint: Extra zeros at the end of decimal fractions, also known as trailing zeros, are omitted in drug dosages because they can easily be misread and lead to errors.

Example 11 ▦   2.2**5** is greater than 2.2 (same as 2.2**0**)

Example 12 ▦   9.7**7** is greater than 9.7 (same as 9.7**0**)

Problems 1.3

Choose the greatest value in each set.

1. a) 0.12   b) 0.15   c) 0.17   _____
2. a) 1.2   b) 1.24   c) 1.23   _____
3. a) 0.37   b) 0.3   c) 0.36   _____
4. a) 3.27   b) 3.25   c) 3.21   _____
5. a) 0.16   b) 0.11   c) 0.19   _____
6. a) 4.23   b) 4.2   c) 4.21   _____
7. a) 3.27   b) 3.21   c) 3.29   _____
8. a) 2.75   b) 2.73   c) 2.78   _____
9. a) 0.31   b) 0.37   c) 0.33   _____
10. a) 0.43   b) 0.45   c) 0.44   _____

Answers   1. c **2.** b **3.** a **4.** a **5.** c **6.** a **7.** c **8.** c **9.** b **10.** b

Now consider the following decimal fractions. Which fraction has the greater value? Check the tenths carefully, regardless of the total of numbers after the decimal point.

0.125   or   0.25

If you chose 0.125, you have just made a serious drug dosage error. Look again at the numbers representing the tenths, and you will see that 0.**2**5 is greater than 0.**1**25. Remember that extra zeros are omitted in decimal fraction dosages because they can lead to errors. In this fraction, 0.25 is the same as 0.250, which is exactly double the value of 0.125.

Example 13 ▦   0.15 (same as 0.150) is greater than 0.125

Example 14 ▦   0.3 (same as 0.30) is greater than 0.15

Example 15 ▦   0.75 (same as 0.750) is greater than 0.325

Example 16 ▦   0.8 (same as 0.80) is greater than 0.16

 Keypoint: The number of figures on the right of the decimal point is not an indication of relative value. Always look at the figure representing the tenths first, and if these are identical, check the hundredths to determine which has the greater value.

This completes your introduction to the relative value of decimals. The key points just reviewed will cover all situations in dosage calculations in which you will have to recognize greater and lesser values. Test yourself more extensively on this information in the following problems.

Problems 1.4

Choose the greatest value in each set.

1. a) 0.24	b) 0.5	c) 0.125	_____
2. a) 0.4	b) 0.45	c) 0.5	_____
3. a) 7.5	b) 6.25	c) 4.75	_____
4. a) 0.3	b) 0.25	c) 0.35	_____
5. a) 1.125	b) 1.75	c) 1.5	_____
6. a) 4.5	b) 4.75	c) 4.25	_____
7. a) 0.1	b) 0.01	c) 0.04	_____
8. a) 5.75	b) 6.25	c) 6.5	_____
9. a) 0.6	b) 0.16	c) 0.06	_____
10. a) 3.55	b) 2.95	c) 3.7	_____

Answers **1.** b **2.** c **3.** a **4.** c **5.** b **6.** b **7.** a **8.** c **9.** a **10.** c

Addition and Subtraction of Decimals

Complex addition and subtraction of decimals should be done with a calculator, but sometimes it is quicker to do simple calculations without one. Also, during a crisis, such as a severe weather event or disaster, calculators may not be available. Let's start by reviewing a few key points that will make manual solution safer.

 Keypoint: When you write down the numbers, line up the decimal points.

Example 1 ■   To add 0.25 and 0.27

$$
\begin{array}{l}
0.25 \\
+0.27 \text{ is safe}
\end{array}
\qquad
\begin{array}{l}
0.25 \\
+0.27 \text{ is unsafe; it could lead to errors.}
\end{array}
$$

 Keypoint: Always add or subtract from right to left.

If you decide to write down the numbers, do not confuse yourself by trying to estimate the answer as this may introduce errors. Also, write any numbers carried or rewrite those reduced by borrowing if you find this helpful.

Example 2 ■   When adding 0.25 and 0.27

$$
\begin{array}{r}
{\scriptstyle 1} \\
0.25 \\
+\underline{0.27} \\
0.52
\end{array}
\qquad
\begin{array}{l}
\text{Add the 5 and 7 first, then the 2, 2, and} \\
\text{the 1 you carried; work from right to left.}
\end{array}
$$

Example 3 ■   When subtracting 0.63 from 0.71

$$
\begin{array}{r}
{\scriptstyle 6\,1} \\
0.71 \\
-\underline{0.63} \\
0.08
\end{array}
\qquad
\begin{array}{l}
\text{Borrow 1 from 7 and rewrite as 6.} \\
\text{Write the borrowed 1; subtract 3 from 11.} \\
\text{Subtract 6 from 6; work from right to left.}
\end{array}
$$

 Keypoint: Add zeros as necessary to make the fractions of equal length.

Adding zeros to make the fractions of equal length does not alter the value of the fractions, and it helps prevent confusion and mistakes.

Example 4 ■   When subtracting 0.125 from 0.25

$$
\begin{array}{l}
0.25 \\
-\underline{0.125}
\end{array}
\quad
\begin{array}{l}
\text{becomes} \\
\text{becomes}
\end{array}
\quad
\begin{array}{l}
0.250 \\
-\underline{0.125}
\end{array}
$$

Answer: 0.125

If you follow these simple rules and make them a habit, you will automatically reduce calculation errors. The following problems will give you an excellent opportunity to practice addition and subtraction.

Problems 1.5

Note: For safety reasons, it is important to develop the habit of using leading zeros and eliminating trailing zeros. In the following problems, if you do not add a zero before the decimal point in answers that do not contain a whole number, or fail to eliminate unnecessary zeros from the end of decimal fractions, your answers will be incorrect.

Add decimals.

1. 0.25 + 0.55 = _____
2. 0.1 + 2.25 = _____
3. 1.74 + 0.76 = _____
4. 1.4 + 0.02 = _____
5. 2.3 + 1.45 = _____

6. 3.75 + 1.05 = _____
7. 6.35 + 2.05 = _____
8. 5.57 + 4.03 = _____
9. 0.33 + 2.42 = _____
10. 1.44 + 3.06 = _____

Subtract decimals.

11. 1.25 − 1.125 = _____
12. 3.25 − 0.65 = _____
13. 2.3 − 1.45   = _____
14. 0.02 − 0.01 = _____
15. 5.5 − 2.5   = _____

16. 7.33 − 4.03 = _____
17. 4.25 − 1.75 = _____
18. 0.07 − 0.035 = _____
19. 0.235 − 0.12 = _____
20. 5.75 − 0.95 = _____

Answers 1. 0.8 **2.** 2.35 **3.** 2.5 **4.** 1.42 **5.** 3.75 **6.** 4.8 **7.** 8.4 **8.** 9.6 **9.** 2.75 **10.** 4.5 **11.** 0.125 **12.** 2.6 **13.** 0.85 **14.** 0.01 **15.** 3 **16.** 3.3 **17.** 2.5 **18.** 0.035 **19.** 0.115 **20.** 4.8

Summary

This concludes the refresher on relative value, addition, and subtraction of simple decimal fractions. The important points to remember from this chapter are:

- If a decimal fraction contains a whole number, the value of the whole number is the first determiner of relative value.

- If a fraction does not include a whole number, a zero is placed in front of the decimal point to emphasize that it is a fractional dosage.

- If there is no whole number, or if the whole numbers are the same, the number representing the tenths in the decimal fraction will be the next determiner of relative value.

- If the tenths in decimal fractions are identical, the number representing hundredths will determine relative value.

- When manually adding or subtracting decimal fractions, first line up the decimal points, then add or subtract from right to left.

▓ Extra zeros on the end of decimal fractions can be a source of error in drug dosages and are routinely eliminated.

▓ When using a calculator, remember to triple-check your answers as it is very easy to enter incorrect data.

Summary Self-Test

Choose the decimal with the greatest value.

1. a) 2.45	b) 2.57	c) 2.19	_____
2. a) 3.07	b) 3.17	c) 3.71	_____
3. a) 0.12	b) 0.02	c) 0.01	_____
4. a) 5.31	b) 5.35	c) 6.01	_____
5. a) 4.5	b) 4.51	c) 4.15	_____
6. a) 0.015	b) 0.15	c) 0.1	_____
7. a) 1.3	b) 1.25	c) 1.35	_____
8. a) 0.1	b) 0.2	c) 0.25	_____
9. a) 0.125	b) 0.1	c) 0.05	_____
10. a) 13.7	b) 13.5	c) 13.25	_____

Use critical thinking to choose the best answer.

11. If you have medication tablets whose strength is 0.1 mg and you must give 0.3 mg, you will need

    a) 1 tab   b) less than 1 tab   c) more than 1 tab   _____

12. If you have tablets with a strength of 0.25 mg and you must give 0.125 mg, you will need

    a) 1 tab   b) less than 1 tab   c) more than 1 tab   _____

13. If you have an order to give a dosage of 7.5 mg and the tablets have a strength of 3.75 mg, you will need

    a) 1 tab   b) less than 1 tab   c) more than 1 tab   _____

14. If the order is to give 0.5 mg and the tablet strength is 0.5 mg, you will give

    a) 1 tab   b) less than 1 tab   c) more than 1 tab   _____

15. The order is to give 0.5 mg and the tablets have a strength of 0.25 mg. You must give

    a) 1 tab   b) less than 1 tab   c) more than 1 tab   _____

Note: Remember, for safety reasons, it is important to develop the habit of using leading zeros and eliminating trailing zeros. For the following problems, if you do not add a zero before the decimal point in answers that do not contain a whole number or fail to eliminate unnecessary zeros from the end of decimal fractions, your answers will be incorrect.

Add the decimals manually.

16. $1.31 + 0.4$ = _____

17. $0.15 + 0.25$ = _____

18. $2.5 + 0.75$ = _____

19. $3.2 + 2.17$ = _____

20. $1.3 + 1.04$ = _____

21. $4.7 + 3.03$ = _____

22. $0.5 + 0.5$ = _____

23. $5.4 + 2.6$ = _____

Use critical thinking to answer the following.

24. You have just given 2 tab with a dosage strength of 3.5 mg each. What was the total dosage administered?   _____

25. You are to give your client 1 tab labeled 0.5 mg and one labeled 0.25 mg. What is the total dosage of these two tablets?   _____

26. If you give 2 tab labeled 0.02 mg each, what total dosage will you administer?   _____

27. You are to give 1 tab labeled 0.8 mg and 2 tab labeled 0.4 mg each. What is the total dosage?   _____

28. You have two tablets: one is labeled 0.15 mg and the other 0.3 mg. What is the total dosage of these two tablets?   _____

Subtract the decimals manually.

29. $4.32 - 3.1$ = _____

30. $2.1 - 1.91$ = _____

31. $3.73 - 1.93$ = _____

32. $5.75 - 4.05$ = _____

33. $1.3 - 0.02$ = _____

34. $0.2 - 0.07$ = _____

35. $3.95 - 0.35$ = _____

36. $1.9 - 0.08$ = _____

Use critical thinking to answer the following.

37. Your client is to receive a dosage of 7.5 mg and you have only 1 tab labeled 3.75 mg. How many more milligrams must you give?   _____

38. You have a tablet labeled 0.02 mg and your client is to receive 0.06 mg. How many more milligrams must you give?   _____

39. The tablet available is labeled 0.5 mg, but you must give a dosage of 1.5 mg. How many more milligrams will you need to obtain the correct dosage?   _____

40. Your client is to receive a dosage of 1.2 mg and you have 1 tab labeled 0.6 mg. What additional dosage in milligrams will you need?   _____

41. You must give your client a dosage of 2.2 mg, but you have only 2 tab labeled 0.55 mg each. What additional dosage in milligrams will you need?   _____

Determine how many tablets will be needed to give the following dosages.

42. Tablets are labeled 0.01 mg. You must give 0.02 mg.   _____

43. Tablets are labeled 2.5 mg. You must give 5 mg.   _____

44. Tablets are labeled 0.25 mg. Give 0.125 mg.   _____

45. Tablets are 0.5 mg. Give 1.5 mg.   _____

46. A dosage of 1.8 mg is ordered. Tablets are 0.6 mg.   _____

47. Tablets available are 0.04 mg. You are to give 0.02 mg.   _____

48. The dosage ordered is 3.5 mg. The tablets available are 1.75 mg.   _____

49. Prepare a dosage of 3.2 mg using tablets with a strength of 1.6 mg.   _____

50. You have tablets labeled 0.25 mg and a dosage of 0.375 mg is
    ordered.   _____

Answers to Summary Self-Test

1. b	**11.** c	**21.** 7.73	**31.** 1.8	**41.** 1.1 mg
2. c	**12.** b	**22.** 1	**32.** 1.7	**42.** 2 tab
3. a	**13.** c	**23.** 8	**33.** 1.28	**43.** 2 tab
4. c	**14.** a	**24.** 7 mg	**34.** 0.13	**44.** ½ tab
5. b	**15.** c	**25.** 0.75 mg	**35.** 3.6	**45.** 3 tab
6. b	**16.** 1.71	**26.** 0.04 mg	**36.** 1.82	**46.** 3 tab
7. c	**17.** 0.4	**27.** 1.6 mg	**37.** 3.75 mg	**47.** ½ tab
8. c	**18.** 3.25	**28.** 0.45 mg	**38.** 0.04 mg	**48.** 2 tab
9. a	**19.** 5.37	**29.** 1.22	**39.** 1 mg	**49.** 2 tab
10. a	**20.** 2.34	**30.** 0.19	**40.** 0.6 mg	**50.** 1½ tab

Multiplication and Division of Decimals

Multiplication and division are integral parts of dosage calculations. As is the case with addition and subtraction, some multiplication and division problems involving dosages can be done manually, so the basic steps in multiplication and division are reviewed in this chapter. In addition, a number of shortcuts will be introduced that can make numbers easier to work with, especially those containing decimal fractions. And for those calculations that are more safely handled with a calculator, safety in calculator use will be discussed.

Clinical Relevance: Decimal fractions are used frequently to order medications. It is important to understand how to interpret decimals and perform calculations. Misplacing a decimal point can result in a tenfold or more increase or decrease in medication dosages. It is important to verify accuracy of your calculations in all situations, including when using a calculator. Rounding is also a critical skill as many medications are administered in syringes that require rounding to the tenth or the hundredth so they can be measured accurately in the syringe or administration device.

Multiplication of Decimals

The main precaution in multiplication of decimals is the placement of the decimal point in the answer, which is called the **product**.

Keypoint: The placement of the decimal point in the product is determined by counting the number of places to the right of the decimal point in each of the multipliers. These are totaled and the decimal point in the product is then placed that many places to the left.

Example 1 ■   Multiply 0.35 by 0.5

It is safer to begin by lining up the numbers to be multiplied on the right side. Then, disregard the decimals during multiplication.

$$
\begin{array}{r}
0.35 \\
\times\ \underline{0.5} \\
175
\end{array}
$$
Line up the numbers on the right.

The product/answer is 175; 0.35 has two numbers after the decimal and 0.5 has one. Place the decimal point three places to the left in the product to make it .175, then add a zero (0) in front of the decimal to emphasize the fraction.

Answer: 0.175

Example 2 ■   Multiply 1.61 by 0.2

$$
\begin{array}{r}
1.61 \\
\times\ \underline{0.2} \\
322
\end{array}
$$
Line up the numbers on the right.

The product is 322; 1.61 has two numbers after the decimal point and 0.2 has one. Place the decimal point three places to the left in the product so that 322 becomes .322, then add a zero in front of the decimal to emphasize the fraction.

Answer: 0.322

Keypoint: If the product contains insufficient numbers for correct placement of the decimal point, add as many zeros as necessary to the left of the product to correct this.

Example 3 ■   Multiply 1.5 by 0.06

$$
\begin{array}{r}
1.5 \\
\times\ \underline{0.06} \\
90
\end{array}
$$
Line up the numbers on the right.

The product is 90; 1.5 has one number after the decimal point and 0.06 has two. To place the decimal three places to the left in the product, a zero must be added, making it .090. Eliminate the excess zero from the end of the fraction and add a zero in front of the decimal point.

Answer: 0.09

Example 4 ◼   Multiply 0.21 by 0.32

$$\begin{array}{r}0.21\\ \times\,0.32\\\hline 42\\ 63\\\hline 672\end{array}$$

     Indent second number multiplication.
     Add the totals.

In this example, 0.21 has two numbers after the decimal point and 0.32 also has two. Add a zero in front of 672 to allow correct placement of the decimal point, making it .0672, then add a zero in front of the fraction to emphasize it.

Answer: 0.0672

Example 5 ◼   Multiply 0.12 by 0.2

$$\begin{array}{r}0.12\\ \times\;\;0.2\\\hline 24\end{array}$$

In this example, there are a total of three numbers after the decimal points in 0.12 and 0.2. Add a zero in front of 24 for correct decimal placement, making it .024, then add a zero in front of .024 to emphasize the fraction.

Answer: 0.024

Problems 2.1

Multiply the decimal fractions without using a calculator.

1. 0.45×0.2 = _____
2. 0.35×0.12 = _____
3. 1.3×0.05 = _____
4. 0.7×0.04 = _____
5. 0.4×0.17 = _____
6. 2.14×0.03 = _____
7. 1.4×0.4 = _____
8. 3.3×1.2 = _____
9. 2.7×2.2 = _____
10. 2.1×0.3 = _____

Answers **1.** 0.09 **2.** 0.042 **3.** 0.065 **4.** 0.028 **5.** 0.068 **6.** 0.0642 **7.** 0.56 **8.** 3.96 **9.** 5.94 **10.** 0.63

Division of Decimal Fractions

A calculator may also be used for division of complex decimal fractions. However, let's start by reviewing the terminology of common fraction division, and three important pre-calculator steps that may make final manual division easier: elimination of decimal points, reduction of the fractions, and reduction of numbers ending in zero. The following is a sample of a common fraction division seen in dosages.

Example ◼ $\dfrac{0.25}{0.125} = \dfrac{\text{numerator}}{\text{denominator}}$

Recall that the top number in a common fraction is called the **numerator**, whereas the bottom number is called the **denominator**. To remember which is which, think of D, for down, for denominator. The denominator is on the bottom. With this basic terminology reviewed, we are now ready to review preliminary math steps that can be used to simplify a fraction or actually solve an equation and eliminate the need for calculator division.

Elimination of Decimal Points

Decimal points can be eliminated from numbers in a decimal fraction without changing its value, if they are moved the same number of places in one numerator and one denominator.

> **Key**point: To eliminate the decimal points from decimal fractions, move them the same number of places to the right in a numerator and a denominator until they are eliminated from both. Zeros may have to be added to accomplish this.

Example 1 ■ $\dfrac{0.25}{0.125}$ becomes $\dfrac{250}{125}$

The decimal point must be moved three places to the right in the denominator 0.125 to make it 125. Therefore, it must be moved three places to the right in the numerator 0.25, which requires the addition of one zero to make it 250.

Example 2 ■ $\dfrac{0.3}{0.15}$ becomes $\dfrac{30}{15}$

The decimal point must be moved two places in 0.15 to make it 15, so it must be moved two places in 0.3, which requires the addition of one zero to become 30.

Example 3 ■ $\dfrac{1.5}{2}$ becomes $\dfrac{15}{20}$

Move the decimal point one place in 1.5 to make it 15; add one zero to 2 to make it 20.

Example 4 ■ $\dfrac{4.5}{0.95}$ becomes $\dfrac{450}{95}$

> **Key**point: As long as both the numerator and denominator are changed, eliminating the decimal points from a decimal fraction before final division does not alter the value of the fraction. By moving the decimal point the same number of places in the numerator and the denominator, the end result is equivalent to multiplying the fraction by 1; therefore, the answer obtained in the final division will not be altered.

Problems 2.2

Eliminate the decimal points from these common fractions.

1. $\dfrac{17.5}{2}$ = _____

2. $\dfrac{0.5}{25}$ = _____

3. $\dfrac{6.3}{0.6}$ = _____

4. $\dfrac{3.76}{0.4}$ = _____

5. $\dfrac{8.4}{0.7}$ = _____

6. $\dfrac{0.1}{0.05}$ = _____

7. $\dfrac{0.9}{0.03}$ = _____

8. $\dfrac{10.75}{2.5}$ = _____

9. $\dfrac{0.4}{0.04}$ = _____

10. $\dfrac{1.2}{0.4}$ = _____

Answers 1. $\dfrac{175}{20}$ 2. $\dfrac{5}{250}$ 3. $\dfrac{63}{6}$ 4. $\dfrac{376}{40}$ 5. $\dfrac{84}{7}$ 6. $\dfrac{10}{5}$ 7. $\dfrac{90}{3}$ 8. $\dfrac{1,075}{250}$ 9. $\dfrac{40}{4}$ 10. $\dfrac{12}{4}$

Reduction of Fractions

Once the decimals are eliminated, a second simplification step is to reduce the numbers as far as possible using common denominators/divisors. The largest number that will evenly divide both a numerator and a denominator should be used.

Keypoint: To further reduce fractions, divide numbers by their greatest common denominator (the largest number that will divide into both a numerator and a denominator).

The **greatest common denominator** is usually 2, 3, 4, 5, or multiples of these numbers, such as 6, 8, 25, and so on.

Example 1 ▪ $\dfrac{175}{20}$ The greatest common denominator is 5

$$\dfrac{\cancel{175}}{\cancel{20}} = \dfrac{35}{4}$$

Example 2 ▪ $\dfrac{63}{6}$ The greatest common denominator is 3

$$\dfrac{\cancel{63}}{\cancel{6}} = \dfrac{21}{2}$$

Example 3 ▪ $\dfrac{1,075}{250}$ The greatest common denominator is 25

$$\dfrac{\cancel{1,075}}{\cancel{250}} = \dfrac{43}{10}$$

There is a second way you could have reduced the fraction in Example 3, and it is equally as correct. Divide by 5, then by 5 again.

$$\dfrac{\cancel{1,075}}{\cancel{250}} = \dfrac{\cancel{215}}{\cancel{50}} = \dfrac{43}{10}$$

Keypoint: If the greatest common denominator is difficult to determine, reduce several times by using smaller common denominators.

Example 4 ■ $\dfrac{376}{40} = \dfrac{47}{5}$ Divide by 8

Or divide by 4, then 2 $\dfrac{376}{40} = \dfrac{94}{10} = \dfrac{47}{5}$

Or divide by 2, then 2, then 2 $\dfrac{376}{40} = \dfrac{188}{20} = \dfrac{94}{10} = \dfrac{47}{5}$

Remember that simple numbers are easiest to work with, and the time spent in extra reductions may be well worth the payoff in safety.

Problems 2.3

Reduce the fractions in preparation for final division.

1. $\dfrac{84}{8}$ = _____

2. $\dfrac{20}{16}$ = _____

3. $\dfrac{250}{325}$ = _____

4. $\dfrac{96}{34}$ = _____

5. $\dfrac{175}{20}$ = _____

6. $\dfrac{40}{14}$ = _____

7. $\dfrac{82}{28}$ = _____

8. $\dfrac{100}{75}$ = _____

9. $\dfrac{50}{75}$ = _____

10. $\dfrac{60}{88}$ = _____

Answers **1.** $\frac{21}{2}$ **2.** $\frac{5}{4}$ **3.** $\frac{10}{13}$ **4.** $\frac{48}{17}$ **5.** $\frac{35}{4}$ **6.** $\frac{20}{7}$ **7.** $\frac{41}{14}$ **8.** $\frac{4}{3}$ **9.** $\frac{2}{3}$ **10.** $\frac{15}{22}$

Reduction of Numbers Ending in Zero

The third type of simplification is not solely related to decimal fractions but is best covered at this time. This concerns reductions in a common fraction when both a numerator and a denominator end with zeros.

 Keypoint: Numbers that end in a zero or zeros may be reduced by crossing off the same number of zeros in both a numerator and a denominator.

Example 1 ■ $\dfrac{800}{250}$

In this fraction, the numerator, 800, has two zeros, but the denominator, 250, has one zero. The number of zeros crossed off must be the same in both numerator and denominator, so only one zero can be eliminated from each.

$$\dfrac{800}{250} = \dfrac{80}{25} \qquad \text{Reduce by } 5 = \dfrac{16}{5}$$

Example 2 ■ $\dfrac{2,4\cancel{00}}{2,0\cancel{00}} = \dfrac{24}{20}$ Reduce by 4 $= \dfrac{6}{5}$

Two zeros can be eliminated from the denominator and the numerator in this fraction.

Example 3 ■ $\dfrac{15,\cancel{000}}{30,\cancel{000}} = \dfrac{15}{30}$ Reduce by 5 $= \dfrac{1}{2}$

In this fraction, three zeros can be eliminated.

Problems 2.4

Reduce the fractions to their lowest terms.

1. $\dfrac{50}{250}$ = _____

2. $\dfrac{120}{50}$ = _____

3. $\dfrac{2,500}{1,500}$ = _____

4. $\dfrac{1,000,000}{750,000}$ = _____

5. $\dfrac{800}{150}$ = _____

6. $\dfrac{110}{100}$ = _____

7. $\dfrac{200,000}{150,000}$ = _____

8. $\dfrac{1,000}{800}$ = _____

9. $\dfrac{60}{40}$ = _____

10. $\dfrac{150}{200}$ = _____

Answers   1. $\frac{1}{5}$ 2. $\frac{12}{5}$ 3. $\frac{5}{3}$ 4. $\frac{4}{3}$ 5. $\frac{16}{3}$ 6. $\frac{11}{10}$ 7. $\frac{4}{3}$ 8. $\frac{5}{4}$ 9. $\frac{3}{2}$ 10. $\frac{3}{4}$

Using a Calculator

Calculators vary in how addition, subtraction, division, and multiplication must be entered, and in the number of fractional numbers displayed after the decimal point. The first precaution in calculator use is to ensure that you know how to use the one available to you. If you must do frequent calculations, it would be wise to buy and use your own. The next precaution—and this is critical—is to enter decimal numbers correctly, which includes entering the decimal points. This is not as easy to remember as it sounds, and this is a step where dosage calculation errors can occur.

 Keypoint: Calculator entry errors tend to be repetitive, so visually check each entry before entering the next.

Expressing to the Nearest Tenth

When a fraction is reduced as much as possible, it is ready for final division. If necessary, this is done using a calculator to divide the numerator by the denominator. Dosage answers are most frequently rounded off and expressed as decimal fractions to the nearest tenth.

Keypoint: To express an answer to the nearest tenth, the division is carried to hundredths (two places after the decimal). When the number representing hundredths is 5 or larger, the number representing tenths is increased by one. If the number representing hundredths is less than 5, the number representing tenths remains unchanged.

Example 1 ▥ $\dfrac{0.35}{0.4} = 0.35 \div 0.4 = 0.87$

          Answer: 0.9

The number representing hundredths is 7, so the number representing tenths is increased by one: 0.87 becomes 0.9.

Example 2 ▥ $\dfrac{0.5}{0.3} = 0.5 \div 0.3 = 1.66 = \mathbf{1.7}$

The number representing hundredths, 6, is larger than 5, so 1.66 becomes 1.7.

Example 3 ▥ $\dfrac{0.16}{0.3} = 0.53 = \mathbf{0.5}$

The number representing hundredths, 3, is less than 5, so the number representing tenths, 5, remains unchanged.

Example 4 ▥ $\dfrac{0.2}{0.3} = 0.66 = \mathbf{0.7}$

Example 5 ▥   An answer of 1.42 remains **1.4**

Example 6 ▥   An answer of 1.86 becomes **1.9**

Problems 2.5

Use a calculator to divide the common fractions. Express answers to the nearest tenth.

1. $\dfrac{5.1}{2.3} =$ _____

2. $\dfrac{0.9}{0.7} =$ _____

3. $\dfrac{3.7}{2} =$ _____

4. $\dfrac{6}{1.3} =$ _____

5. $\dfrac{1.5}{2.1} =$ _____

6. $\dfrac{2.7}{1.1} =$ _____

7. $\dfrac{4.2}{5} =$ _____

8. $\dfrac{0.5}{2.5} =$ _____

9. $\dfrac{5.2}{0.91} =$ _____

10. $\dfrac{2.4}{2.7} =$ _____

Answers **1.** 2.2 **2.** 1.3 **3.** 1.9 **4.** 4.6 **5.** 0.7 **6.** 2.5 **7.** 0.8 **8.** 0.2 **9.** 5.7 **10.** 0.9

Expressing to the Nearest Hundredth

Some drugs are administered in dosages carried to the nearest hundredth. This is common in pediatric dosages and in drugs that alter a vital function of the body—for example, heart rate.

> **Key**point: To express an answer to the nearest hundredth, the division is carried to thousandths (three places after the decimal point). When the number representing thousandths is 5 or larger, the number representing hundredths is increased by one. If the number representing thousandths is less than 5, the number representing hundredths remains unchanged.

Example 1 ▪   0.736   becomes   **0.74**

The number representing thousandths, 6, is larger than 5, so the number representing hundredths, 3, is increased by one to become 4.

Example 2 ▪   0.777   becomes   **0.78**

Example 3 ▪   0.373   remains   **0.37**

The number representing thousandths, 3, is less than 5, so the number representing hundredths, 7, remains unchanged.

Example 4 ▪   0.934   remains   **0.93**

Problems 2.6

Express the numbers to the nearest hundredth.

1. 0.175 = _____
2. 0.344 = _____
3. 1.853 = _____
4. 0.306 = _____
5. 3.015 = _____
6. 2.154 = _____
7. 1.081 = _____
8. 1.327 = _____
9. 0.739 = _____
10. 0.733 = _____
11. 2.072 = _____
12. 0.089 = _____

Answers **1.** 0.18 **2.** 0.34 **3.** 1.85 **4.** 0.31 **5.** 3.02 **6.** 2.15 **7.** 1.08 **8.** 1.33 **9.** 0.74 **10.** 0.73 **11.** 2.07 **12.** 0.09

Summary

This concludes the chapter on multiplication and division of decimals. The important points to remember from this chapter are:

▪   When decimal fractions are multiplied manually, the decimal point is placed the same number of places to the left in the product as the total of numbers after the decimal points in the fractions multiplied.

▢ Zeros must be placed in front of a product if it contains insufficient numbers for the correct placement of the decimal point.

▢ Excess trailing zeros are eliminated in dosages.

▢ To simplify fractions for final division, the preliminary steps of eliminating decimal points, reducing the numbers by common denominators, and reducing numbers ending in zeros can be used.

▢ To express to tenths, increase the answer by one if the number representing the hundredths is 5 or larger. If the number representing the hundredths is less than 5 there is no change to the number in the tenths place.

▢ To express to hundredths, increase the answer by one if the number representing the thousandths is 5 or larger. If the number representing the thousandths is less than 5 there is no change to the number in the hundredths place.

▢ Practice using a calculator until proficiency is achieved.

▢ All calculator entries and answers must be triple-checked to ensure accuracy.

▢ Calculator running totals should be disregarded because they can cause confusion.

▢ A personal calculator is a must if frequent calculations are necessary.

Summary Self-Test

Multiply the decimals. A calculator may be used. Do not round your answers.

1. $1.49 \times 0.05 =$ _____

2. $0.15 \times 3.04 =$ _____

3. $0.025 \times 3.5 =$ _____

4. $0.55 \times 2.5 \ =$ _____

5. $1.31 \times 2.07 =$ _____

6. $5.3 \times 1.02 \ =$ _____

7. $0.35 \times 1.25 =$ _____

8. $4.32 \times 0.05 =$ _____

9. $0.2 \times 0.02 \ =$ _____

10. $0.4 \times 1.75 \ =$ _____

Use critical thinking to answer the following.

11. You are to administer 4 tab with a dosage strength of 0.04 mg each. What total dosage are you giving? _____

12. You have given 2½ (2.5) tab with a strength of 1.25 mg per tablet. What total dosage is this? _____

13. The tablets your client is to receive are labeled 0.1 mg, and you are to give 3½ (3.5) tab. What total dosage is this? _____

14. You gave your client 3 tab labeled 0.75 mg each, and they were to receive a total of 2.25 mg. Did they receive the correct dosage? _____

15. The tablets available for your client are labeled 12.5 mg, and you are to give 4½ (4.5) tab. What total dosage will this be? _____

16. Your client is to receive a dosage of 4.5 mg. The tablets available are labeled 3.5 mg, and there are 2½ tab in their medication drawer. Is this a correct dosage? _____

Divide the fractions. Express answers to the nearest tenth. A calculator may be used.

17. $\dfrac{1.3}{0.7}$ = _____

18. $\dfrac{1.9}{3.2}$ = _____

19. $\dfrac{32.5}{9}$ = _____

20. $\dfrac{0.04}{0.1}$ = _____

21. $\dfrac{1.45}{1.2}$ = _____

22. $\dfrac{250}{1,000}$ = _____

23. $\dfrac{0.8}{0.09}$ = _____

24. $\dfrac{2,000,000}{1,500,000}$ = _____

25. $\dfrac{4.1}{2.05}$ = _____

26. $\dfrac{7.3}{12}$ = _____

27. $\dfrac{150,000}{120,000}$ = _____

28. $\dfrac{0.15}{0.08}$ = _____

29. $\dfrac{2,700}{900}$ = _____

30. $\dfrac{0.25}{0.15}$ = _____

Divide the fractions. Express answers to the nearest hundredth. A calculator may be used.

31. $\dfrac{900}{1,700}$ = _____

32. $\dfrac{0.125}{0.3}$ = _____

33. $\dfrac{1,450}{1,500}$ = _____

34. $\dfrac{65}{175}$ = _____

35. $\dfrac{0.6}{1.35}$ = _____

36. $\dfrac{0.04}{0.12}$ = _____

37. $\dfrac{750}{10,000}$ = _____

38. $\dfrac{0.65}{0.8}$ = _____

39. $\dfrac{3.01}{4.2}$ = _____

40. $\dfrac{4.5}{6.1}$ = _____

41. $\dfrac{0.13}{0.25}$ = _____

42. $\dfrac{0.25}{0.7}$ = _____

43. $\dfrac{3.3}{5.1}$ = _____

44. $\dfrac{0.19}{0.7}$ = _____

45. $\dfrac{1.1}{1.3}$ = _____

46. $\dfrac{3}{4.1}$ = _____

47. $\dfrac{62}{240}$ = _____

48. $\dfrac{280,000}{300,000}$ = _____

49. $\dfrac{115}{255}$ = _____

50. $\dfrac{10}{14.3}$ = _____

Answers to Summary Self-Test				
1. 0.0745	**11.** 0.16 mg	**21.** 1.2	**31.** 0.53	**41.** 0.52
2. 0.456	**12.** 3.125 mg	**22.** 0.3	**32.** 0.42	**42.** 0.36
3. 0.0875	**13.** 0.35 mg	**23.** 8.9	**33.** 0.97	**43.** 0.65
4. 1.375	**14.** yes	**24.** 1.3	**34.** 0.37	**44.** 0.27
5. 2.7117	**15.** 56.25 mg	**25.** 2	**35.** 0.44	**45.** 0.85
6. 5.406	**16.** no	**26.** 0.6	**36.** 0.33	**46.** 0.73
7. 0.4375	**17.** 1.9	**27.** 1.3	**37.** 0.08	**47.** 0.26
8. 0.216	**18.** 0.6	**28.** 1.9	**38.** 0.81	**48.** 0.93
9. 0.004	**19.** 3.6	**29.** 3	**39.** 0.72	**49.** 0.45
10. 0.7	**20.** 0.4	**30.** 1.7	**40.** 0.74	**50.** 0.7

Solving Common Fraction Equations

The majority of clinical drug dosage calculations involve solving an equation containing one to five common fractions. Two examples are:

$$\frac{2}{5} \times \frac{3}{4} \quad \text{and} \quad \frac{20}{1} \times \frac{1,000}{60,000} \times \frac{1,200}{1} \times \frac{1}{60}$$

Two options are available to solve common fraction equations: calculator use throughout, or initial fraction reduction followed by calculator use for final division. Both options are presented in this chapter, and you may use whichever you wish, or whichever your instructor requires.

 Keypoint: Common fraction equations are solved by dividing the numerators by the denominators.

It is important that you do the calculations for each example and then compare them with the math provided. Just reading the examples will not teach you the calculation skills you need. The examples and problems provided incorporate all the content covered in the first two chapters. They represent the full range of calculations you will be doing on a continuing basis.

 Keypoint: Calculator solution of equations is most safely done by concentrating only on the entries being made, not the numbers that register and change throughout the calculation. Remember, when using a calculator, it is important to triple-check data to ensure accuracy.

Clinical Relevance: The use of fractions is common in the calculation of dosages. For this reason, it is imperative to understand how to interpret a fraction and perform calculations that involve fractions. Remember that a fraction such as $\frac{125}{250}$ is read as 125 divided by 250. It is helpful to determine if the fraction has an overall value greater than or equal to 1.

Objectives

The learner will:

1. solve equations containing whole numbers.
2. solve equations containing decimal numbers.
3. solve equations containing multiple numbers.

Prerequisites

Chapters 1 and 2

For example, the fraction $\frac{125}{250}$ has a value less than one, whereas $\frac{350}{125}$ has a value greater than one. When working with a formula that includes a fraction, this concept will be helpful for critical thinking.

When performing calculations that involve several fractions in an equation, it is important to multiply all the numerators first and then divide by the denominators to obtain your answer. Your answer should then be rounded according to guidelines of the clinical setting and the equipment that is available for medication administration. This allows for the greatest accuracy.

Whole-Number Equations

The fractions used in dosage calculation may include whole numbers or decimals. Some equations will involve fractions composed completely of whole numbers, whereas others will contain decimals or a combination of decimals and whole numbers. We will discuss whole number fractions first.

Example 1 ■   **Option 1: Calculator Use Throughout**

$$\frac{2}{5} \times \frac{3}{4}$$

$2 \times 3 \div 5 \div 4$ Multiply the numerators, 2 and 3, and then divide by the denominators, 5 then 4, in continuous entries.

$= 0.3$

Answer: 0.3 (tenth)

Option 2: Initial Reduction of Fractions

$$\frac{2}{5} \times \frac{3}{4}$$

$$\frac{{}^1\cancel{2}}{5} \times \frac{3}{\cancel{4}_2}$$ Divide the numerator, 2, and the denominator, 4, by 2 (to become 1 and 2).

$3 \div 5 \div 2$ Use the calculator to divide the remaining numerator, 3, by the remaining denominators, 5 and 2.

$= 0.3$

Answer: 0.3 (tenth)

 Keypoint: Initial reduction of fractions in an equation can simplify final calculator entries, especially if the numbers are large or contain decimal fractions or zeros.

Example 2 ■   **Option 1: Calculator Use Throughout**

$$\frac{250}{175} \times \frac{150}{325}$$

$$250 \times 150 \div 175 \div 325$$

Multiply the numerators, 250 and 150, then divide by the denominators, 175 and 325.

$$= 0.659$$

Answer: 0.7 (tenth) or 0.66 (hundredth)

Option 2: Initial Reduction of Fractions

$$\frac{250}{175} \times \frac{150}{325}$$

$$\frac{\overset{10}{250}}{\underset{7}{175}} \times \frac{\overset{6}{150}}{\underset{13}{325}}$$

Divide the numerator, 250, and the denominator, 175, by 25 (to become 10 and 7); divide the numerator, 150, and the denominator, 325, by 25 (to become 6 and 13).

$$10 \times 6 \div 7 \div 13$$

Use the calculator to multiply the numerators, 10 and 6, then divide by the denominators, 7 and 13.

$$= 0.659$$

Answer: 0.7 (tenth) or 0.66 (hundredth)

Example 3 ■

Option 1: Calculator Use Throughout

$$\frac{7}{50} \times \frac{25}{3} \times \frac{120}{32}$$

$$7 \times 25 \times 120 \div 50 \div 3 \div 32$$

Multiply the numerators, 7, 25, and 120, then divide by the denominators, 50, 3, and 32.

$$= 4.375$$

Answer: 4.4 (tenth) or 4.38 (hundredth)

Option 2: Initial Reduction of Fractions

$$\frac{7}{50} \times \frac{25}{3} \times \frac{120}{32}$$

$$\frac{7}{\underset{2}{50}} \times \frac{\overset{1}{25}}{3} \times \frac{\overset{15}{120}}{\underset{4}{32}}$$

Divide 25 and 50 by 25, then divide 120 and 32 by 8.

$$7 \times 15 \div 2 \div 3 \div 4$$

$$= 4.375$$

Answer: 4.4 (tenth) or 4.38 (hundredth)

Example 4 ■

Option 1: Calculator Use Throughout

$$\frac{20}{1} \times \frac{1,000}{60,000} \times \frac{1,200}{1} \times \frac{1}{60}$$

$$20 \times 1,000 \times 1,200 \div 60,000 \div 60$$

$$= 6.666$$

Answer: 6.7 (tenth) or 6.67 (hundredth)

Option 2: Initial Reduction of Fractions

$$\frac{20}{1} \times \frac{1{,}000}{60{,}000} \times \frac{1{,}200}{1} \times \frac{1}{60}$$

This will take several steps to reduce the fractions.

$$\frac{20}{1} \times \frac{\overset{1}{1{,}\cancel{000}}}{\underset{60}{\cancel{60{,}000}}} \times \frac{\overset{120}{1{,}\cancel{200}}}{1} \times \frac{1}{\underset{6}{\cancel{60}}}$$

First, eliminate the zeros in the 1,000 and 60,000 and one zero in the 1,200 and 60.

$$\frac{\overset{1}{\cancel{20}}}{1} \times \frac{1}{\underset{3}{\cancel{60}}} \times \frac{\overset{20}{\cancel{120}}}{1} \times \frac{1}{\underset{1}{\cancel{6}}}$$

You can then reduce the numerator 20 and the denominator 60 by dividing both by 20; and then reduce the numerator 120 and the denominator 6 by dividing both by 6.

$$20 \div 3$$

$$= 6.666$$

Answer: 6.7 (tenth) or 6.67 (hundredth)

Example 5 ▪

Option 1: Calculator Use Throughout

$$\frac{2{,}000}{1{,}500} \times \frac{2{,}500}{3{,}000}$$

$$2{,}000 \times 2{,}500 \div 1{,}500 \div 3{,}000$$

$$= 1.111$$

Answer: 1.1 (tenth) or 1.11 (hundredth)

Option 2: Initial Reduction of Fractions

$$\frac{2{,}000}{1{,}500} \times \frac{2{,}500}{3{,}000}$$

$$\frac{\overset{2}{2{,}\cancel{000}}}{\underset{15}{1{,}\cancel{500}}} \times \frac{\overset{25}{2{,}\cancel{500}}}{\underset{3}{3{,}\cancel{000}}}$$

Eliminate the same number of zeros in the numerators and denominators. Eliminate three zeros in the numerator 2,000 and three zeros in the denominator 3,000. Then eliminate two zeros in the numerator 2,500 and the denominator 1,500.

$$2 \times 25 \div 15 \div 3$$

$$= 1.111$$

Answer: 1.1 (tenth) or 1.11 (hundredth)

Problems 3.1

Solve the equations. Express answers to the nearest tenth and hundredth. A calculator may be used.

1. $\dfrac{3}{8} \times \dfrac{6}{3}$ = _____ _____

2. $\dfrac{3}{4} \times \dfrac{10}{2}$ = _____ _____

3. $\dfrac{3}{5} \times \dfrac{1,050}{40}$ = _____ _____

4. $\dfrac{10}{1} \times \dfrac{750}{40,000} \times \dfrac{1,000}{1} \times \dfrac{1}{60}$ = _____ _____

5. $\dfrac{12}{1} \times \dfrac{500}{2,700} \times \dfrac{2,000}{1} \times \dfrac{1}{60}$ = _____ _____

6. $\dfrac{1,500}{750} \times \dfrac{350}{600}$ = _____ _____

7. $\dfrac{1,000}{2,700} \times \dfrac{1,300}{500} \times \dfrac{70}{50}$ = _____ _____

8. $\dfrac{15}{1} \times \dfrac{2,500}{20,000} \times \dfrac{1,000}{1} \times \dfrac{1}{60}$ = _____ _____

9. $\dfrac{8}{1} \times \dfrac{1,000}{5,000} \times \dfrac{100}{1} \times \dfrac{1}{60}$ = _____ _____

10. $\dfrac{750}{500} \times \dfrac{250}{300}$ = _____ _____

Answers 1. 0.8; 0.75 **2.** 3.8; 3.75 **3.** 15.8; 15.75 **4.** 3.1; 3.13 **5.** 74.1; 74.07 **6.** 1.2; 1.17 **7.** 1.3; 1.35 **8.** 31.3; 31.25 **9.** 2.7; 2.67 **10.** 1.3; 1.25

Decimal Fraction Equations

Decimal fraction equations raise an instant warning flag in calculations because it is where most dosage errors occur. As with whole-number equations, simplifying the numbers by eliminating decimal points and reducing the numbers is an optional first step. If you elect to do the entire calculation with a calculator, be sure to enter the decimal points carefully. Triple-check all calculator entries and answers.

 Keypoint: Particular care must be taken with calculator entry of decimal numbers to include the decimal point. Each entry and answer must be routinely triple-checked.

Example 1 ■   **Option 1: Calculator Use Throughout**

$$\dfrac{0.3}{1.65} \times \dfrac{2.5}{1}$$

$0.3 \times 2.5 \div 1.65$ Multiply 0.3 by 2.5, then divide by 1.65.

$= 0.454$

Answer: 0.5 (tenth) or 0.45 (hundredth)

Option 2: Initial Elimination of Decimal Points and Reduction of Fractions

$$\dfrac{0.3}{1.65} \times \dfrac{2.5}{1}$$

$$\dfrac{30}{165} \times \dfrac{25}{10}$$ Move the decimal point two places in 0.3 and 1.65 (to become 30 and 165) and one place in 2.5 and 1 (to become 25 and 10).

$$\frac{\overset{3}{\cancel{30}}}{\underset{33}{\cancel{165}}} \times \frac{\overset{5}{\cancel{25}}}{\underset{1}{\cancel{10}}}$$ Divide 30 and 10 by 10, then divide 25 and 165 by 5.

$$\frac{\overset{1}{\cancel{3}}}{\underset{11}{\cancel{33}}} \times \frac{5}{1}$$ Divide 3 and 33 by 3.

$5 \div 11$ Divide the remaining numerator, 5, by the denominator, 11.

$= 0.454$

Answer: 0.5 (tenth) or 0.45 (hundredth)

Example 2 ▪ **Option 1: Calculator Use Throughout**

$$\frac{0.3}{1.2} \times \frac{2.1}{0.15}$$

$0.3 \times 2.1 \div 1.2 \div 0.15$ Multiply 0.3 by 2.1, then divide by 1.2 and 0.15.

$= 3.5$

Answer: 3.5 (tenth) or 3.5 (hundredth)

Option 2: Initial Elimination of Decimal Points and Reduction of Fractions

$$\frac{0.3}{1.2} \times \frac{2.1}{0.15}$$

$$\frac{3}{12} \times \frac{210}{15}$$ Eliminate the decimal points by moving them one place in 0.3 and 1.2 (to become 3 and 12) and two places in 2.1 and 0.15 (to become 210 and 15).

$$\frac{\overset{1}{\cancel{3}}}{\underset{4}{\cancel{12}}} \times \frac{\overset{42}{\cancel{210}}}{\underset{3}{\cancel{15}}}$$ Divide 3 and 12 by 3, then divide 210 and 15 by 5.

$$\frac{1}{\underset{2}{\cancel{4}}} \times \frac{\overset{21}{\cancel{42}}}{3}$$ Divide 42 and 4 by 2.

$21 \div 2 \div 3$ Use a calculator to divide the numerator, 21, by 2 and then by 3.

$= 3.5$

Answer: 3.5 (tenth) or 3.5 (hundredth)

Example 3 ▪ **Option 1: Calculator Use Throughout**

$$\frac{0.15}{0.17} \times \frac{3.1}{2}$$

$0.15 \times 3.1 \div 0.17 \div 2$ Multiply 0.15 by 3.1, divide by 0.17, and then divide by 2.

$= 1.367$

Answer: 1.4 (tenth) or 1.37 (hundredth)

Option 2: Initial Elimination of Decimal Points and Reduction of Fractions

$$\frac{0.15}{0.17} \times \frac{3.1}{2}$$

$\dfrac{15}{17} \times \dfrac{31}{20}$	Move the decimal point two places in 0.15 and 0.17 and one place in 3.1 and 2 (requires adding a zero to 2).

$\dfrac{\overset{3}{\cancel{15}}}{17} \times \dfrac{31}{\underset{4}{\cancel{20}}}$	Divide 15 and 20 by 5.

$3 \times 31 \div 17 \div 4$	Complete this with a calculator.

$$= 1.367$$

Answer: 1.4 (tenth) or **1.37 (hundredth)**

Example 4 ■   **Option 1: Calculator Use Throughout**

$$\frac{2.5}{1.5} \times \frac{1.2}{1.1}$$

$$2.5 \times 1.2 \div 1.5 \div 1.1$$

$$= 1.818$$

Answer: 1.8 (tenth) or **1.82 (hundredth)**

Option 2: Initial Elimination of Decimal Points and Reduction of Fractions

$$\frac{2.5}{1.5} \times \frac{1.2}{1.1}$$

$\dfrac{25}{15} \times \dfrac{12}{11}$	Move the decimal point one place in 2.5 and 1.5 and one place in 1.2 and 1.1.

$\dfrac{\overset{5}{\cancel{25}}}{\underset{3}{\cancel{15}}} \times \dfrac{12}{11}$	Divide 25 and 15 by 5.

$\dfrac{5}{\underset{1}{\cancel{3}}} \times \dfrac{\overset{4}{\cancel{12}}}{11}$	Divide 12 and 3 by 3.

$$5 \times 4 \div 11$$

$$= 1.818$$

Answer: 1.8 (tenth) or **1.82 (hundredth)**

Problems 3.2

Solve the equations. Express answers to the nearest tenth and hundredth. A calculator may be used.

1. $\dfrac{2.1}{1.15} \times \dfrac{0.9}{1.2} =$ _____ _____

2. $\dfrac{3.1}{2.7} \times \dfrac{2.2}{1.4} =$ _____ _____

3. $\dfrac{0.3}{1.2} \times \dfrac{3}{2.1} =$ _____ _____

4. $\dfrac{0.17}{0.3} \times \dfrac{2.5}{1.5} =$ _____ _____

5. $\dfrac{1.75}{0.95} \times \dfrac{1.5}{2} =$ _____ _____

6. $\dfrac{0.75}{1.15} \times \dfrac{3}{1.25} =$ _____ _____

7. $\dfrac{10.2}{1.5} \times \dfrac{2}{5.1} =$ _____ _____

8. $\dfrac{0.125}{0.25} \times \dfrac{2.5}{1.5} =$ _____ _____

9. $\dfrac{0.9}{0.3} \times \dfrac{1.2}{1.4} =$ _____ _____

10. $\dfrac{0.35}{1.7} \times \dfrac{2.5}{0.7} =$ _____ _____

Answers 1. 1.4; 1.37 **2.** 1.8; 1.8 **3.** 0.4; 0.36 **4.** 0.9; 0.94 **5.** 1.4; 1.38 **6.** 1.6; 1.57 **7.** 2.7; 2.67 **8.** 0.8; 0.83 **9.** 2.6; 2.57 **10.** 0.7; 0.74

Multiple-Number Equations

The calculation steps just practiced are also used for multiple-number equations, which occur frequently in advanced clinical calculations. Reduction of numbers may be of particular benefit here because calculations of this type sometimes have numbers that cancel and/or reduce dramatically. Answers are expressed to the nearest whole number in the examples and problems that follow to replicate actual clinical calculations.

Example 1 ■   **Option 1: Calculator Use Throughout**

$$\frac{60}{1} \times \frac{1,000}{4} \times \frac{1}{1,000} \times \frac{6}{1}$$

$60 \times 1,000 \times 6 \div 4 \div 1,000$ Multiply 60 by 1,000, then by 6; divide by 4 and 1,000.

$= 90$

Answer: 90

Option 2: Initial Reduction of Fractions

$$\frac{60}{1} \times \frac{1,000}{4} \times \frac{1}{1,000} \times \frac{6}{1}$$

$$\frac{60}{1} \times \frac{\overset{1}{1,000}}{\underset{2}{4}} \times \frac{1}{\underset{1}{1,000}} \times \frac{\overset{3}{6}}{1}$$ Eliminate 1,000 from a numerator and denominator, then divide 6 and 4 by 2.

$60 \times 3 \div 2$ Multiply 60 by 3, then divide by 2.

$= 90$

Answer: 90

Example 2 ■

Option 1: Calculator Use Throughout

$$\frac{20}{1} \times \frac{75}{1} \times \frac{1}{60}$$

$20 \times 75 \div 60$ Multiply 20 by 75, then divide by 60.

$= 25$

Answer: 25

Option 2: Initial Reduction of Fractions

$$\frac{20}{1} \times \frac{75}{1} \times \frac{1}{60}$$

$$\frac{\overset{1}{\cancel{20}}}{1} \times \frac{\overset{25}{\cancel{75}}}{1} \times \frac{1}{\underset{\underset{1}{3}}{\cancel{60}}}$$ Divide 20 and 60 by 20 to become 1 and 3, then divide 75 and 3 by 3 to become 25 and 1.

$= 25$

Answer: 25   The answer is obtained by cancellation alone.

Example 3 ■

Option 1: Calculator Use Throughout

$$\frac{2}{0.5} \times \frac{1}{100} \times \frac{275}{1}$$

$2 \times 275 \div 0.5 \div 100$ Multiply 2 by 275, then divide by 0.5 and 100.

$= 11$

Answer: 11

Option 2: Initial Reduction of Fractions

$$\frac{2}{0.5} \times \frac{1}{100} \times \frac{275}{1}$$

$$\frac{20}{5} \times \frac{1}{100} \times \frac{275}{1}$$ Eliminate the decimal point by moving it one place in 0.5 and one place in 2, which requires adding a zero to 2 (to become 5 and 20).

$$\frac{\overset{1}{\cancel{20}}}{\underset{1}{\cancel{5}}} \times \frac{1}{\underset{5}{\cancel{100}}} \times \frac{\overset{55}{\cancel{275}}}{1}$$ Divide 20 and 100 by 20, then divide 275 and 5 by 5.

$$\frac{1}{\underset{1}{\cancel{5}}} \times \frac{\overset{11}{\cancel{55}}}{1}$$ Divide 5 and 55 by 5.

$= 11$

Answer: 11   The answer is obtained by cancellation alone.

Example 4 ■

Option 1: Calculator Use Throughout

$$\frac{1}{60} \times \frac{1}{12} \times \frac{10}{1} \times \frac{750}{1}$$

$10 \times 750 \div 60 \div 12$

$= 10.4$

Answer: 10

Option 2: Initial Reduction of Fractions

$$\frac{1}{60} \times \frac{1}{12} \times \frac{10}{1} \times \frac{750}{1}$$

$$\frac{1}{\underset{6}{60}} \times \frac{1}{\underset{6}{12}} \times \frac{\overset{1}{\cancel{10}}}{1} \times \frac{\overset{375}{\cancel{750}}}{1}$$ Divide 60 and 10 by 10 to become 6 and 1; then divide 12 and 750 by 2 to become 6 and 375.

$$375 \div 6 \div 6$$

$$= 10.4$$

Answer: 10

Problems 3.3

Solve the equations. Express answers to the nearest whole number.

1. $\frac{15}{1} \times \frac{350}{5} \times \frac{1}{60}$ = _____

2. $\frac{1}{32} \times \frac{60}{1} \times \frac{7.5}{3.1}$ = _____

3. $\frac{10}{1} \times \frac{2,500}{24} \times \frac{1}{60}$ = _____

4. $\frac{1.7}{2.3} \times \frac{15.3}{12.1} \times \frac{6.2}{0.3}$ = _____

5. $\frac{20}{1} \times \frac{1,200}{16} \times \frac{1}{60}$ = _____

6. $\frac{5}{1} \times \frac{320}{1.5} \times \frac{1}{60}$ = _____

7. $\frac{100}{1} \times \frac{1,750}{200} \times \frac{1}{60}$ = _____

8. $\frac{60}{1} \times \frac{1,150}{200} \times \frac{1}{100}$ = _____

9. $\frac{25}{4} \times \frac{1,000}{8} \times \frac{1}{60}$ = _____

10. $\frac{18}{10} \times \frac{120}{7} \times \frac{9}{17}$ = _____

Answers **1.** 18 **2.** 5 **3.** 17 **4.** 19 **5.** 25 **6.** 18 **7.** 15 **8.** 3 **9.** 13 **10.** 16

Summary

This concludes the chapter on solving common fraction equations. The important points to remember from this chapter are:

- Most clinical calculations consist of an equation containing 1 to 5 common fractions.

- In solving equations, all the numerators are multiplied, and then divided by the denominators.

- Numbers in an equation may initially be reduced using common denominators/divisors to simplify final multiplication and division.

- Zeros may be eliminated from the same number of numerators and denominators without altering the value.

- Triple-check all calculator entries and answers.

▨   Answers may be expressed as whole numbers, or to the nearest tenth or hundredth, depending on the calculation being done.

▨   It is important to follow the guidelines of the clinical setting or your instructor with rounding. In most cases it is important to perform the calculation completely prior to rounding, so that only the final answer is rounded.

Summary Self-Test

Solve the equations. Express answers to the nearest tenth and hundredth. A calculator may be used.

1. $\dfrac{0.8}{0.65} \times \dfrac{1.2}{1}$ = _____ _____

2. $\dfrac{350}{1,000} \times \dfrac{4.4}{1}$ = _____ _____

3. $\dfrac{0.35}{1.3} \times \dfrac{4.5}{1}$ = _____ _____

4. $\dfrac{0.4}{1.5} \times \dfrac{2.3}{1}$ = _____ _____

5. $\dfrac{1}{75} \times \dfrac{500}{1}$ = _____ _____

6. $\dfrac{0.15}{0.12} \times \dfrac{1.45}{1}$ = _____ _____

7. $\dfrac{100,000}{80,000} \times \dfrac{1.7}{1}$ = _____ _____

8. $\dfrac{1.45}{2.1} \times \dfrac{1.5}{1}$ = _____ _____

9. $\dfrac{1,550}{500} \times \dfrac{0.5}{1}$ = _____ _____

10. $\dfrac{4}{0.375} \times \dfrac{0.25}{1}$ = _____ _____

11. $\dfrac{0.08}{0.1} \times \dfrac{2.1}{1}$ = _____ _____

12. $\dfrac{1.5}{1.25} \times \dfrac{1.45}{1}$ = _____ _____

13. $\dfrac{0.5}{0.15} \times \dfrac{0.35}{1}$ = _____ _____

14. $\dfrac{300,000}{200,000} \times \dfrac{1.7}{1}$ = _____ _____

15. $\dfrac{13.5}{10} \times \dfrac{1.8}{1}$ = _____ _____

16. $\dfrac{1,000,000}{800,000} \times \dfrac{1.4}{1}$ = _____ _____

17. $\dfrac{1.3}{0.2} \times \dfrac{0.25}{1}$ = _____ _____

18. $\dfrac{1.5}{0.1} \times \dfrac{0.25}{1}$ = _____ _____

19. $\dfrac{1.9}{3.5} \times \dfrac{3.2}{1.4}$ = _____ _____

20. $\dfrac{15{,}000}{7{,}500} \times \dfrac{3.5}{1.2}$ = _____ _____

21. $\dfrac{4.7}{1.3} \times \dfrac{50}{20} \times \dfrac{4}{25} \times \dfrac{8.2}{2.1}$ = _____ _____

22. $\dfrac{40}{24} \times \dfrac{250}{5} \times \dfrac{0.375}{7.5}$ = _____ _____

23. $\dfrac{6.9}{21.6} \times \dfrac{250}{5} \times \dfrac{0.75}{2.1}$ = _____ _____

24. $\dfrac{1}{60} \times \dfrac{1}{25} \times \dfrac{10}{1} \times \dfrac{1{,}000}{1}$ = _____ _____

25. $\dfrac{50.5}{22.75} \times \dfrac{4.7}{6.3} \times \dfrac{31.7}{10.2}$ = _____ _____

Solve the equations. Express answers to the nearest whole number. A calculator may be used.

26. $\dfrac{104}{95} \times \dfrac{20}{15} \times \dfrac{63}{1.6}$ = _____

27. $\dfrac{40{,}000}{10{,}000} \times \dfrac{30}{1} \times \dfrac{3.7}{12.5}$ = _____

28. $\dfrac{60}{1} \times \dfrac{500}{50} \times \dfrac{1}{1{,}000} \times \dfrac{116}{1}$ = _____

29. $\dfrac{1.5}{0.6} \times \dfrac{10}{14} \times \dfrac{3.2}{5.3} \times \dfrac{100}{2}$ = _____

30. $\dfrac{60}{1} \times \dfrac{50}{250} \times \dfrac{1}{100} \times \dfrac{455}{1}$ = _____

31. $\dfrac{33.7}{15.9} \times \dfrac{19.2}{2.6} \times \dfrac{2.9}{3.85}$ = _____

32. $\dfrac{20}{4} \times \dfrac{100}{88} \times \dfrac{1{,}200}{250} \times \dfrac{10}{30}$ = _____

33. $\dfrac{14}{7.9} \times \dfrac{88}{8}$ = _____

34. $\dfrac{10}{1} \times \dfrac{325}{1.5} \times \dfrac{1}{60}$ = _____

35. $\dfrac{60}{1} \times \dfrac{300}{400} \times \dfrac{1}{800} \times \dfrac{400}{1}$ = _____

36. $\dfrac{3.7}{1.3} \times \dfrac{12}{8} \times \dfrac{3.1}{7.4} \times \dfrac{5}{1}$ = _____

37. $\dfrac{20}{2} \times \dfrac{125}{25} \times \dfrac{2}{750} \times \dfrac{216}{1}$ = _____

38. $\dfrac{4}{3} \times \dfrac{45}{1} \times \dfrac{22.5}{37.8}$ = _____

39. $\dfrac{7.5}{12.3} \times \dfrac{55}{5} \times \dfrac{23.2}{1.2}$ = _____

40. $\dfrac{1,000}{1} \times \dfrac{50}{250} \times \dfrac{20}{1} \times \dfrac{1}{60}$ = _____

41. $\dfrac{15}{1} \times \dfrac{1,000}{4,000} \times \dfrac{800}{1} \times \dfrac{1}{60}$ = _____

42. $\dfrac{15}{1} \times \dfrac{500}{3} \times \dfrac{1}{60}$ = _____

43. $\dfrac{25}{3} \times \dfrac{750}{8} \times \dfrac{0.1}{1}$ = _____

44. $\dfrac{40}{2} \times \dfrac{250}{50} \times \dfrac{1}{800} \times \dfrac{154}{1}$ = _____

45. $\dfrac{33}{4} \times \dfrac{75}{40} \times \dfrac{2}{150} \times \dfrac{432}{1}$ = _____

46. $\dfrac{22.5}{7} \times \dfrac{100}{5} \times \dfrac{1}{700} \times \dfrac{3}{80} \times \dfrac{3,150}{1}$ = _____

47. $\dfrac{100}{250} \times \dfrac{50}{1} \times \dfrac{27.5}{1.375}$ = _____

48. $\dfrac{2.2}{0.25} \times \dfrac{3.6}{1} \times \dfrac{3.7}{7.1}$ = _____

49. $\dfrac{1.3}{0.21} \times \dfrac{0.3}{2} \times \dfrac{10.1}{0.75}$ = _____

50. $\dfrac{27.5}{10} \times \dfrac{40}{7} \times \dfrac{8.5}{1.9}$ = _____

Answers to Summary Self-Test

1. 1.5; 1.48	**11.** 1.7; 1.68	**21.** 5.6; 5.65	**31.** 12	**41.** 50
2. 1.5; 1.54	**12.** 1.7; 1.74	**22.** 4.2; 4.17	**32.** 9	**42.** 42
3. 1.2; 1.21	**13.** 1.2; 1.17	**23.** 5.7; 5.7	**33.** 19	**43.** 78
4. 0.6; 0.61	**14.** 2.6; 2.55	**24.** 6.7; 6.67	**34.** 36	**44.** 19
5. 6.7; 6.67	**15.** 2.4; 2.43	**25.** 5.1; 5.15	**35.** 23	**45.** 89
6. 1.8; 1.81	**16.** 1.8; 1.75	**26.** 57	**36.** 9	**46.** 11
7. 2.1; 2.13	**17.** 1.6; 1.63	**27.** 36	**37.** 29	**47.** 400
8. 1; 1.04	**18.** 3.8; 3.75	**28.** 70	**38.** 36	**48.** 17
9. 1.6; 1.55	**19.** 1.2; 1.24	**29.** 54	**39.** 130	**49.** 13
10. 2.7; 2.67	**20.** 5.8; 5.83	**30.** 55	**40.** 67	**50.** 70

Introduction to Drug Measures

Metric/International (SI) System

Objectives

The learner will:

1. list the commonly used units of measure in the metric system.

2. express metric weights and volumes using correct notation rules.

3. convert metric weights and volumes within the system.

4. identify errors in metric/SI notation and transcription.

Prerequisites

Familiarity with the metric system.

You are probably already familiar with the metric system, which is the major system of weights and measures used in medicine. The metric system is sometimes referred to as the International System of Units (SI system), which is derived from the French Système International. The strength of the metric system lies in its simplicity because all units of measure differ from each other in powers of ten (10). Conversions between units in the system are accomplished by simply moving a decimal point.

> **Key**point: A major strength of the metric system is that all its units of measure differ from each other in powers of ten (10), and conversions between the units can be made by simply moving the decimal point.

This is also one of the metric system's greatest hazards. This is because a misplaced decimal point alters the value of a number by a multiple of at least 10. It is not necessary for you to memorize the entire metric system to administer medications safely, but you must understand its basic structure and become familiar with the units of measure you will be using in the clinical setting.

> **Key**point: The greatest hazard of the metric system in drug dosages is that a misplaced decimal point will alter a dosage by a multiple of at least 10.

Clinical Relevance: The metric system is used extensively in medicine, especially in medication prescriptions and administration. It is important to understand the basic units of measure in the metric system and how they relate to one another. Misplacement of a decimal point or overlooking a decimal point can result in a tenfold or more increase or decrease in a medication dose and can have catastrophic results. Clearly document decimal points in numbers and clarify any numbers that are difficult to read.

There are units of measure for length, weight, and volume; but measurements of weight and volume will be the most frequently used in medication administration. For weight, from greater to lesser value, the units are kg, g, mg, mcg; for volume, the units are L, mL. It is important to understand the relationships between the units of measure. As the unit of measure decreases in size (g → mg), the quantity will increase (1 g → 1,000 mg). As the unit of measure increases in size (mg → g), the quantity will decrease (100 mg → 0.1 g). Understanding this relationship can be beneficial in avoiding errors in decimal point placement and ultimately avoiding errors in medication administration.

Basic Units of the Metric/SI System

Three types of metric measures are in common clinical use: those for length, volume (or capacity), and weight. The basic units of these measures are:

length — **meter**
volume — **liter**
weight — **gram**

Memorize the basic units if you do not already know them. In addition to the basic units, there are both larger and smaller units of measure for length, volume, and weight. Let's compare this concept with something familiar. The pound is a unit of weight that we use every day. A smaller unit of measure is the ounce; a larger, the ton. However, all are units measuring weight.

In the same way, there are smaller and larger units than the basic meter, liter, and gram. Prefixes are used to indicate the unit of measure. Prefixes, such as micro-, milli-, centi-, kilo- will be used. There is one very important advantage in the metric system: all other units, whether larger or smaller than the basic units, have the name of the basic unit incorporated in them following the prefix. So, when you see a unit of metric measure, there is no doubt what it is measuring: meter—length, liter—volume, and gram—weight.

Problems 4.1

Identify the metric measures with their appropriate category of weight, length, or volume.

1. milligram _____
2. centimeter _____
3. milliliter _____
4. millimeter _____
5. kilogram _____
6. microgram _____
7. kilometer _____
8. kiloliter _____

Answers **1.** weight **2.** length **3.** volume **4.** length **5.** weight **6.** weight **7.** length **8.** volume

Metric/SI Prefixes

Let's explore further the prefixes that are used in combination with the names of the basic units of measure. The same prefixes are used with all three measures. Therefore, there is a kilo*meter*, kilo*gram*, and a kilo*liter*.

Prefixes also change the value of each of the basic units by the same amount. For example, the prefix "**kilo**" identifies a unit of measure that is larger than (or multiplies) the basic unit by 1,000.

1 kilometer	=	1,000 meters
1 kilogram	=	1,000 grams
1 kiloliter	=	1,000 liters

Kilo is the only prefix you will be using in the clinical setting that identifies a measure larger than the basic unit. Kilograms are frequently used as a measure for body weight.

You will see only three measures smaller than the basic unit in common clinical use. The prefixes for these are:

centi—1/100th as in centimeter

milli—1/1,000th as in milligram

micro—1/1,000,000th as in microgram

Therefore, you will primarily be working with only four prefixes: kilo, which identifies a larger unit of measure than the basic measure; and centi, milli, and micro, which identify smaller units than the basic measure.

Problems 4.2

Answer the following questions related to Metric/SI prefixes.

1. Identify the prefix that represents 1/100th of the basic unit of measure.

   _____

2. Does the prefix milli represent a smaller or larger unit of measure when compared to the basic unit of measure?

   _____

3. Which prefix represents a unit of measure that is 1,000 times larger than the basic unit of measure?

   _____

Answers 1. centi 2. smaller 3. kilo

Metric/SI Abbreviations

In clinical use, units of metric measure are abbreviated. The basic units are abbreviated to their first initial and printed in lowercase letters, except for liter, which is capitalized:

meter is abbreviated as **m**

gram is abbreviated as **g**

liter is abbreviated as **L**

> **Key**point: The abbreviations for the prefixes used in combination with the basic units are all printed using lowercase letters:
>
>   kilo is k (as in kilogram—kg)
>   centi is c (as in centimeter—cm)
>   milli is m (as in milligram—mg)
>   micro is mc (as in microgram—mcg)

Micro has an additional abbreviation, the symbol μ, but its use has been discontinued in medication dosages. This became necessary because medication errors were made when handwritten μg was misread as mg, a dosage 1,000 times the mcg dosage ordered.

> **Key**point: Micro is always abbreviated using the prefix mc rather than the symbol μ, which has an inherent safety risk.

In combination, liter remains capitalized. Therefore, milliliter is mL and kiloliter is kL.

Problems 4.3

Abbreviate the following metric units.

1. microgram   _____
2. liter   _____
3. kilogram   _____
4. milliliter   _____
5. centimeter   _____
6. milligram   _____
7. meter   _____
8. kiloliter   _____
9. millimeter   _____
10. gram   _____

Answers **1.** mcg **2.** L **3.** kg **4.** mL **5.** cm **6.** mg **7.** m **8.** kL **9.** mm **10.** g

Metric/SI Notation Rules

To remember the rules of metric notations, in which a unit of measure is expressed with a quantity, it is helpful to memorize some prototypes (examples) that incorporate all the rules. For the metric system, the notations for one-half, one, and one and one-half milliliters incorporate all the official notation rules.

Prototype Notations: 0.5 mL   1 mL   1.5 mL

Rule 1   The quantity is written in Arabic numerals: 1, 2, 3, 4, and so forth.

   Example: 0.5   1   1.5

Rule 2   The numerals representing the quantity are placed in front of the abbreviations.

   Example: 0.5 mL   1 mL   1.5 mL   (*not* mL 0.5, mL 1, mL 1.5)

Rule 3   A full space is used between the numeral and the abbreviation.

   Example: 0.5 mL   1 mL   1.5 mL   (*not* 0.5mL, 1mL, 1.5mL)

Rule 4   Fractional parts of a unit are expressed as decimal fractions.

Example: 0.5 mL   1.5 mL   (*not* ½ mL, 1½ mL)

Rule 5   A zero is placed in front of the decimal when it is not preceded by a whole number, to emphasize the decimal point.

Example: 0.5 mL   (*not* .5 mL)

Rule 6   Excess zeros following a decimal fraction are eliminated.

Example: 0.5 mL   1 mL   1.5 mL   (*not* 0.50 mL, 1.0 mL, 1.50 mL)

Problems 4.4

Write the metric measures using official abbreviations and notation rules.

1. two grams   _____

2. five hundred milliliters   _____

3. five-tenths of a liter   _____

4. two-tenths of a milligram   _____

5. five-hundredths of a gram   _____

6. two and five-tenths kilograms   _____

7. one hundred micrograms   _____

8. two and three-tenths milliliters   _____

9. seven-tenths of a milliliter   _____

10. three-tenths of a milligram   _____

11. two and four-tenths liters   _____

12. seventeen and five-tenths kilograms   _____

13. nine-hundredths of a milligram   _____

14. ten and two-tenths micrograms   _____

15. four-hundredths of a gram   _____

Answers 1. 2 g **2.** 500 mL **3.** 0.5 L **4.** 0.2 mg **5.** 0.05 g **6.** 2.5 kg **7.** 100 mcg **8.** 2.3 mL **9.** 0.7 mL **10.** 0.3 mg **11.** 2.4 L **12.** 17.5 kg **13.** 0.09 mg **14.** 10.2 mcg **15.** 0.04 g

Conversion Between Metric/SI Units

When you administer medications, you will be routinely converting units of measure within the metric system; for example, g to mg and mg to mcg. Learning the relative value of the units with which you will be working is the first prerequisite for accurate conversions.

There are only four metric weights commonly used in medicine. From greater to lesser value, these are:

kg	=	kilogram
g	=	gram
mg	=	milligram
mcg	=	microgram

Only two units of volume are frequently used. From greater to lesser value, these are:

L	=	liter
mL	=	milliliter

Keypoint: Each of these clinical metric measures differs from the next by 1,000.

1 kg	=	1,000 g
1 g	=	1,000 mg
1 mg	=	1,000 mcg
1 L	=	1,000 mL

To reiterate, the ordering of units for weight, from greater to lesser value, is: kg—g—mg—mcg; for volume: L—mL. Each unit differs in value from the next by 1,000 and all conversions will be between sequential units of measure; for example, g to mg, mg to mcg, and L to mL.

Problems 4.5

Choose true (T) or false (F) for each conversion.

1. T   F   1,000 mL   =   1,000 L
2. T   F   1,000 mg   =   1 g
3. T   F   1,000 g   =   1 kg
4. T   F   1,000 mg   =   1 mcg
5. T   F   1,000 mcg =   1 g
6. T   F   1 kg   =   1,000 g
7. T   F   1 mg   =   1,000 g
8. T   F   1,000 mcg =   1 mg
9. T   F   1 g   =   100 mcg
10. T   F   1,000 L   =   1 kL

Answers **1.** F **2.** T **3.** T **4.** F **5.** F **6.** T **7.** F **8.** T **9.** F **10.** T

Because the metric system is a decimal system, conversions between the units are accomplished by moving the decimal point. Also, each unit of measure in clinical use differs from the next by 1,000. If you know one conversion, you know them all.

How far do you move the decimal point? There is a simple rule that can be used with all metric conversions. There are three zeros in 1,000. The decimal point moves three places, the same number of places as the zeros in the conversion.

Keypoint: In metric conversions between sequential units of clinical measures differing by 1,000 (for example, g to mg), the decimal point is moved three places, the same as the number of zeros in 1,000.

This rule holds true for all decimal conversions in the metric system. If the difference in value was 10, which has one zero, it would move only one place. If the difference was 100, which has two zeros, it would move two places. When the difference is 1,000, as in clinical conversions, which has three zeros, the decimal point moves three places.

Which way do you move the decimal point? If you are converting to a smaller unit of measure—for example, g to mg or L to mL—the quantity must get larger. The decimal point must move three places to the right.

Example 1 ■   0.5 g = _____ mg

In this example, you are converting to smaller units of measure, from g to mg, so the quantity will be larger. Move the decimal point three places to the right. To do this, you must add two zeros to the end of the quantity and eliminate the zero in front of it.

0.5 g = 500 mg

Answer: 500 mg   The larger quantity indicates that you have moved the decimal point in the correct direction.

Example 2 ■   2.5 L = _____ mL

In this example, you are converting to smaller units of measure, so the quantity will be larger. Move the decimal point three places to the right. To do this, you must add two zeros.

2.5 L = 2,500 mL

Answer: 2,500 mL   The larger quantity indicates that you have moved the decimal point in the correct direction.

Problems 4.6

Convert the metric measures.

1. 7 mg = _____ mcg

2. 1.7 L = _____ mL

3. 3.2 g = _____ mg

4. 0.03 kg = _____ g

5. 0.4 mg = _____ mcg

6. 1.5 mg = _____ mcg

7. 0.7 g = _____ mg

8. 0.3 L = _____ mL

9. 7 kg = _____ g

10. 0.01 mg = _____ mcg

Answers   1. 7,000 mcg   **2.** 1,700 mL   **3.** 3,200 mg   **4.** 30 g   **5.** 400 mcg   **6.** 1,500 mcg   **7.** 700 mg   **8.** 300 mL   **9.** 7,000 g   **10.** 10 mcg

In metric conversions from smaller to larger units of measurement, such as mL to L and mcg to mg, the quantity will be smaller. The decimal point is moved three places to the left.

Example 3 ▨   200 mL = _____ L

In this example, you are converting to a larger unit of measure, mL to L, so the quantity will be smaller. Move the decimal point three places to the left.

$$.200, \text{mL} = .200 \text{ L}$$

Eliminate the two unnecessary zeros at the end of the quantity, making it .2, then add a zero in front of the decimal point to correctly write the dosage as 0.2 L.

Answer: 0.2 L

Example 4 ▨   1,500 mcg = _____ mg

In this example, you are converting to a larger unit of measure, so the quantity will be smaller. Move the decimal point three places to the left. Place a decimal point in front of the 5, and then eliminate the two zeros after the 5.

$$1,500. \text{ mcg} = 1.500 \text{ mg}$$

Answer: 1.5 mg

Example 5 ▨   300 mcg = _____ mg

In this example, you are converting to a larger unit of measure, mcg to mg, so the quantity will be smaller. Move the decimal point three places to the left.

$$.300, \text{ mcg} = .300 \text{ mg}$$

Two zeros will need to be eliminated from the end of this decimal fraction, making it .3, and a zero must be placed in front of the decimal point to complete the decimal fraction.

Answer: 0.3 mg

Problems 4.7

Convert the metric measures.

1. 3,500 mL	= _____ L		6. 250 mcg	= _____ mg
2. 520 mg	= _____ g		7. 1,200 mg	= _____ g
3. 1,800 mcg	= _____ mg		8. 600 mL	= _____ L
4. 750 mL	= _____ L		9. 100 mg	= _____ g
5. 150 mg	= _____ g		10. 950 mcg	= _____ mg

Answers 1. 3.5 L **2.** 0.52 g **3.** 1.8 mg **4.** 0.75 L **5.** 0.15 g **6.** 0.25 mg **7.** 1.2 g **8.** 0.6 L **9.** 0.1 g
10. 0.95 mg

Common Errors in Metric/SI Dosages

Most errors in the metric system occur because orders are not written using correct notation rules, or they are not transcribed correctly. Errors usually involve decimal fractions. Even though you have just finished learning metric notation rules, let's review the most common errors.

One error is the failure to enter a zero in front of a decimal point; for example, .2 mg instead of 0.2 mg. Regardless of the presence of a zero in front of the decimal in a written order, one must be added when the order is transcribed to a medication administration record.

 Keypoint: Fractional dosages in the metric system are transcribed with a zero in front of the decimal point.

Another common error is including zeros where they should not be; for example, 2.0 mg instead of 2 mg, or 0.20 mg instead of 0.2 mg. Each error can be misread as 20 mg, a dosage that greatly exceeds the intended dosage.

 Keypoint: Unnecessary zeros are eliminated when metric dosages are transcribed.

Errors are also more likely to occur in calculations that include decimal fractions. The presence of a decimal fraction in a calculation is an indication to slow down and triple-check all math. Use your critical thinking abilities. If a decimal is misplaced, the answer will be a minimum of 10 times too large or 10 times too small. Question quantities that seem unreasonable. A 1.5 mL IM injection dosage makes sense, but a 0.15 mL or 15 mL does not, and this is the type of error you might encounter.

 Keypoint: Question orders and calculations that seem unreasonably large or small.

Additional errors to be aware of are in conversions within the metric system. Errors in conversions can be eliminated by thinking "three." All conversions between the weight measures (kg, g, mg, and mcg) and the volume measurements (L and mL) are accomplished by moving the decimal point three places.

Listing the weight measures from left to right in order of largest to smallest unit of measure—**kg, g, mg, mcg**—will help you determine the direction to move the decimal point. For example, when converting from kg to g, move the decimal point three places to the right, just as the units of measure are listed left to right from largest to smallest. When converting from a smaller to a larger unit of measure, mcg to mg for example, move the decimal point to the left three places; just as the order of measures of weight are listed.

This concept will also apply to measures of volume—when converting from a larger unit of measure to a smaller unit of measure, such as L to mL, move the decimal point to the right three places. Converting from a smaller unit of measure to a larger unit of measure, such as mL to L, the decimal point is moved three places to the left.

Keypoint: Recalling the units of measure for weight from left to right in order of greatest to smallest—kg, g, mg, mcg—will help you determine the direction to move the decimal point when you convert. The decimal point will always move three places and the direction can be identified by looking at the order. If you convert mg to mcg, you will move the decimal point to the right three places as mcg is to the right of mg. Converting g to kg will result in moving the decimal point to the left three places as kg is listed to the left of g.

Problems 4.8

Correct the following errors in Metric/SI notation.

1. .2 mg   _____

2. 0.400 mcg   _____

3. 6.0 g   _____

Identify the direction the decimal point will be moved in the following conversions.

4. 25 mg to mcg   _____

5. 100 g to kg   _____

6. 0.5 g to mg   _____

Answers 1. 0.2 mg (missing a zero in front of the decimal point) **2.** 0.4 mcg (trailing zeros are not needed) **3.** 6 g (decimal and trailing zero are not needed) **4.** Right three places (25,000 mcg) **5.** Left three places (0.1 kg) **6.** Right three places (500 mg)

Summary

This concludes the refresher on the metric system. The important points to remember from this chapter are:

- The meter (m), liter (L), and gram (g) are the basic units of metric measure.
- Only liter is capitalized, L.
- Larger and smaller units than the basics are identified by prefixes.
- The prefixes are printed using lowercase letters.
- The one larger unit you will encounter is kilo (k).
- The smaller units you will be seeing are centi (c), milli (m), and micro (mc).
- Each prefix changes the value of a basic unit by the same amount.
- Converting from one unit to another within the system is accomplished by moving a decimal point.
- Conversions between the units of measure for weight and volume will require moving the decimal point three places.

- When you convert from larger to smaller units of measurement, the quantity will increase.

- To convert from larger to smaller units, the decimal point is moved to the right.

- When you convert from smaller to larger units of measurement, the quantity will get smaller.

- To convert from smaller to larger units, the decimal point is moved to the left.

- Fractional dosages are transcribed with a zero in front of the decimal point.

- Unnecessary zeros are eliminated from dosages.

Summary Self-Test

List the basic units of measure of the metric system and the measure they are used for.

1. _____   _____

   _____   _____

   _____   _____

Which of the following are official metric/SI abbreviations?

2. a) L
   b) g
   c) kL
   d) mgm
   e) mg
   f) kg
   g) mL
   h) G

   _____

Use official metric abbreviations and notation rules to express the following measurements as numerals.

3. Six-hundredths of a milligram   _____

4. Three hundred and ten milliliters   _____

5. Three-tenths of a kilogram   _____

6. Four-tenths of a milliliter   _____

7. One and five-tenths grams   _____

8. One-hundredths of a gram   _____

9. Four thousand milliliters   _____

10. One and two-tenths milligrams   _____

List the four commonly used clinical units of weight and the two of volume from greater to lesser value.

11. Weight _____   _____

                   _____   _____

    Volume _____   _____

Convert the following metric measures.

12. 160 mg	=	_____ g	27. 300 mg	=	_____ g
13. 10 kg	=	_____ g	28. 2.5 mg	=	_____ mcg
14. 1,500 mcg	=	_____ mg	29. 1 kL	=	_____ L
15. 750 mg	=	_____ g	30. 3 L	=	_____ mL
16. 200 mL	=	_____ L	31. 2 L	=	_____ mL
17. 0.3 g	=	_____ mg	32. 0.7 mg	=	_____ mcg
18. 0.05 g	=	_____ mg	33. 4 g	=	_____ mg
19. 0.15 g	=	_____ mg	34. 1,000 mL	=	_____ L
20. 1.2 L	=	_____ mL	35. 2,500 mL	=	_____ L
21. 1,800 mL	=	_____ L	36. 1,000 mg	=	_____ g
22. 2 mg	=	_____ mcg	37. 0.2 mg	=	_____ mcg
23. 900 mcg	=	_____ mg	38. 2,000 g	=	_____ kg
24. 2.1 L	=	_____ mL	39. 1.4 g	=	_____ mg
25. 475 mL	=	_____ L	40. 0.5 L	=	_____ mL
26. 0.9 L	=	_____ mL			

Answers to Summary Self-Test

1. gram-weight; liter-volume; meter-length	**11.** kg, g, mg, mcg, L, mL	**21.** 1.8 L	**31.** 2,000 mL
2. a, b, c, e, f, g	**12.** 0.16 g	**22.** 2,000 mcg	**32.** 700 mcg
3. 0.06 mg	**13.** 10,000 g	**23.** 0.9 mg	**33.** 4,000 mg
4. 310 mL	**14.** 1.5 mg	**24.** 2,100 mL	**34.** 1 L
5. 0.3 kg	**15.** 0.75 g	**25.** 0.475 L	**35.** 2.5 L
6. 0.4 mL	**16.** 0.2 L	**26.** 900 mL	**36.** 1 g
7. 1.5 g	**17.** 300 mg	**27.** 0.3 g	**37.** 200 mcg
8. 0.01 g	**18.** 50 mg	**28.** 2,500 mcg	**38.** 2 kg
9. 4,000 mL	**19.** 150 mg	**29.** 1,000 L	**39.** 1,400 mg
10. 1.2 mg	**20.** 1,200 mL	**30.** 3,000 mL	**40.** 500 mL

Chapter

5

Unit, Percentage, Milliequivalent, Ratio, and Household Measures

Objectives

The learner will:

1. identify dosages measured in international units and units.

2. identify dosages measured as percentages.

3. identify dosages measured in milliequivalents.

4. identify dosages using ratio strengths.

5. identify dosages measured in household measures.

Although metric measures predominate in medication administration, other measures are frequently used in the prescribing and administration of medications. In addition, while the apothecary system has become obsolete, you may still encounter several measures in the household system. This chapter covers alternate measures that designate medication strength as well as the most frequently used measures in the household system.

Clinical Relevance: When working with medications in the clinical setting, you will notice that there are other measurements used that are not part of the metric system. Some of the measures, such as units and milliequivalents, will be supplied and ordered as units and milliequivalents. For example, a medication order may read "heparin 5,000 units," and the supply you have will be labeled "10,000 units per mL." It is important to recognize that units and milliequivalents do not need conversions. Other measures, such as percentages and ratios, are equivalent to a concentration of medication in the solution. While household measures are not used often in the clinical setting, it is possible that you will have to relay information to patients using household measures.

International Units and Units

The terms *international units* and *units* are often used interchangeably. Hormones, vitamins, and enzymes are types of substances that may be measured as international units or units. Specific medications that are measured as units or international units include insulin, penicillin, vitamins, and heparin. A unit measures a drug in terms of its action, not its physical weight. The word *units* is not abbreviated as the abbreviation is on The Joint Commission's (TJC's) Do Not Use List. It is written in lowercase letters using Arabic numerals in front of the measure, with a space between; for example, 2,000 units or 1,000,000 units. Refer to Figure 5-1 for a medication label showing units. There are varying thoughts on whether a comma should be used in numbers greater than 999. However, since many medication labels include commas with numbers greater than 999, we will utilize commas for consistency.

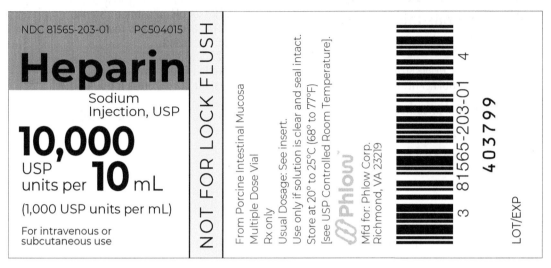

▲ **Figure 5-1**

Problems 5.1

Express the unit dosages in numerals.

1. Two hundred and fifty thousand units   _____

2. Ten units   _____

3. Five thousand units   _____

4. Forty-four units   _____

5. Forty thousand units   _____

6. One million units   _____

7. One thousand units   _____

8. Twenty-five hundred units   _____

9. Thirty-four units   _____

10. One hundred units   _____

Answers   **1.** 250,000 units   **2.** 10 units   **3.** 5,000 units   **4.** 44 units   **5.** 40,000 units   **6.** 1,000,000 units   **7.** 1,000 units   **8.** 2,500 units   **9.** 34 units   **10.** 100 units

Percentage (%) Measures

Percentage strengths are used extensively in intravenous solutions. They are less commonly used for a variety of other medications, including eye and topical (for external use) ointments. Percentage (%) means parts per hundred and the greater the percentage strength, the stronger the solution or ointment. For example, 3% is stronger than 1%. Fractional percentages are expressed as decimal fractions; for example, 0.45%. Notice that, unlike other written dosages, percentages are generally written with no space between the quantity and percentage sign. Refer to Figure 5-2 for the label of a medication expressed as a percent.

NDC 0409-1159-09 *Preservative-Free*   30 mL Single-dose Teartop Vial   Rx only

0.25% Bupivacaine
Hydrochloride Injection, USP
75 mg/30 mL (2.5 mg/mL)

For INFILTRATION, NERVE BLOCK,
CAUDAL and EPIDURAL ANESTHESIA.

Not for spinal anesthesia.

LOT ##-###-AA
EXP DMMMYYYY

Each mL contains bupivacaine HCl, anhydrous
2.5 mg; sodium chloride 8.6 mg. May contain
NaOH and/or HCl for pH adjustment. Sterile,
nonpyrogenic. Usual dosage and route of
administration: See insert.
Store at 20 to 25°C (68 to 77°F).
[see USP Controlled Room Temperature.]
Dist. by Hospira, Inc., Lake Forest, IL 60045 USA

novaplus✝   RL-7562

▲ **Figure 5-2**

 Keypoint: In solutions, percent represents the number of grams of drug per 100 mL of solution.

Example 1 ▪   100 mL of a 1% solution will contain 1 g of drug.

Example 2 ▪   100 mL of a 2.5% solution will contain 2.5 g of drug.

Example 3 ▪   100 mL of a 10% solution will contain 10 g of drug.

Example 4 ▪   100 mL of a 0.9% solution will contain 0.9 g of drug.

 Keypoint: These examples are included to point out that percentage solutions contain a significant amount of drug or other solute, and that reading percentage labels requires the same care as that used with other drug dosages.

Problems 5.2

Answer the following questions related to percentages.

1. Which of the following percentages is the strongest?
   3.5%, 35%, 0.35%   _____

2. Identify the equivalent of a 5% solution by identifying
   the number of grams in 100 mL of solution.   _____

3. Identify the equivalent of a 5.5% solution by identifying
   the number of grams in 100 mL of solution.   _____

Answers 1. 35% is the strongest **2.** 5 grams in 100 mL **3.** 5.5 grams in 100 mL

Milliequivalent (mEq) Measures

To understand a milliequivalent, you must first understand what an equivalent is. An **equivalent** is the amount of a substance that reacts with a certain number of hydrogen ions. A **milliequivalent (mEq)** is one-thousandth of a chemical equivalent. There are no conversions to memorize for milliequivalents. The measure of milliequivalent is used primarily with electrolytes such as potassium, chloride, and sodium.

Dosages expressed in milliequivalents will be written with Arabic numbers followed by mEq. For example, a medication order may read, "Potassium chloride 20 mEq by mouth stat." The medication will be supplied using a measure of milliequivalents so no conversion will be needed. Figure 5-3 shows a medication label using mEq as the measure.

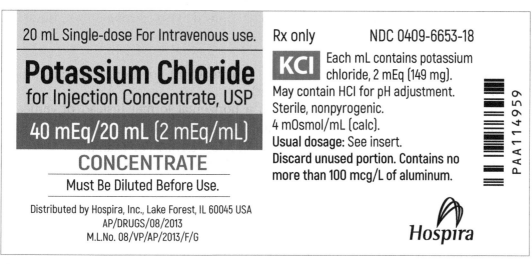

▲ **Figure 5-3**

Problems 5.3

Express the milliequivalent dosages in numerals.

1. Sixty milliequivalents   _____

2. Fifteen milliequivalents   _____

3. Forty milliequivalents   _____

4. One milliequivalent   _____

5. Fifty milliequivalents   _____

6. Eighty milliequivalents   _____

7. Fifty-five milliequivalents   _____

8. Seventy milliequivalents   _____

9. Thirty milliequivalents   _____

10. Twenty milliequivalents   _____

Answers **1.** 60 mEq **2.** 15 mEq **3.** 40 mEq **4.** 1 mEq **5.** 50 mEq **6.** 80 mEq **7.** 55 mEq **8.** 70 mEq **9.** 30 mEq **10.** 20 mEq

Ratio Measures

Ratio strengths are used primarily to identify concentration of solutions. They represent parts of drug per parts of solution and usually represent grams of the medication in milliliters of solution. Some examples follow:

Example 1 ▪   A 1:100 strength solution has 1 gram drug in 100 mL solution.

Example 2 ▪   A 1:5 solution contains 1 gram drug in 5 mL solution.

Example 3 ▪   A solution that is 1 gram drug in 2 mL solution would be written 1:2.

 Keypoint: The less solution a drug is dissolved in, the stronger the solution.

For example, a ratio strength of 1:10 (1 gram drug to 10 mL solution) is much stronger than a 1:100 (1 gram drug in 100 mL solution).

Ratios are actually fractions written in a horizontal format instead of vertically. Therefore 1:5 could also be written as $\frac{1}{5}$. Just as fractions are written in lowest terms, ratio strengths should be expressed in their simplest terms. For example, 2:10 would be incorrect because it can be reduced to 1:5. Notice that ratio dosages are written separated by a colon, and no space before or after the colon, as shown in Figure 5-4.

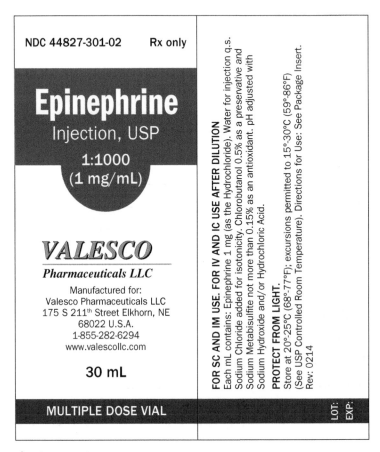

▲ **Figure 5-4**

Dosages using ratio strengths are not common, but you do need to know what they represent. The Food and Drug Administration (FDA) has revised its standards for drug labeling and is requiring removal of ratio expressions from the labeling of single ingredient medications, such as epinephrine.[1] Instead, the agency is recommending that the strength be expressed as weight per volume. For example, instead of a label that indicates a ratio of 1:1000 (meaning 1 gram in 1000 mL), the label would instead indicate 1 mg per 1 mL.

Problems 5.4

Express as ratios.

1. 1 part drug to 200 parts solution _____

2. 1 part drug to 4 parts solution _____

3. 1 part drug to 7 parts solution _____

Identify the strongest solution.

4. a) 1:20   b) 1:200   c) 1:2   _____

5. a) 1:50   b) 1:20   c) 1:100   _____

6. a) 1:1000   b) 1:5000   c) 1:2000   _____

Answers   1. 1:200   **2.** 1:4   **3.** 1:7   **4.** c   **5.** b   **6.** a

Household and Apothecary Measures

Household measures are rarely used. They are primarily used in the home care setting, and their clinical use is becoming less frequent. The measures you may occasionally encounter include the ounce, tablespoon, teaspoon, and drop. Abbreviations and/or names for all these measures, except the drop, still appear on many disposable medication cups and must not be confused with metric dosages. It is quite possible that these measures will be eliminated in the future because the health care industry has been moving rapidly to improve dosage labeling and medication abbreviation guidelines to reduce the possibility of errors.

The various abbreviations for household dosages and their metric equivalents are listed in Table 5-1.

Table 5-1 Household Measures and Metric Equivalents

Household Measure	Abbreviation	Metric Equivalent
ounce	oz	30 mL
tablespoon	T, TBS, tbs	15 mL
teaspoon	t, TSP, tsp	5 mL
drop	gtt	volume varies

---

[1] "Single Entity Injectable Drug Products," U.S. Food and Drug Administration (June 23, 2017), www.fda.gov/drugs /information-drug-class/single-entity-injectable-drug-products

Keypoint: The volume of a drop depends on the size of the dropper being used.

A drop is such an inaccurate and variable measure that medication droppers are now often included with small-volume liquid medication preparations, as shown in Figure 5-5. The dropper is specific to that medication. The use of drops is largely restricted to eye and ear drop use. Exceptions include small-volume pediatric liquid medications and liquid concentrates, which are prepared with medicine droppers included with the medication and which are calibrated by volume, or by actual dosage.

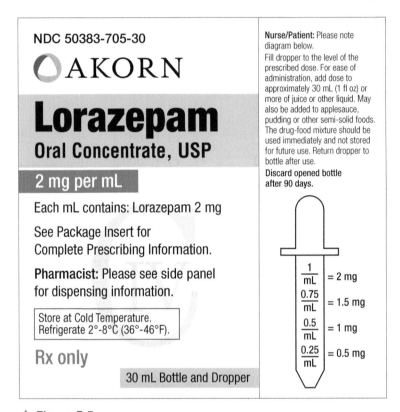

▲ **Figure 5-5**

Apothecary measures are officially obsolete. The grain was the measure for weight. The grain was originally based on the weight of a grain of wheat, which exposes its inaccuracy, and why this measure is now obsolete. Appendix A includes some additional information on this obsolete system in the event your instructor feels it necessary for you to learn.

Summary

This concludes your introduction to the additional measures you will see used in dosages and in solutions. The important points to remember from this chapter are:

- International units measure a drug by its action rather than its weight.

- The abbreviation for units and international units is on The Joint Commission Do Not Use List. These measures are written in full in lowercase letters.

- Percentage (%) strengths are frequently used in solutions and ointments.

- Percent represents grams of drug per 100 mL of solution.

- The greater the percentage strength, the stronger the solution.

- Milliequivalent is abbreviated mEq and is primarily used in measurements of electrolytes, such as potassium, chloride, and sodium.

- Ratio strengths represent parts of drug per parts of solution.

- If the number representing parts of drug are the same, the solution with the smaller volume will be more concentrated. For example, 1:10 is more concentrated than 1:100.

- T, TBS, or tbs is the abbreviation for tablespoon (15 mL), and t, TSP, or tsp is the abbreviation for teaspoon (5 mL).

- The abbreviation gtt is used for drop, and oz for ounce.

Summary Self-Test

Express the dosages using the official symbols/abbreviations.

1. Three hundred thousand units _____

2. Forty-five units _____

3. Ten percent _____

4. Two and a half percent _____

5. Forty milliequivalents _____

6. A one in two thousand ratio _____

7. A one in ten ratio _____

8. One percent _____

9. One drop _____

10. Two thousand units _____

11. Five milliequivalents _____

12. Nine-tenths percent _____

13. Ten units _____

14. A one in two ratio _____

15. Five percent _____

16. Twenty milliequivalents _____

17. Fourteen units _____

18. Twenty percent _____

19. Two million units _____

20. One hundred thousand units _____

Answers to Summary Self-Test

1. 300,000 units	**6.** 1:2000	**11.** 5 mEq	**16.** 20 mEq
2. 45 units	**7.** 1:10	**12.** 0.9%	**17.** 14 units
3. 10%	**8.** 1%	**13.** 10 units	**18.** 20%
4. 2.5%	**9.** 1 gtt	**14.** 1:2	**19.** 2,000,000 units
5. 40 mEq	**10.** 2,000 units	**15.** 5%	**20.** 100,000 units

Preparing for Medication Administration

Safe Medication Administration

Objectives

The learner will:

1. identify medications to be administered according to the MAR/eMAR.

2. explain the components of necessary documentation on the MAR/eMAR.

3. list the components of a medication order.

4. discuss the six rights of medication administration.

5. list common causes of dosage errors.

6. explain "partnering with the client" in medication administration.

7. list the steps to take when a dosage error occurs.

8. list major safety concerns addressed by TJC and ISMP.

In this chapter you will be introduced to a sample Medication Administration Record (MAR) and the Electronic Medication Administration Record (eMAR) that may be used to prepare, administer, and chart medications. Additional instruction will include the elements of a medication order, the six rights of medication administration, the basic guidelines for all medication administration, information on the most common sources of medication errors, and the actions that you must take when errors occur. You will also be introduced to transcription guidelines for medication dosages and abbreviations that have been addressed by the major watchdog organizations for medication safety: The Joint Commission (TJC) and The Institute for Safe Medication Practices (ISMP).

Clinical Relevance: Safe medication administration is accomplished by following the guidelines in this chapter. Major factors in medication administration errors are distraction and fatigue. In the clinical setting, it is important to limit distractions during preparation and administration of medications; prepare only one client's medications at a time; and ensure that all the rights of safe medication administration are practiced every time you prepare and administer medications. If a client questions you about the medication you are prepared to give, it is important for you to take the time to investigate their concerns. This could help you avoid a serious medication error. Medication administration will become a routine nursing function for you, but it is important not to consider it so routine that you skim over the basic principles of safe medication administration. You must always exercise caution with medication administration. Medication administration should never become "just a task." Engaging in critical thinking throughout the process of medication preparation and administration will help you avoid errors. Regardless of the reason for the error, if you give a wrong medication or dosage, you are legally responsible and must hold yourself accountable.

Medication Administration Records

The eMAR uses the bar code medication administration (BCMA) system to scan medication package bar codes prior to administration. This system was developed to decrease the risk of medication errors. Even with this system, you must still ask the client their name and birthdate, as well as verify drug and dose accuracy. This is not a perfect system. Concerns that have been identified include cost, lack of continuous training, technical malfunctions/loss of internet, and nurse complaints of spending more time on documentation than with the client.

Physicians insert medication orders directly into the electronic system. After being verified by the pharmacy, the medication orders will appear on the eMAR.

The MAR is, simply stated, a paper record of all medications a client is receiving and has received. Physician orders are written and transcribed to the MAR by a nurse, pharmacist, or another qualified healthcare professional. The focus of this section is to familiarize you with a sample MAR and eMAR so that you will understand the many features each contains. Your instructors will orient you to the MARs/eMARs you will use in your clinical experiences, and you will quickly discover that there is no universal system in use. Each clinical facility using MARs/eMARs makes its own determination on the particular format that suits its needs.

Regardless of which medication administration system is used, each one will contain similar features. These would include the drug name (generic/trade), dosage, frequency, actual times of administration, and precautions related to administration, such as checking blood pressure, pulse, or body weight. These precautions are important because some will include parameters such as an order to hold blood pressure medication for systolic less than 100 mm Hg. In addition, the MAR will also have a separate section for PRN medications.

Refer to the sample MAR in Figure 6-1 on the next page to view the following column headings and entries.

Column 1 Labeled "Start" (date for medication to begin) and "Stop" (discontinuation of the medication). The three drugs listed are being given on a continuing basis. They were started on "5-3." None has been discontinued.

Column 2 Labeled "Medication and Dose." The first drug listed is digoxin including its trade name, Lanoxin®. The dosage, "0.25 mg," and frequency, "daily," is next. There is a precautionary designation to "Check apical pulse."

Column 3 Labeled "Schedule." Gives the actual time each medication is scheduled to be administered. For digoxin, this is 8 am. On the MAR you may see standard or international time, but not both on the same MAR.

Column 4 This column has two designations: "Route," which is oral or PO for digoxin and furosemide, and IV route for ciprofloxacin. The Nurse space, which "GJ" has initialed, identifies the transcriber of these medication orders. The bottom of the MAR identifies GJ as G Jennings.

Column 5 There are three designations here: Time, the actual hour the drug is given (i.e., "8 am"); Site if the drug is parenteral; and Initials, where the nurse who gave the drug, "BPP," verified administration. The apical pulse, 64, is recorded next to the 8 am digoxin dosage. The bottom of the MAR identifies the nurse, BPP, as BP Prentiss.

Start Stop	Medication and Dose	Schedule	Route Nurse		Date 5-3					Date 5-4					Date 5-5					Date 5-6				
5-3	Digoxin (Lanoxin) 0.25 mg daily. Check apical pulse. Hold for apical pulse < 60.	8am	PO GJ	Time Site Initials	8 P64 BPP																			
5-3	Furosemide (Lasix) 20 mg twice daily. Record daily weight in patient records.	8am 4pm	PO GJ	Time Site Initials	8 BPP	4 GJ																		
5-3	Ciprofloxacin (Cipro) 500 mg twice daily.	6am 6pm	IV GJ	Time Site Initials	6 BPP	6 GJ																		
				Time Site Initials																				
				Time Site Initials																				
				Time Site Initials																				
				Time Site Initials																				

Initials	Signature	Initials	Signature	Initials	Signature	Initials	Signature
BPP	BP Prentiss RN						
GJ	G JENNINGS RN						

Allergies Latex, Tetracyclines	Physician Dr. R. Swartz
Room # 204 Name Susan Smith	

MEDICATION ADMINISTRATION RECORD

▲ **Figure 6-1** Medication Administration Record (MAR)

This particular MAR covers only four days of medications, "5-3" through "5-6." However, most MARs provide for longer periods of up to a month.

Problems 6.1

Refer to the MAR in Figure 6-1 to answer the following questions.

1. List the two medications that are due to be given at 8 am.

   _____   _____

2. Who administered the 4 pm dosage of furosemide?

   _____   _____

3. Ciprofloxacin is administered twice a day. Identify the hours this drug is to be given, and identify the route.

   _____   _____

Answers **1.** digoxin 0.25 mg, furosemide 20 mg **2.** G. Jennings **3.** 6 am and 6 pm, IV route

The eMAR also utilizes columns for each category in medication administration. Refer to Figure 6-2. These columns will appear after scanning the client ID band. But, prior to scanning the ID band, you will retrieve the medications from a storage unit in the designated medication room. Compare the eMAR medication list to the medication labels following the order of the medications on the eMAR screen. This will be the first check for drug accuracy, and following the order of the medications on the eMAR will prevent errors. This process should be followed during all checks of the medication. The three checks of medication administration will be discussed in the Right Drug section later in the chapter. After taking the eMAR to the client's room, you will scan the client ID band and ask the client their name and date of birth. The ID band scan will activate the BCMA system and the medication list will appear on the eMAR screen. Utilizing the eMAR screen, match the medication labels with the screen. This will be the second medication check for accuracy. Do not skip this step and rely on the eMAR to be perfect. The final check, and prior to administration, is to scan each medication bar code in order as it appears on the screen. Once the medications are administered, the final step is to click *submit* to ensure confirmation of the medication administration. Once *submit* is clicked, the current medication time and list will disappear from the screen, and the next medication times will appear.

ELECTRONIC MEDICATION ADMINISTRATION RECORD

Patient: John Jones Gender: M DOB: 8/14/1950 Age: 71 Room: 312

Admitted: 2/12/2022

Attending Physician: Dr. B. Miller

Allergies: Shellfish, Vancomycin

SCHEDULED

TIME	DRUG NAME - GENERIC	ALTERNATE DRUG NAME	DOSE	ROUTE	FREQUENCY	DIRECTIONS
0800	INSULIN ASPART PEN	NOVOLOG PEN	10 UNITS	SUBQ	TID WITH MEALS	Hold for blood sugar < 80
0800	METFORMIN	GLUCOPHAGE	500 MG = 1 TAB	PO	BID WITH MEALS	Hold if NPO or contrast
0900	CEFEPIME	MAXIPIME	1 GM	IV	DAILY	
0900	FUROSEMIDE	LASIX	40 MG = 1 TAB	PO	DAILY	
0900	NYSTATIN 500,000 UNITS	MYCOSTATIN LIQUID	5 ML	PO	QID	SWISH AND SWALLOW
0900	LISINOPRIL	PRINIVIL	10 MG = 1 TAB	PO	DAILY	Hold for systolic BP < 110
1200	INSULIN ASPART PEN	NOVOLOG PEN	10 UNITS	SUBQ	TID WITH MEALS	Hold for blood sugar < 80

PRN

TIME ADMIN	DRUG NAME	ALTERNATE DRUG NAME	DOSE	ROUTE	FREQUENCY	DIRECTIONS	START DATE
0945	MORPHINE	MORPHINE	2 MG = 1 ML	IV	Q 2 HOURS PRN	PAIN	2/12/22
	ONDANSETRON	ZOFRAN ODT	4 MG = 1 TAB	PO	Q 4 HOURS PRN	NAUSEA OR VOMITING	2/12/22
	LORAZEPAM	ATIVAN	0.5 MG = 1 TAB	PO	Q 6 HOURS PRN	ANXIETY	2/12/22
0945	ACETAMINOPHEN	TYLENOL	650 MG = 2 TAB	PO	Q 4 HOURS PRN	FEVER	2/12/22

▲ **Figure 6-2** Electronic Medication Administration Record (eMAR)

Problems 6.2

Refer to the eMAR in Figure 6-2 to answer the following questions.

1. What medications are due at 0800?

   _____

2. What is the direction for giving nystatin (Mycostatin® liquid)?

   _____

3. Why would the medication lisinopril (Prinivil®) be held?

   _____

4. Which PRN medications were given at 0945?

   _____

5. What medication would the client receive for nausea/vomiting?

   _____

Answers 1. Insulin Aspart pen (Novolog®), metformin (Glucophage®) **2.** Swish and Swallow **3.** lisinopril (Prinivil®) will be held if the systolic blood pressure (BP) is less than 110 mm Hg **4.** Morphine and acetaminophen (Tylenol®) **5.** Ondansetron (Zofran ODT®)

Components of a Medication Order

When a physician writes a medication order, and prior to the transcription of the order to the MAR/eMAR, you must ensure the medication order is complete. This will also confirm that the six rights of medication administration have been incorporated into the medication orders. The elements of a complete medication order include the six rights and the prescriber's signature, as shown below:

1. Client name and birthdate
2. Date and time of order
3. Name of medication
4. Dose of medication
5. Route of medication
6. Time/frequency of administration
7. Prescriber signature

The Six Rights of Medication Administration

The six rights of medication administration consist of the right person, the right drug, the right dosage, the right route, the right time, and the right documentation of a dosage when it is administered. These rights will be covered in more detail in your fundamentals text, but it is appropriate to discuss them briefly here.

Right Person

Administering medications to the right person sounds simple enough, but errors can still occur. All MARs/eMARs include the client's room number. However, this should not be used in the identification process. The current identification procedure for an MAR or eMAR is to ask an individual their name and birthdate, then check the response against the wrist identification band (ID band). According to the 2022 Joint Commission National Patient Safety Goals (NPSGs), you must use at least two person-specific identifiers, prioritizing name and birthdate. The ID band is scanned in the eMAR system. Once the client's ID band is scanned, the client's medications will appear on the computer screen. If a person is unable to verbalize their name and birthdate, you must verify identity by comparing their name band to the MAR/eMAR. In facilities where ID bands are not used, follow the facility policy for client identification methods.

Of considerable concern is the possibility of having two people with the same surname on the same floor or even, though more rarely, in the same room. Duplicate names are a source of errors, so read both surname, first name, and birthdate on each ID band. Do this every time you give a medication. No exceptions. Once a drug is administered, there is no way to get it back.

Right Drug

When preparing dosages, the drug order and drug label are routinely checked against each other three times: once when you locate the drug, once just before you open or pour it, and then immediately before you administer it. There are three specific safety reminders related to reading labels that need to be revisited. The first is that a drug may be ordered by trade name but be available only in a generic so make sure you have the drug that was ordered. The second concern is that many drug names, particularly generic, are very similar and must be identified carefully. And, finally, because it is easy to miss the special initials that follow a drug name—a familiar example is isosorbide/Dilatrate-SR® for sustained release—look for and identify these. When doing the three required order and label cross checks, all these precautions to locate the correct drug apply.

Right Dosage

The MAR/eMAR may not tell you how many tablets, capsules, or milliliters to administer. You will need to calculate this yourself. Dosage is a particular concern in metric dosages containing a decimal. Recall your instruction in conversions between the different units of metric measure containing decimals. You know that in conversions with metric equivalents used for dosages, the decimal point will always move three places. If you are converting from a greater to a lesser unit: g to mg or mg to mcg, the number will become larger; if you are converting from a lesser to a greater unit: mcg to mg or mg to g, the number will become smaller. If you inadvertently convert in the wrong direction, the numbers often don't make sense: 0.25 mg cannot be 250 g; and 2 mg cannot be 0.002 mcg.

Medications are prepared and calculated in dosages that reflect a reasonable number of tablets and capsules. Ask yourself if the conversion makes sense, and recognize when it does not. Learn to question orders for more than three tablets or capsules. Although some drugs require multiple tablets, most do not. Remember to always triple-check your calculations for accuracy.

 Keypoint: An unusual number of tablets or capsules could be a warning of an error in prescribing, transcribing, or calculating.

Right Route

Oral medications are swallowed. This is not always easy for clients to do, and this is why many children's medications are prepared as liquids. This means you must watch the client actually take oral medications. If you have any doubt that the medications have been swallowed, check the client's mouth thoroughly.

Oral disintegrating tablets (ODT) make it easier for clients with swallowing difficulties. They dissolve within seconds and there is no need for additional fluids. A common ODT tablet is ondansetron (Zofran ODT®) for nausea/vomiting.

An additional oral route is **sublingual**, or under the tongue. There has been a considerable increase in the number of sublingual drugs in use, so this route designation is one to carefully identify. A swallowed sublingual drug will not have the desired effect, if it has any at all, because the acid of the stomach will destroy it.

Drops are another administration route, and eye, nose, and ear drops are quite common. Eye medications are also prepared as ointments, and, understandably, they are clearly labeled for their intended **ophthalmic** use. Read the label carefully to ensure the medication is designated for ophthalmic use.

An increasing number of **topical** drugs is in use. These may include ointments, creams, lotions, and so on, that are applied to the skin. The amount of the topical drug to be used is specific. Refer to the physician's order for directions for cleansing the site, as well as whether the site should be covered after application.

Currently, **transdermal patches** are widely used. The precautions in their use relate to where the patch must be applied, how long it is to stay on, and examination for local skin reaction to the adhesive that secures the patch. Unfortunately, many people are sensitive to transdermal patch adhesives. A rash may appear when a patch is used for the first time, or even after repeated use. Inflamed skin will not absorb the medication well, and inflammation can cause acute discomfort.

A large number of inhalation medications are in common use. These medications are usually self-administered. Your responsibility will be to make sure that the client understands how to use the inhalation device, how many activations each dosage requires, and how many times a day to use the medication. It is also your responsibility to be familiar with any precautions related to the use of inhalation medications.

The creams and suppositories used for the genitorectal systems provide another method of direct medication application. These are very clearly labeled and recognizable. It is very important to administer these medications in the correct site.

Finally, there are the **parenterals**, which are medications that are not administered via the intestinal tract. The **intravenous (IV)** route is the primary parenteral route, with **intramuscular (IM)** and **subcutaneous (SUBQ)** coming in second, and **intradermal (ID)** a distant third. Most injectable drugs are site-specific and are labeled for IV, IM, or subcutaneous use. You will be reading many drug labels that identify specific parenteral site routes in the balance of this text.

As a nurse, you are not qualified to change the route of a drug. For example, if a client has an IV site, but the order is for an IM injection, the client may ask you to inject the medication into the IV line to avoid pain from the IM injection. You would need a physician's order for an IV route of this drug in order to comply with the client's request.

Right Time

The time each drug is to be given is often critical. Rapid-acting and short-acting insulins have a very short onset, and must be given immediately before a meal. Drugs may be ordered at specific hours during the day or only at bedtime. Some drugs must be given before or after specific blood tests. PRN medications are time sensitive and must be given as soon as possible. These medications are given as needed and must be given before symptoms become more severe. These medications are typically ordered for pain, fever, nausea or vomiting, anxiety, high blood pressure, and more. The client's list of ordered PRN medications are typically on a separate list on the MAR/eMAR. It is crucial that the nurse looks at the previous administered time of a PRN drug before preparing it for the client. You should be aware of what is available for the client on the PRN list.

Each clinical facility designates routine administration times; however, twice a day may mean 9 am and 5 pm or 9 am and 9 pm, depending on the action of the drug being given. Each MAR identifies two time-related specifics: frequency—for example, "twice a day"—then specific hours—for example, 9 (am) and 5 (pm) or, in international/military time, 0900 and 1700.

A clinical facility will use either standard or international/military time, but not both. International/military time uses a 24-hour clock, starting with 0001 for one minute after midnight, to 2400 for midnight of the same day. To convert from standard to international/military time, add 12 hours to each hour beginning with 1 pm standard time. For example, 2 pm plus 12 hours is 1400; 4 pm plus 12 (hours) is 1600. If you are unfamiliar with using international time, it will initially require careful thought. Refer to the inside front cover for a complete time conversion chart.

Right Documentation

If an administered drug is not charted, it can be given again in error. There is an absolute rule that a drug given must be recorded immediately. It is also necessary to record and report unusual reactions to a medication, such as nausea or dizziness, or a client's refusal to take a medication. In such an occurrence, record and report the incident immediately, and include the reason for refusal.

If you give a parenteral medication other than by IV, the injection site must be recorded, so that a different site can be used next time. In actual practice, sites are chosen by the condition of the tissues at acceptable sites, because previous injection sites are generally easy to see and must be avoided. Some medications will have preferred sites for injection.

Other Considerations for Medication Administration

Partnering with the client is an important concern. The client is one of your best assets in preventing errors. Consider the following, not uncommon, verbal reports: "I just had my medication." Or, "My doctor told me they were stopping this drug." Or, "The doctor said I needed a bigger dose." Or, "This pill doesn't look the same as the one I had before." Or, "Where is my . . . pill?" Or, "This pill made me sick the last time I took it." Or, "At home, my pill is white. This one is pink." Learn to listen very carefully and consider the client correct until proven otherwise.

You will also be responsible for educating the client about the drugs and dosages they are taking, what they are for, what time they must be taken, and how they must be taken. Most individuals will be discharged with medications, so the sooner they can learn what they are taking, the better. If the client is not deemed responsible, the caretaker must be educated about the drugs and dosages. Clients and/or caretakers must also learn about common side effects and, if particularly relevant, what untoward effects they should report to the healthcare provider.

 Keypoint: An important safety precaution is recognition of the client as a full partner in medication administration.

There are other considerations to think about. Checking for medication allergies is one consideration. This may include checking the list of allergies on the MAR/eMAR, or even asking the client. If the physician orders a medication that appears on the allergy list, it is your responsibility to question the order. A second consideration is the right of the client to refuse a medication. All information necessary to understand the consequences of the refusal must be provided to the client. If the client continues to refuse the medication, this must be documented. Another consideration is your responsibility to recognize any nursing implications for assessment prior to giving the medication. For example, blood pressure should be taken prior to the administration of an antihypertensive medication. Following administration of a medication, it is your responsibility to reassess your client and determine the effects of the medication.

> **Key**point: For safety reasons, never leave medications unattended. It is not a safe practice to leave the medications with the client to take independently. Never ask another nurse to give a medication you prepared. Never give medication that another nurse prepared.

Common Medication Errors

Prescription drugs are the cause of death to more than 100,000 people a year in the United States, although not all these deaths are hospital based. Medication errors happen, and they will continue to happen in all three of the modalities related to drug orders: the **prescribing** (done by a licensed practitioner), the **transcribing/verifying** on a MAR/eMAR (done by a person who specializes in this responsibility, frequently the pharmacy staff), or the **administering** (primarily a nursing responsibility).

There has been a concerted international effort in recent years to identify the source of, and take active steps to reduce, the incidence of medication errors caused by the use of administration abbreviations. The Joint Commission, formerly known as the Joint Commission on Accreditation of Healthcare Organizations, and the Institute for Safe Medication Practices (ISMP) are leaders in this endeavor.

Errors in Abbreviations and Drug Names

A number of abbreviations designating the frequency and routes of medication administration have been eliminated and Figure 6-3, the Official "Do Not Use" List, identifies these changes. For example, the abbreviations Q.D., QD, q.d., and qd used for a single daily dose and Q.O.D., QOD, q.o.d., and qod used for a dosage given every other day are no longer used. Instead, they are now clearly written as daily or every other day. Similarly, qhs, formerly used for nightly and misread as every hour, is now written as nightly; SC or sub q used for subcutaneous has been changed to SUBQ or subcutaneous; the use of per os for by mouth has been eliminated in favor of PO, by mouth, or orally. An additional abbreviation, q2h or q2hr (or any specific hour) is now clearly written as every 2 hours. Another deletion is the use of a lowercase u or uppercase U or IU for units. As you have already learned, *units* is not abbreviated but is written as units. A current list of acceptable administration abbreviations is available on the inside front cover of this text and Appendix B, but do keep in mind that there may be future changes in this evolving area of concern.

Common examples of confusing drug name abbreviations are MS for morphine sulfate and MSO_4 or $MgSO_4$ for magnesium sulfate. These drugs are now identified using their complete names.

Errors in Writing Metric Dosages

All the correct rules for writing metric dosages have been covered in previous chapters. But let's review common areas for mistakes, which are also identified in Figure 6-3. The first error is in placing a decimal and a zero (0) following a whole number dosage (called a trailing zero); for example, 4.0 g instead of 4 g. The decimal could easily be missed and 10 times the ordered dosage, 40 g, administered. The second error is failing to place a zero in front of a decimal fraction (referred to as lack of a leading zero); for example, .5 mg instead of 0.5 mg. Once again, the decimal could be missed and 5 mg administered.

Official "Do Not Use" List[1]

Do Not Use	Potential Problem	Use Instead
U, u (unit)	Mistaken for "0" (zero), the number "4" (four) or "cc"	Write "unit"
IU (International Unit)	Mistaken for IV (intravenous) or the number 10 (ten)	Write "International Unit"
Q.D., QD, q.d., qd (daily)	Mistaken for each other	Write "daily"
Q.O.D., QOD, q.o.d, qod (every other day)	Period after the Q mistaken for "I" and the "O" mistaken for "I"	Write "every other day"
Trailing zero (X.0 mg)* Lack of leading zero (.X mg)	Decimal point is missed	Write X mg Write 0.X mg
MS	Can mean morphine sulfate or magnesium sulfate	Write "morphine sulfate" Write "magnesium sulfate"
MSO$_4$ and MgSO$_4$	Confused for one another	

[1] Applies to all orders and all medication-related documentation that is handwritten (including free-text computer entry) or on preprinted forms.

*Exception: A "trailing zero" may be used only where required to demonstrate the level of precision of the value being reported, such as for laboratory results, imaging studies that report size of lesions, or catheter/tube sizes. It may not be used in medication orders or other medication-related documentation.

▲ **Figure 6-3** Official "Do Not Use" list of medical abbreviations

Additional changes have been recommended by ISMP and are listed in Appendix B. These lists are for reference only and do not need to be memorized.

Action Steps When Errors Occur

The goal is safe medication administration throughout your career. Following the considerations outlined in this chapter will afford you the best opportunity for safe practice related to medication administration. However, because you are human, there may be instances where medication errors will occur. It is important for you to understand the action steps that you must take if an error occurs. First and foremost, you must ensure the safety of the client. Assess your client for any untoward effects from the error, and act to keep them safe. After you have ensured the safety of your client, you will need to complete the following steps:

Step 1　Errors must be reported as soon as they are discovered.

Step 2　Necessary remedial measures must be instituted immediately.

Step 3　The reason for the error must be determined.

Step 4　An incident/accident report must be prepared.

Step 5　Corrective policies/procedures must be instituted, if possible, to prevent the error from recurring.

Reporting the error is extremely important. If an error isn't reported, no action can be taken. Keep in mind that an error is an accident, and it is not necessarily a reflection on competency, nor will reporting an error terminate your career. There are several factors that contribute to medication errors, including distraction and fatigue. When in stressful situations, you must be particularly aware and vigilant so that you do not become the person making an error. Medication administration should never become so routine that the principles of safe medication administration are not followed.

Summary

This completes your introduction to safe medication administration. The important points to remember from this chapter are:

- Identification of the right person begins with asking the client their name and birthdate, followed by comparing the identification band to the MAR/eMAR.

- When identifying a drug, be sure to complete three checks of the medication label to the order prior to administering the medication.

- When identifying dosages, take special precautions with metric dosages containing a decimal.

- Most dosages of tablets or capsules consist of ½ to 3 tablets (1 to 3 capsules, which cannot be broken in half). An unusual number of tablets or capsules may indicate an error.

- The route of administration is critical to medication safety and effectiveness.

- The time of administration is an important consideration particularly for PRN medications that are given to a client based on symptoms that are present, such as pain, nausea or vomiting, anxiety, high blood pressure, to name a few.

- The time of administration will also be critical for certain medications with a rapid action, such as insulin and heart medications.

- Listening to the concerns of the client or caretaker is very important in the administration of medications.

- Using only standard abbreviations and avoiding troublesome abbreviations will increase safety in the clinical setting.

- If a medication error occurs, client safety must be ensured and the error must be reported immediately.

- The MAR/eMAR is the reference for medication administration. It is extremely important to keep them current and compare them to the physician orders if there are any questions.

- Medication administration must never become routine and "just a task."

Summary Self-Test

Answer the questions as briefly as possible.

1. List the six rights of medication administration. _____

_____

2. What consideration was stressed regarding reading generic names? _____
_____

3. What might extra initials following a drug name identify? _____
_____
_____

4. List the two major transcribing considerations for metric dosages containing a decimal. _____
_____
_____

5. Your dosage of a drug calculates to give the client 10 tablets. What will you consider before you prepare this medication for the client?
_____
_____

6. Name and discuss two time-sensitive medications that are identified in this chapter.
_____
_____

7. How will you ensure you have the right client prior to medication administration?
_____
_____

8. What will you do if a client refuses a medication? _____
_____

9. List the steps you must take when a medication error occurs. _____
_____
_____
_____

10. List your responsibilities in educating a client about their medication.
_____
_____
_____

Answers to Summary Self-Test

1. Drug, dosage, route, person, time, and documentation. **2.** Read carefully; they are often similar. **3.** Additional medications in a preparation or special action. **4.** Use a zero in front of a decimal to draw attention to it; no decimal or zero following a whole-number dosage. **5.** An unusual number of oral tablets or capsules or excessively large mL volumes must be questioned. **6.** PRN medications—give before symptoms become more severe; rapid-acting/short-acting insulin—administer immediately before a meal. **7.** Ask the client for his or her name and birthdate; check response against the ID band. For the eMAR system, scan the ID band while asking for name and birthdate. **8.** Ask why, educate the client on the reason for the ordered drug, record it, report it. **9.** After ensuring the safety of the client, report the error, take remedial measures as necessary, determine the cause, complete an incident report, and institute a policy to prevent a repeat. **10.** Review all medications by asking the client to explain the dosage, frequency, time, and route of administration for each. Review these again as necessary, including side effects and precautions.

Interpreting Drug Labels

Objectives

The learner will:

1. identify generic and trade names on medication labels.

2. locate dosage strength on the medication label.

3. identify the form of the drug from the label.

4. locate the total quantity on a medication label.

5. identify the administration route on a medication label.

6. identify the medications on the combination drug label.

7. identify information on a label which would indicate a controlled substance.

8. identify the instructions on a label for mixing or reconstituting a drug.

9. recognize other important components on a drug label.

In this chapter, you will be introduced to labels of medications for both oral and parenteral use. Medication labels include various pieces of information that will be important as you calculate dosages, and prepare and administer medications. The type of information included on medication labels is similar, regardless of the preparation; however, the information may be difficult to decipher due to the small print on labels and amount of information included on the label. Therefore, it is important that you have an understanding of the information available to you on a medication label. As we discussed in Chapter 6, the provider will order the medication and dosage to be administered; the medication label will provide us with the information to perform the calculations necessary to administer the ordered medication. We will begin by looking at the information that is common on all medication labels.

Clinical Relevance: The ability to interpret the information on labels is critical to the process of preparing and administering medications. The label will have much information, and sometimes the printing will be small and difficult to read. It is important to understand the types of information you need from the label in order to prepare and administer medications safely. If you have difficulty reading the information on the label at any point, it is imperative that you seek assistance and clarification to ensure you are interpreting the information correctly. Correct interpretation of the information on the label is critical to avoid medication errors and protect the client from potential harm. Correctly interpreting the label information also protects your license and decreases the chance of criminal charges due to malpractice.

Generic and Trade Names

Medication labels will include the name of the medication. The generic name, or official name, is traditionally in lowercase letters, but not always. There is only one generic name for a medication, and the generic name must be included on the medication label, as shown in Figure 7-1. The trade name, or brand name, may be more prominent on a medication label. Uppercase letters may be used, especially to start the medication name. The trade name is followed with ® to indicate that the medication is registered with that trade name. The trade name is provided by the manufacturer who makes the medication; therefore, there may be more than one trade name for medications. For example, the generic medication ibuprofen may have a trade name of Motrin® or Advil®, depending on the manufacturer. Most labels do contain **both** the trade name and the generic name in parentheses, as shown in Figure 7-2. Drugs may be ordered by either name depending on hospital policy or prescriber preference, although the current trend is to use generic names. The eMAR always lists the generic name first. You will frequently need to cross-check trade and generic names for accurate drug identification.

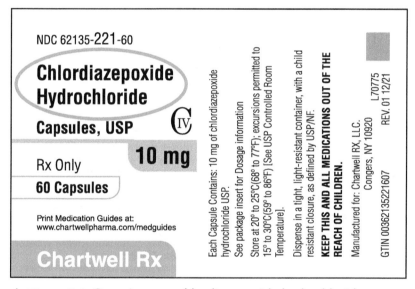

▲ **Figure 7-1** Generic name chlordiazepoxide hydrochloride

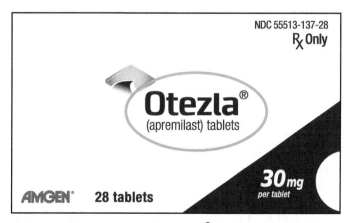

▲ **Figure 7-2** Trade name Otezla® and generic name apremilast

Dosage Strength

The dosage strength is also found on a medication label, as shown in Figures 7-3 and 7-4. This will be identified in terms of weight and will almost always use the metric system. However, recall from Chapter 5 that some medications are identified as units or milliequivalents. For example, insulin will have units as the dosage strength, and not gram, milligram, or microgram.

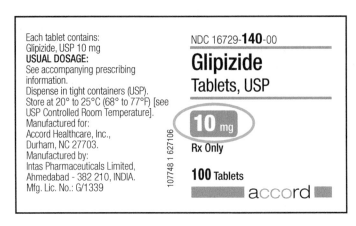

▲ **Figure 7-3** Dosage Strength 10 mg

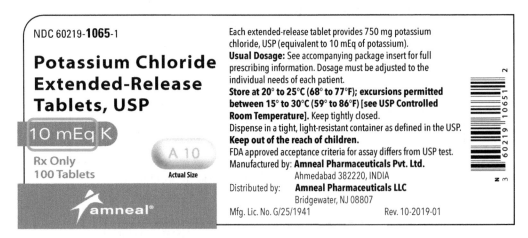

▲ **Figure 7-4** Dosage strength 10 mEq

Form

The form of the drug is the way the drug is designed to be administered. For oral preparations, the form may be tablets, capsules, or liquids/suspensions. Refer to Figure 7-5 for different types of oral preparations.

The solid forms of oral preparations can include various types of tablets and capsules. Note that some tablets are **scored**, or divided, with a line so they can be split in half. This information will be important to know as you learn dosage calculation in preparation for medication administration.

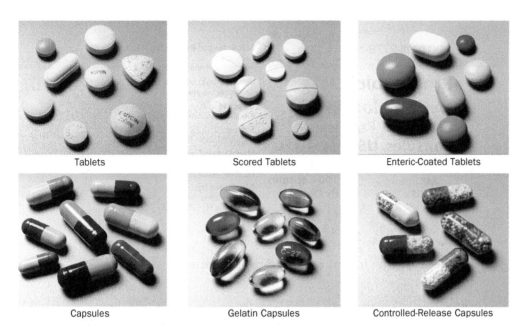

Tablets   Scored Tablets   Enteric-Coated Tablets

Capsules   Gelatin Capsules   Controlled-Release Capsules

▲ **Figure 7-5**

For injectable preparations, the form will be liquid. For liquid forms, the designation may be milliliters, teaspoons, or even tablespoons, especially for over-the-counter (OTC) medications that lay people may obtain for use, such as acetaminophen. Some oral and injectable preparations may be supplied as powders, which must be reconstituted into a liquid prior to use. Reconstitution directions on labels will be discussed later in this chapter and in Chapter 13.

Although oral and injectable forms of medications are the most common, other medication forms include suppositories, ointments, and transdermal patches, shown in Figure 7-6, or extended-release capsules, shown in Figure 7-7, to name a few.

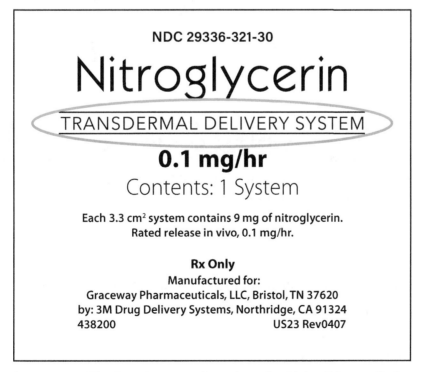

NDC 29336-321-30

Nitroglycerin

TRANSDERMAL DELIVERY SYSTEM

0.1 mg/hr

Contents: 1 System

Each 3.3 cm^2 system contains 9 mg of nitroglycerin.
Rated release in vivo, 0.1 mg/hr.

Rx Only
Manufactured for:
Graceway Pharmaceuticals, LLC, Bristol, TN 37620
by: 3M Drug Delivery Systems, Northridge, CA 91324
438200   US23 Rev0407

▲ **Figure 7-6** The form is a transdermal patch which will be applied to the skin.

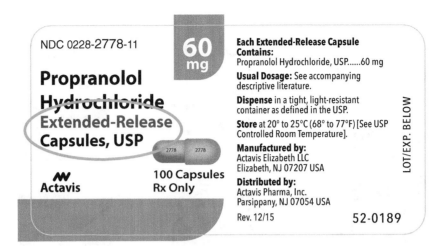

▲ **Figure 7-7** The form is extended-release capsule.

 Keypoint: The dosage strength and form together, shown in Figure 7-8, will provide the information for your supply when you learn to calculate dosages. You need to become very familiar with locating this information on the drug label.

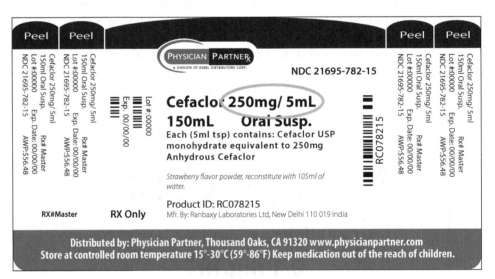

▲ **Figure 7-8** This dosage strength and form (250 mg per 5 mL) will be your supply when you begin to calculate dosages.

Problems 7.1

Refer to the label in Figure 7-9 below to answer the following questions.

1. What is the generic name? _____

2. What is the trade name? _____

3. What is the form of the drug? _____

4. What is the dosage strength? _____

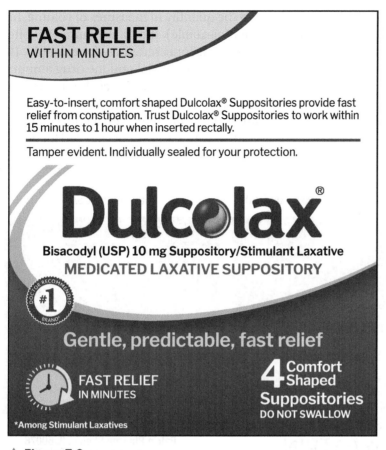

▲ **Figure 7-9**

Total Quantity

Medications may be supplied in unit dose containers or multiple dose containers. In unit dose packages of tablets or capsules, the total quantity is understood to be 1, as there is only 1 tablet or capsule in the package. In a multiple-dose container of tablets or capsules, you may see the total quantity of tablets written on the label. For example, 10 tablets would be the total quantity. Refer to Figure 7-10.

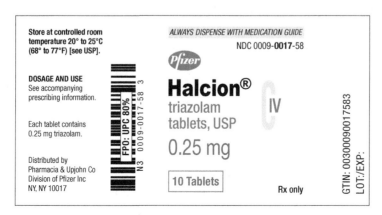

▲ **Figure 7-10** Total quantity – 10 tablets

Liquid medications will identify the quantity in measures of volume. In a unit dose of a liquid medication (injectable or noninjectable), the total volume will often accompany the dosage strength and will be written as a concentration—for example, 100 mg per mL. This would indicate there is 1 mL in the unit dose vial and the drug amount in that mL is 100 mg. In a multiple dose container, many times you will see the concentration, as well as the total volume. In Figure 7-11 for example, the label identifies a medication with a concentration of 5 mg in 5 mL in a multiple dose container with a total volume of 500 mL. It is important not to confuse the total volume with the numbers needed for dosage calculation.

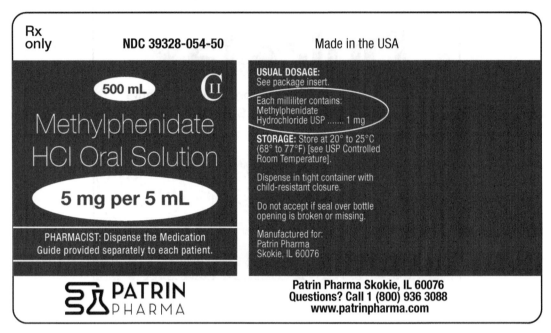

▲ **Figure 7-11** This label shows 5 mg per 5 mL as the concentration. It also reduces it to 1 mg per mL, as shown. The total volume is 500 mL.

Remember that the dosage strength on the label of a tablet or capsule will be the amount in 1 tablet or capsule, regardless of the total quantity in the container. The concentration of a liquid medication will be identified as a unit of weight per unit of volume. In addition to this concentration, the total volume will be on the label. Refer to Figures 7-12 and 7-13 for additional examples.

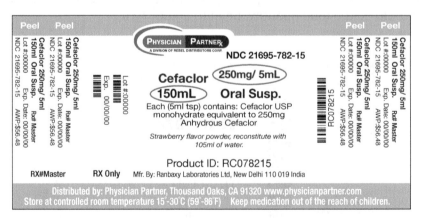

▲ **Figure 7-12** This label shows the concentration of this medication as the dosage strength and form or 250 mg/5 mL and shows a total volume of 150 mL.

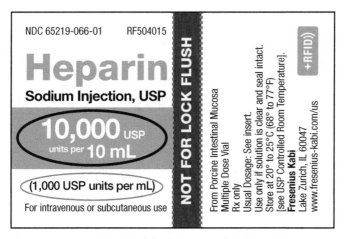

▲ **Figure 7-13** On this label, the total volume is present (10,000 units/10mL). The final concentration is 1,000 units per mL.

Administration Route

Medication labels will include the administration route. Often, however, if it is a capsule or tablet, the administration route is understood to be oral, unless another route such as sublingual, is identified. Liquids will be identified as oral use, injectable use, or specific routes, such as intravenous, intramuscular, and subcutaneous. Refer to Figure 7-14. If the medication is not labeled for a specific route, it cannot be administered via the route. For example, if the medication indicates intravenous route, it cannot be given intramuscularly or subcutaneously. Ointments and creams will be identified as topical use or the site for application such as the eye or for ophthalmic use, as shown in Figure 7-15. Major routes of administration include oral, enteral (usually administered through a tube into the stomach or intestine), ophthalmic, topical, intravenous, intramuscular, subcutaneous (Figure 7-16), as well as others.

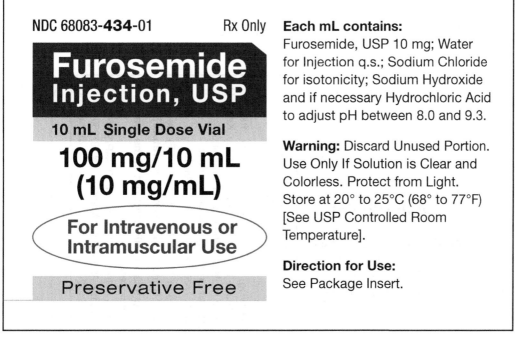

▲ **Figure 7-14** Route is intravenous or intramuscular use.

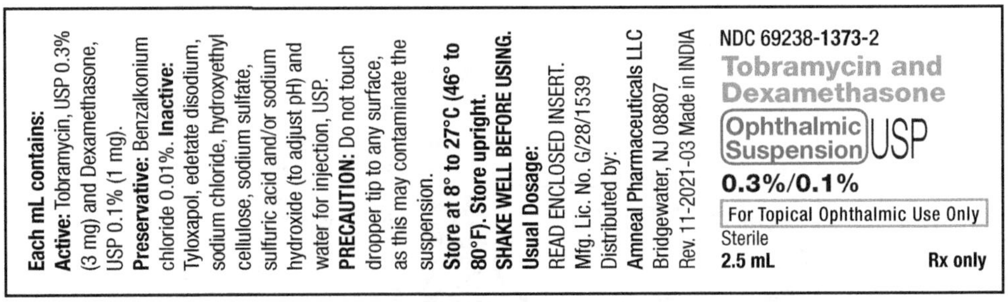

Each mL contains:
Active: Tobramycin, USP 0.3% (3 mg) and Dexamethasone, USP 0.1% (1 mg).
Preservative: Benzalkonium chloride 0.01%. **Inactive:** Tyloxapol, edetate disodium, sodium chloride, hydroxyethyl cellulose, sodium sulfate, sulfuric acid and/or sodium hydroxide (to adjust pH) and water for injection, USP.
PRECAUTION: Do not touch dropper tip to any surface, as this may contaminate the suspension.
Store at 8° to 27°C (46° to 80°F). Store upright.
SHAKE WELL BEFORE USING.
Usual Dosage:
READ ENCLOSED INSERT.
Mfg. Lic. No. G/28/1539
Distributed by:
Amneal Pharmaceuticals LLC
Bridgewater, NJ 08807
Rev. 11-2021-03 Made in INDIA

NDC 69238-1373-2
Tobramycin and Dexamethasone
Ophthalmic Suspension USP
0.3%/0.1%
For Topical Ophthalmic Use Only
Sterile
2.5 mL Rx only

▲ **Figure 7-15** Route–Ophthalmic suspension (eye drops)

NDC 63323-568-83
FK562883
Rx Only
Enoxaparin Sodium Injection
30 mg/ 0.3 mL
SINGLE DOSE SYRINGES WITH AUTOMATIC SAFETY DEVICE
FOR SUBCUTANEOUS INJECTION
FRESENIUS KABI
Ten 0.3 mL Syringes

▲ **Figure 7-16** Route–subcutaneous injection

Problems 7.2

Refer to the label in Figure 7-17 below to answer the following questions.

1. What is the total quantity in this medication container? _____
2. What is the dosage strength and form written together? _____
3. By what route should this medication be administered? _____
4. Is nitroglycerin the trade name or the generic name of the medication? _____

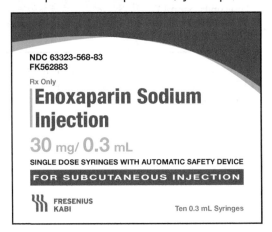

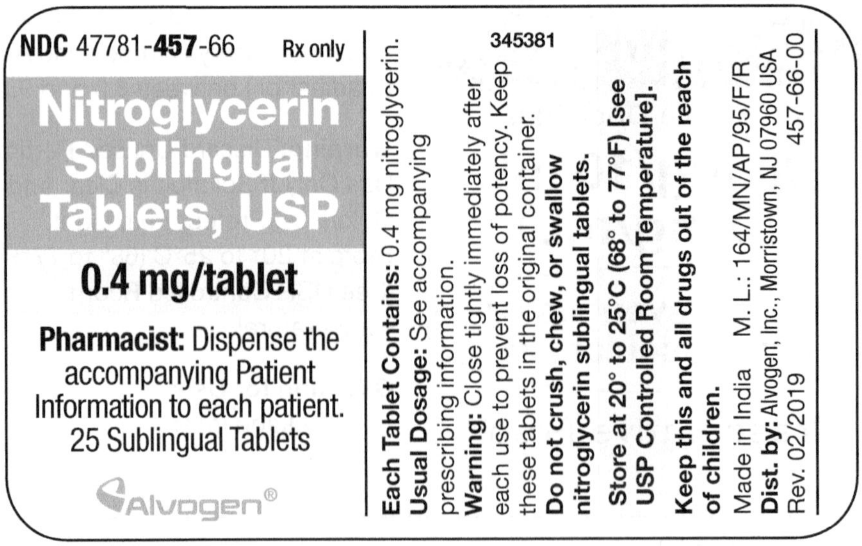

NDC 47781-**457**-66   Rx only   345381
Nitroglycerin Sublingual Tablets, USP
0.4 mg/tablet
Pharmacist: Dispense the accompanying Patient Information to each patient.
25 Sublingual Tablets
Alvogen®

Each Tablet Contains: 0.4 mg nitroglycerin.
Usual Dosage: See accompanying prescribing information.
Warning: Close tightly immediately after each use to prevent loss of potency. Keep these tablets in the original container.
Do not crush, chew, or swallow nitroglycerin sublingual tablets.
Store at 20° to 25°C (68° to 77°F) [see USP Controlled Room Temperature].
Keep this and all drugs out of the reach of children.
Made in India   M. L.: 164/MN/AP/95/F/R
Dist. by: Alvogen, Inc., Morristown, NJ 07960 USA
457-66-00
Rev. 02/2019

▲ **Figure 7-17**

Combination Drug Labels

A combination drug has two or more medications within one drug. These medications will typically be ordered by the number of tablets, capsules, milliliters, and inhalations, rather than the dosage strength. The dosage strength of each drug will appear on the label, as shown in Figure 7-18. Combination inhalers come as either aerosol or dry powder. Medications treating heart disease and diabetes lead the list of combination drugs. Refer to Figures 7-19 and 7-20 for additional examples.

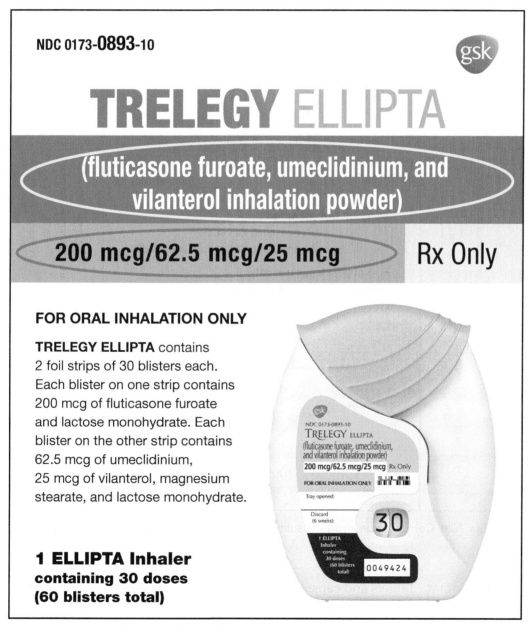

NDC 0173-**0893**-10

gsk

TRELEGY ELLIPTA

(fluticasone furoate, umeclidinium, and vilanterol inhalation powder)

200 mcg/62.5 mcg/25 mcg   Rx Only

FOR ORAL INHALATION ONLY

TRELEGY ELLIPTA contains 2 foil strips of 30 blisters each. Each blister on one strip contains 200 mcg of fluticasone furoate and lactose monohydrate. Each blister on the other strip contains 62.5 mcg of umeclidinium, 25 mcg of vilanterol, magnesium stearate, and lactose monohydrate.

1 ELLIPTA Inhaler containing 30 doses (60 blisters total)

▲ **Figure 7-18** Combination drug – fluticasone furoate/umeclidinium/vilanterol inhalation powder

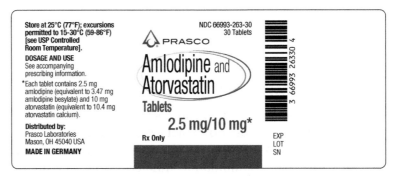

▲ **Figure 7-19** Combination drug – Amlodipine 2.5 mg and Atorvastatin 10 mg

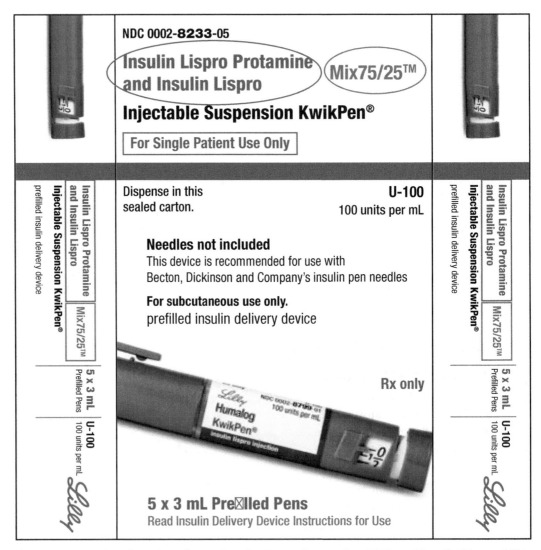

▲ **Figure 7-20** Combination drug – Insulin Lispro Protamine 75% and Insulin Lispro 25%

Keypoint: Tablets and capsules that contain more than one drug are usually ordered by number of tablets or capsules to be given, rather than by dosage.

Problems 7.3

Refer to the labels in Figures 7-21 and 7-22 to answer the following questions.

1. The physician orders the inhaler Advair.® Looking at Figure 7-21 you know that this medication is a combination medication and includes which medications?

    _____

2. Percocet® is a combination medication. The physician orders 1 tablet of this medication. When looking at the label in Figure 7-22, what medications are included in this tablet and how much of each medication is present?

    _____

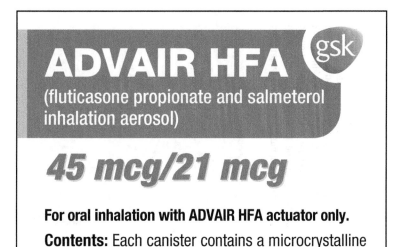

▲ **Figure 7-21**

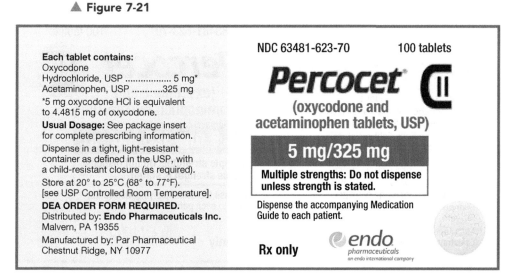

▲ **Figure 7-22**

Controlled Substance Labels

Medications that are considered controlled substances are classified into schedules. The United States Drug Enforcement Administration (DEA) enforces the controlled substance laws. The Controlled Substances Act (CSA) places all substances that are regulated under existing federal law into one of five schedules. Controlled substances are ranked according to the potential risk of physical and psychological dependence. On drug labels, controlled substances are identified by the letter C surrounding the schedule Roman numeral as shown in Figures 7-23 and 7-24. Refer to Table 7-1 for the symbol, description, and examples of each.

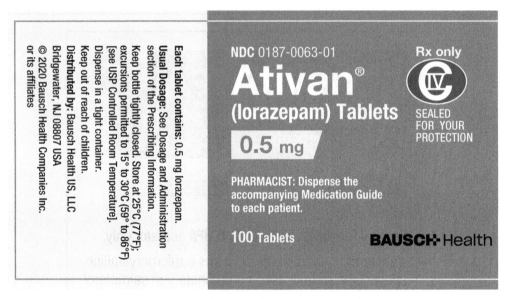

▲ **Figure 7-23** Controlled substance–Schedule IV (4).

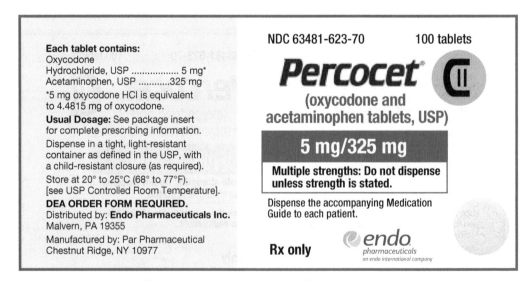

▲ **Figure 7-24** Controlled substance–Schedule II (2).

Schedule	Symbol	Description	Examples
Schedule I	C I	Drugs, substances, or chemicals that have a high potential for abuse and have no currently accepted medical use.	Heroin, LSD, Ecstasy
Schedule II	C II	Drugs, substances, or chemicals that have a high potential for abuse, and may potentially lead to severe psychological or physical dependence. Also considered dangerous.	hydrocodone (Vicodin®), hydromorphone (Dilaudid®), oxycodone (OxyContin®), methylphenidate (Ritalin®)
Schedule III	C III	Drugs, substances, or chemicals that have a low to moderate potential for physical and psychological dependence. Abuse potential is less than Schedules I and II.	acetaminophen (Tylenol®) with Codeine (containing less than 90 mg of codeine), ketamine (Ketalar®), testosterone (Depo-Testosterone®)
Schedule IV	C IV	Drugs, substances, or chemicals that have a low potential for abuse and dependence.	lorazepam (Ativan®), alprazolam (Xanax®), diazepam (Valium®), zolpidem (Ambien®)
Schedule V	C V	Drugs, substances, or chemicals with a lower potential for abuse than Schedule IV. This list consists of drugs with a limited quantity of certain narcotics.	diphenoxylate/atropine (Lomotil®), pregabalin (Lyrica®), antitussive (anti-cough) medications that contain no more than 200 mg of codeine per 100 mL

Table 7-1 Controlled Substance Schedule

Problems 7.4

1. Referring to Table 7-1, identify the controlled substance schedule that includes substances that are dangerous and have a potential for severe psychological and physical dependence.

_____

Refer to the labels in Figures 7-25 and 7-26 to answer the following questions.

2. Why does the medication shown in Figure 7-25 qualify as a Schedule V controlled substance?

_____

3. Referring to Figure 7-26 and Table 7-1, identify the controlled substance schedule that includes this medication.

_____

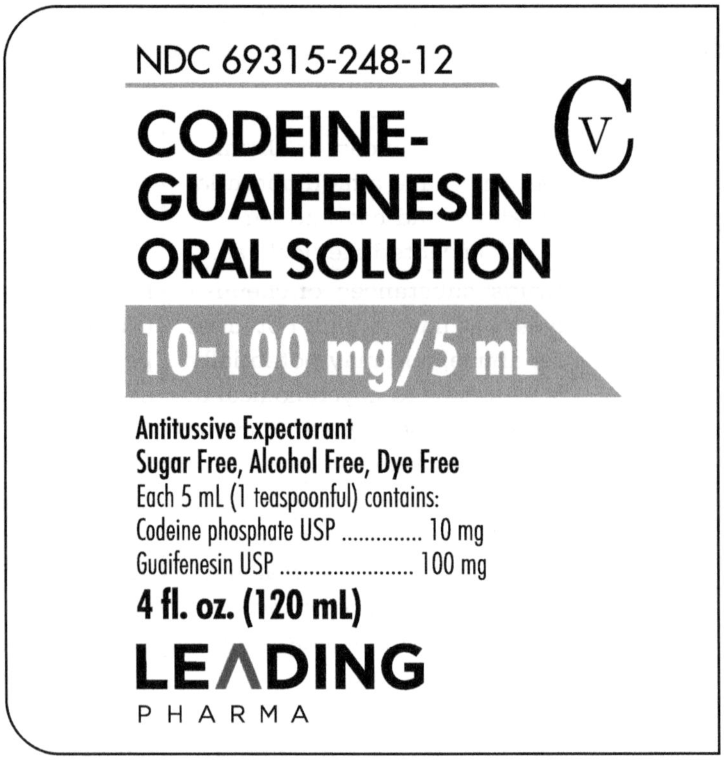
NDC 69315-248-12
CODEINE-
GUAIFENESIN
ORAL SOLUTION
CV
10-100 mg/5 mL
Antitussive Expectorant
Sugar Free, Alcohol Free, Dye Free
Each 5 mL (1 teaspoonful) contains:
Codeine phosphate USP .... 10 mg
Guaifenesin USP .... 100 mg
4 fl. oz. (120 mL)
LEADING
PHARMA

▲ **Figure 7-25**

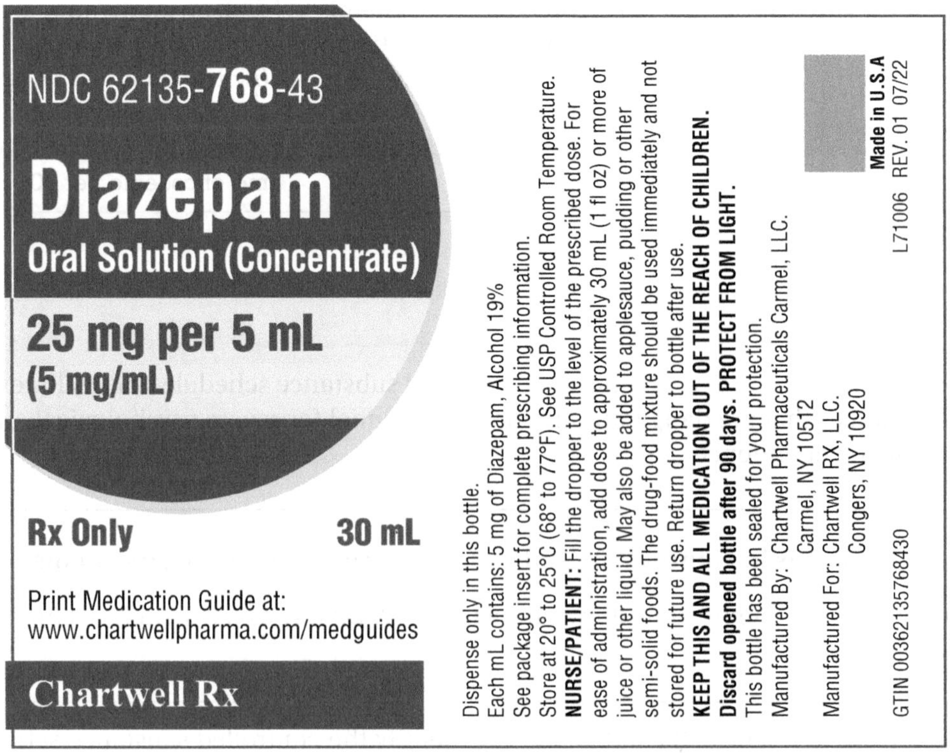
NDC 62135-768-43
Diazepam
Oral Solution (Concentrate)
25 mg per 5 mL
(5 mg/mL)
Rx Only
30 mL
Print Medication Guide at:
www.chartwellpharma.com/medguides
Chartwell Rx
Dispense only in this bottle.
Each mL contains: 5 mg of Diazepam, Alcohol 19%
See package insert for complete prescribing information.
Store at 20° to 25°C (68° to 77°F). See USP Controlled Room Temperature.
NURSE/PATIENT: Fill the dropper to the level of the prescribed dose. For ease of administration, add dose to approximately 30 mL (1 fl oz) or more of juice or other liquid. May also be added to applesauce, pudding or other semi-solid foods. The drug-food mixture should be used immediately and not stored for future use. Return dropper to bottle after use.
KEEP THIS AND ALL MEDICATION OUT OF THE REACH OF CHILDREN.
Discard opened bottle after 90 days. PROTECT FROM LIGHT.
This bottle has been sealed for your protection.
Manufactured By: Chartwell Pharmaceuticals Carmel, LLC.
Carmel, NY 10512
Manufactured For: Chartwell RX, LLC.
Congers, NY 10920
Made in U.S.A
GTIN 00362135768430
L71006 REV. 01 07/22

▲ **Figure 7-26**

Answers **1.** Schedule II **2.** According to the label, there are 10 mg of codeine in 5 mL. Schedule V cough medications cannot exceed 200 mg of codeine in 100 mL. If you multiply 10 mg times 20 (equals 200 mg), and 5 mL times 20 (equals 100 mL), the amount is equal to 200 mg in 100 mL, and this qualifies it as a schedule V controlled drug. **3.** Schedule IV

Directions for Mixing Or Reconstituting

Many parenteral drugs are packaged in powder form because they are not stable in a liquid form. These drugs must be reconstituted with an appropriate and compatible solution or diluent. You may also see the terms *constitute* or *dilute* on the label or package insert to describe reconstitution instructions. Directions for reconstituting will be on the vial label or on the package insert. There may be one instruction for multiple routes (Figure 7-27), or different instructions for an intramuscular injection versus an intravenous injection/ infusion (Figure 7-28). It is very important that these directions be followed very closely.

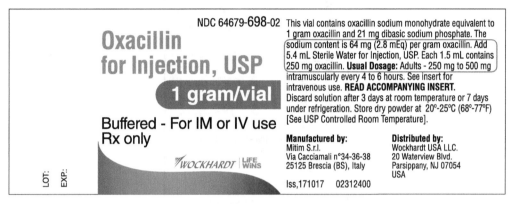

▲ **Figure 7-27** Instructions for reconstitution–One instruction for IM and IV routes- Add 5.4 mL sterile water for injection, USP.

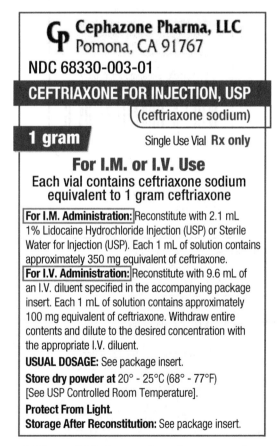

▲ **Figure 7-28** Instructions for reconstitution – Different instructions for IM and IV.

Calculations with a reconstituted drug may become challenging because you will reconstitute the entire container, but only be administering a partial amount of the medication. This will be discussed more thoroughly in Chapter 13. The most common reconstitution solution is normal saline (0.9% sodium chloride) for parenteral medications, but there are exceptions. For oral medications that need reconstituted, tap water, distilled water, or sterile water is used. See Figures 7-29 and 7-30 for additional labels with reconstitution directions.

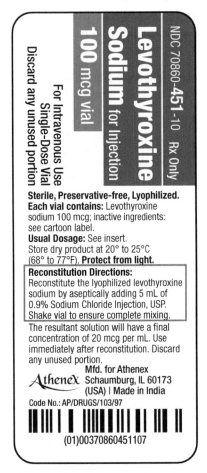

▲ **Figure 7-29** Instructions for reconstitution – IV reconstitution directions.

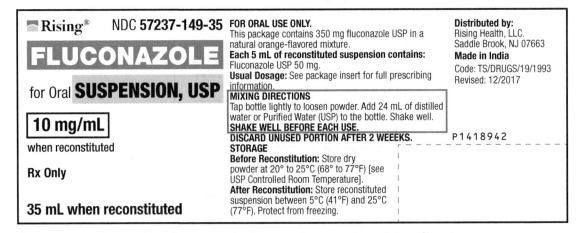

▲ **Figure 7-30** Instructions for reconstitution – oral suspension mixing directions.

Problems 7.5

Refer to the following figures to answer the following questions.

1. According to Figure 7-31, cefazolin, how many milliliters of diluent will be added to this vial to mix this medication for an IM injection?

_____

2. According to Figure 7-32, Solumedrol®, what solution will be used for reconstitution?

_____

3. According to Figure 7-32, Solumedrol®, what is the final concentration after reconstitution?

_____

4. *True or False*: The drug in Figure 7-33, Augmentin®, must be mixed with a total of 125 mL of water.

_____

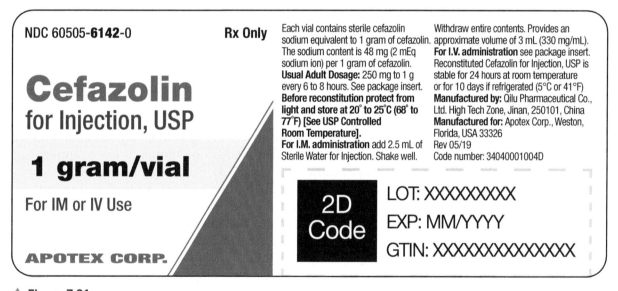

▲ Figure 7-31

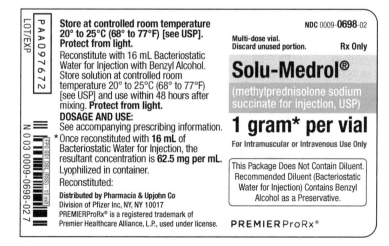

▲ Figure 7-32

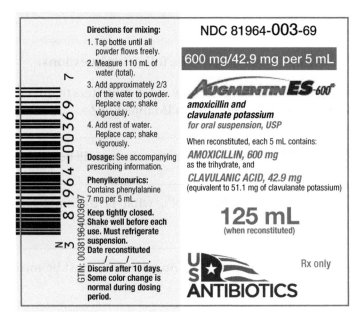

▲ Figure 7-33

Additional Components of a Drug Label

Drug acronyms are used to describe the drug delivery system of a medication and are identified by capital letters at the end of many medication names. Some examples are: ER/XR/XL (extended-release) as shown in Figure 7-34, SR (sustained-release) as shown in Figure 7-35, CR (controlled-release), and LA (long-acting). Medications with these letters release the drug into the bloodstream over a period of time, and should never be chewed, crushed, or broken in half. This would alter the action and release of this drug.

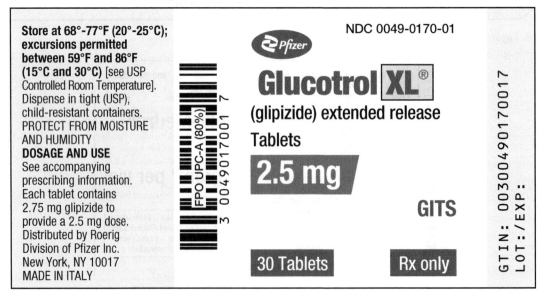

▲ **Figure 7-34** XL – Extended release

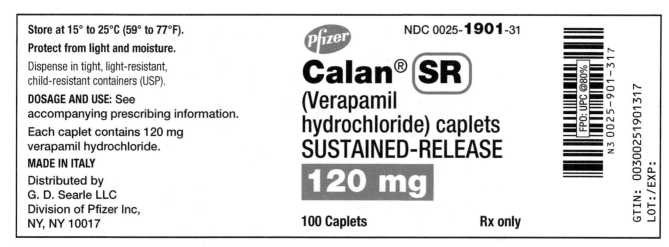

▲ **Figure 7-35** SR – Sustained-release

The **expiration date** of a drug will always be on the label, as shown in Figure 7-36, and must be checked prior to medication preparation. According to information from United States Pharmacopeia (USP—General Chapter 7), manufacturers are required to use a four-digit year for the expiration date. This requirement was initiated in 2023. This will prevent confusion between other numbers on the label. If the drug is expired, it must be sent back to pharmacy and replaced. Also, check expiration dates on intravenous (IV) bags. The Food and Drug Administration (FDA) requires stability testing when a drug approval application is submitted. This testing guarantees that the drug will meet the standards of strength, quality, and purity throughout the shelf-life of the drug. Appropriate studies must be submitted to the FDA that will provide confidence of the expiration date.

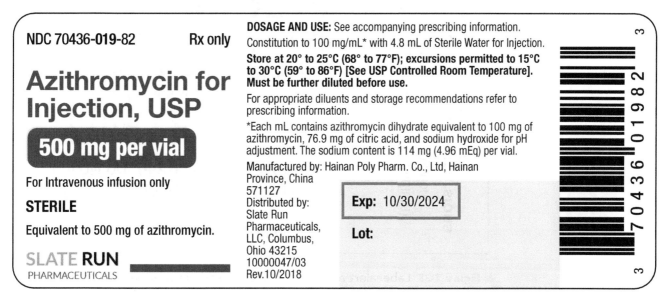

▲ **Figure 7-36** Expiration date – 10/30/2024

Label alerts are items on a drug label that may include precautions or warnings from the manufacturer as well as from the pharmacy. These alerts may include: protect from the light, store at a certain temperature, swallow the tablet whole, and do not chew, crush, or cut in half. Refer to Figures 7-37 and 7-38 for examples of label alerts.

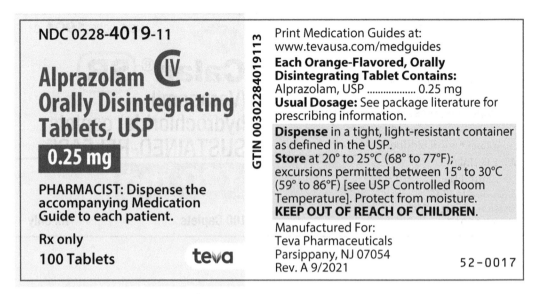

▲ **Figure 7-37** Label alerts

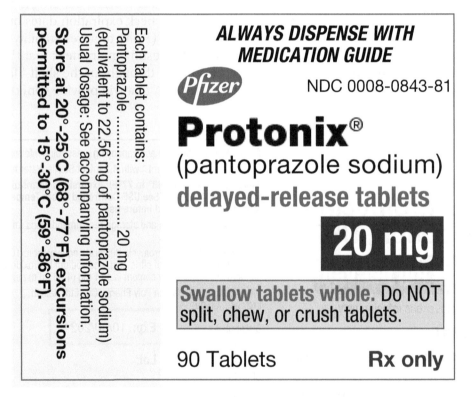

▲ **Figure 7-38** Label alert related to medication administration

The **bar code** on the label, as shown in Figure 7-39, has many purposes. In medication administration, the bar code is scanned to determine and validate the correct drug on the eMAR screen. Other reasons for the bar code include: meeting FDA regulations, recording health data, tracing drugs in case of contamination, and preventing tampering and counterfeiting.

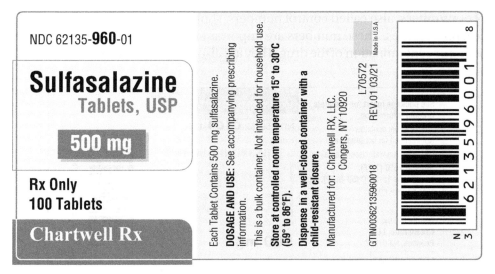

▲ **Figure 7-39** Bar code

Codes indicating official national approved lists of drugs. The United States Pharmacopeia (USP), National Formulary (NF), and the National Drug Code Directory (NDC) are all directories and official publications that describe the guidelines for the composition, dosage, and preparation of medications. All drugs are assigned an NDC. The USP code is typically next to the generic name of the drug, as shown in Figure 7-40.

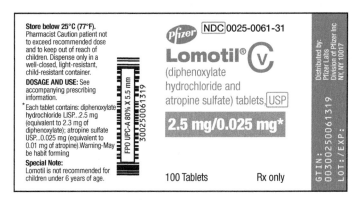

▲ **Figure 7-40** NDC and USP

The **name of the manufacturer** appears on all medication labels as shown in Figure 7-41. There may be a name of subsidiary manufacturer as well.

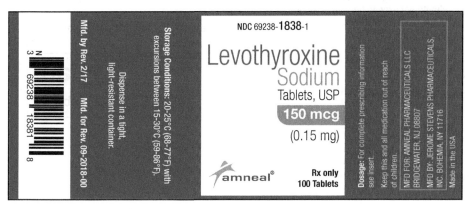

▲ **Figure 7-41** Manufacturer

    Lot numbers, also called control numbers, shown in Figure 7-42, are required on all medication packages. These numbers are important to identify the medication in cases of tampering or contamination of the drug. They are also useful for adverse reaction reporting.

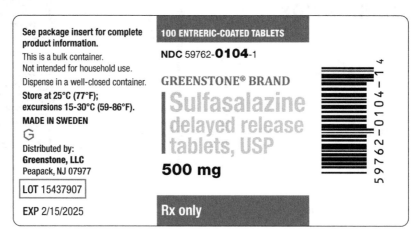

▲ **Figure 7-42** Lot number

Problems 7.6

Refer to Figure 7-43 to answer the following questions.

1. What is the NDC code on the clozapine label? _____

2. Who is the manufacturer shown on this label? _____

3. The initials USP follow the name clozapine on the far left of the label. What does USP stand for? _____

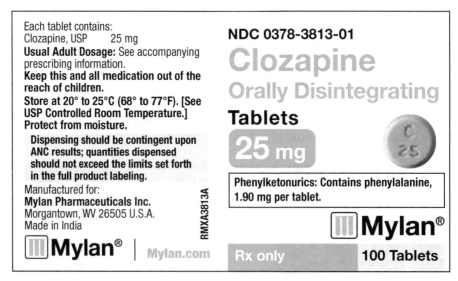

▲ **Figure 7-43**

Summary

This concludes the chapter on reading medication labels. The important points to remember from this chapter are:

- Most labels contain both generic and trade names.

- Dosage strengths are clearly printed on the label, including preparations containing multiple drugs.

- Combined dosage tablets and capsules may be ordered by generic or trade name and number of tablets/capsules to be given and may include dosages.

- Become familiar with controlled substance designations.

- Carefully read reconstitution directions to ensure the correct route, and the correct amount of solution is used to mix the powder.

- The letters USP (United States Pharmacopeia) and NF (National Formulary) on drug labels identify their official generic listings.

- Additional letters that follow a drug name are used to identify the preparation or a special action of the drug.

- Check expiration dates on labels before use.

Summary Self-Test

Refer to Figure 7-44 to answer questions 1 through 5.

1. What is the trade name on the label? _____

2. What is the form of the medication? _____

3. What controlled substance category is this medication in? _____
_____

4. What is the manufacturer of this medication? _____

5. What is the dosage strength of the medication? _____

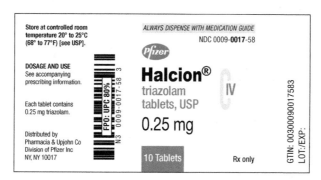

▲ **Figure 7-44**

Refer to Figure 7-45 to answer questions 6 through 9.

6. What two medications are combined to make Lotrel®? _____
_____

7. What are the storage instructions on this label? _____
_____

8. What is the form of this medication? _____

9. What is the NDC code? _____

NDC 0078-0405-05

Lotrel® **5 mg */10 mg**

amlodipine and benazepril
hydrochloride capsules

*each capsule contains 6.9 mg of
amlodipine besylate

100 capsules
Rx only

℧ NOVARTIS

Recommended Dosage: See Prescribing Information.
Store at 20°C to 25°C (68°F to 77°F); excursions permitted
between 15°C to 30°C (59°F to 86°F).
[See USP controlled room temperature.] Protect from moisture.
Dispense in tight container (USP).
Keep this and all drugs out of the reach of children.
Mfd. by: Eon Labs Inc.
Wilson, NC 27893
Dist. by: Novartis Pharmaceuticals Corp.
East Hanover, New Jersey 07936
©Novartis   GTIN: 00300780405058
                EXP/LOT   46192916 US

REV0521

▲ **Figure 7-45**

Refer to Figure 7-46 to answer questions 10 through 13.

10. What is the trade name of this medication? _____

11. What does LA mean following the medication name? _____
_____

12. What is the total quantity of capsules? _____

13. What is the dosage strength? _____

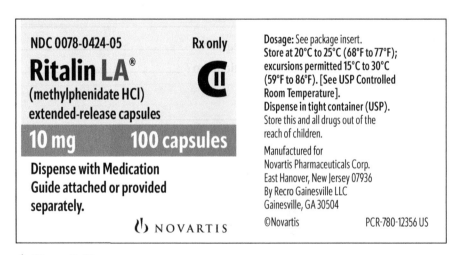

NDC 0078-0424-05   **Rx only**

Ritalin LA®
(methylphenidate HCl)
extended-release capsules

C II

10 mg   100 capsules

**Dispense with Medication
Guide attached or provided
separately.**

℧ NOVARTIS

Dosage: See package insert.
Store at 20°C to 25°C (68°F to 77°F);
excursions permitted 15°C to 30°C
(59°F to 86°F). [See USP Controlled
Room Temperature].
Dispense in tight container (USP).
Store this and all drugs out of the
reach of children.

Manufactured for
Novartis Pharmaceuticals Corp.
East Hanover, New Jersey 07936
By Recro Gainesville LLC
Gainesville, GA 30504

©Novartis   PCR-780-12356 US

▲ **Figure 7-46**

Refer to Figure 7-47 to answer questions 14 through 18.

14. What are the reconstitution directions for this medication? _____
_____

15. If this medication is reconstituted on September 1, 2024 at 0800 when should it be

    discarded according to the information on the label? _____

16. What is the route for administration for this medication? _____

    _____

17. Using household measures, what volume will contain 100 mg? _____

    _____

18. What is the dosage strength using metric measures? _____

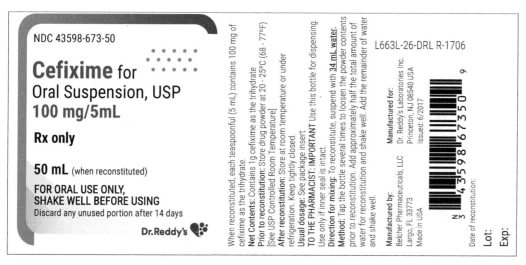

▲ **Figure 7-47**

Refer to Figure 7-48 to answer questions 19 through 22.

19. What is the route of administration for this medication? _____

    _____

20. What is the dosage strength in 1 mL? _____

21. How many doses will this pen deliver? _____

22. Who is the manufacturer? _____

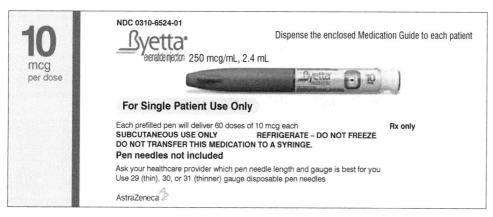

▲ **Figure 7-48**

Refer to Figure 7-49 to answer questions 23 through 26.

23. What is the generic name for this medication? _____

24. What is the warning printed on this label? _____

_____

25. What is the route of administration? What does this mean? _____
_____

26. What is the dosage strength of each tablet? _____

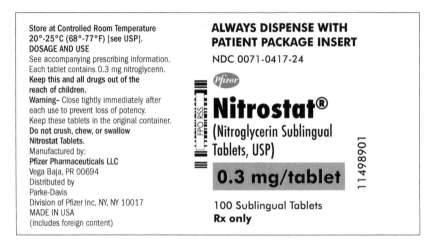

Store at Controlled Room Temperature
20°-25°C (68°-77°F) [see USP].
DOSAGE AND USE
See accompanying prescribing information.
Each tablet contains 0.3 mg nitroglycerin.
**Keep this and all drugs out of the
reach of children.**
Warning- Close tightly immediately after
each use to prevent loss of potency.
Keep these tablets in the original container.
**Do not crush, chew, or swallow
Nitrostat Tablets.**
Manufactured by:
Pfizer Pharmaceuticals LLC
Vega Baja, PR 00694
Distributed by
Parke-Davis
Division of Pfizer Inc, NY, NY 10017
MADE IN USA
(includes foreign content)

**ALWAYS DISPENSE WITH
PATIENT PACKAGE INSERT**
NDC 0071-0417-24
Pfizer
Nitrostat®
(Nitroglycerin Sublingual
Tablets, USP)
0.3 mg/tablet
100 Sublingual Tablets
Rx only

▲ **Figure 7-49**

Refer to Figure 7-50 to answer questions 27 through 30.

27. What directions are on this package regarding discard? _____
_____

28. According to the image of the dropper, how many milligrams of this medication are
present in 0.5 mL? _____
_____

29. There is a controlled substance image on this package. Using this image, as well as
the information in Table 7-1, what schedule is this medication part of?
_____

30. What is the route for this medication? _____

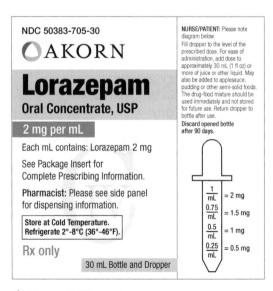

NDC 50383-705-30
◯AKORN
Lorazepam
Oral Concentrate, USP
2 mg per mL
Each mL contains: Lorazepam 2 mg
See Package Insert for
Complete Prescribing Information.
Pharmacist: Please see side panel
for dispensing information.
**Store at Cold Temperature.
Refrigerate 2°-8°C (36°-46°F).**
Rx only
30 mL Bottle and Dropper

NURSE/PATIENT: Please note
diagram below.
Fill dropper to the level of the
prescribed dose. For ease of
administration, add dose to
approximately 30 mL (1 fl oz) or
more of juice or other liquid. May
also be added to applesauce,
pudding or other semi-solid foods.
The drug-food mixture should be
used immediately and not stored
for future use. Return dropper to
bottle after use.
**Discard opened bottle
after 90 days.**

$\frac{1}{mL}$ = 2 mg
$\frac{0.75}{mL}$ = 1.5 mg
$\frac{0.5}{mL}$ = 1 mg
$\frac{0.25}{mL}$ = 0.5 mg

▲ **Figure 7-50**

Critical Thinking Questions

Refer to Figure 7-51 to answer the following question.

1. The physician has ordered Heparin 2,500 units IM once daily for a client. When the nurse starts to prepare the drug and reviews the label, the nurse should:

   a. prepare the drug as ordered.
   b. call the physician concerning the order.
   c. administer the drug as ordered.
   d. identify the client.

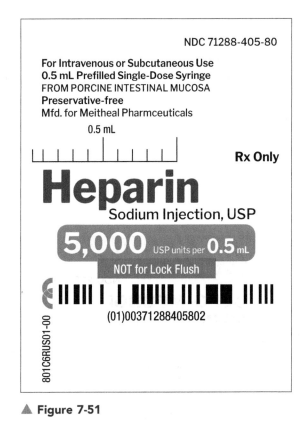

▲ Figure 7-51

Refer to Figure 7-52 to answer the following question.

2. A client is ordered a Byetta® (exenatide) subcutaneous 10 mcg injection on 9/23/2024, before breakfast, to manage type 2 diabetes mellitus. The nurse

reviews the label against the order and is preparing the medication. Prior to administering the medication, the nurse should:

a. put the medication into a syringe.
b. ensure the medication was kept in the freezer.
c. call the pharmacy regarding information on the label.
d. check the lot number.

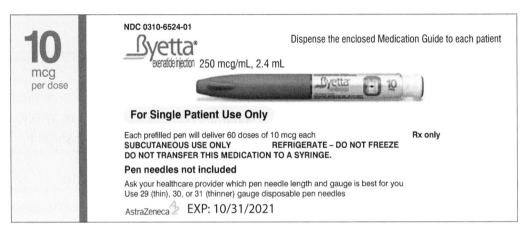

▲ **Figure 7-52**

Refer to Figure 7-53 to answer the following question.

3. The nurse is preparing Depo-Medrol® (methylprednisolone acetate) injection for a client. After reviewing the label, the nurse identifies the concentration of the medication as:

a. 200 mg/1 mL
b. 40 mg/1 mL
c. 40 mg/5 mL
d. 200 mg/5 mL

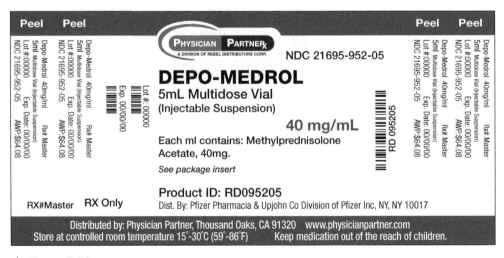

▲ **Figure 7-53**

Refer to Figure 7-54 to answer the following question.

4. Cefazolin 500 mg IV has been ordered every 8 hours for a client with pneumonia. The vial will need reconstituted. The nurse should:

  a. reconstitute the vial with 3 mL of sterile water.
  b. read the package insert.
  c. reconstitute the vial with 2.5 mL of sterile water.
  d. contact the pharmacy.

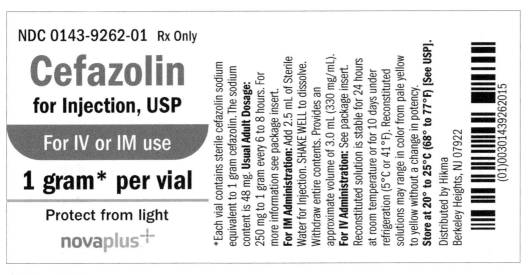

▲ Figure 7-54

Refer to Figure 7-55 to answer the following question.

5. A client has returned from abdominal surgery and is ordered enoxaparin injection 30 mg daily to prevent deep venous thrombosis. After reviewing the label, the nurse will inject the medication by which route?

  a. The medication may be given by any injection route
  b. The intravenous route
  c. The intramuscular route
  d. The subcutaneous route

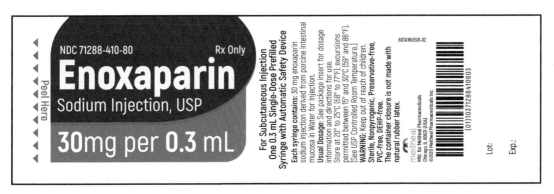

▲ Figure 7-55

Refer to Figure 7-56 to answer the following question.

6. Health care professionals are working in a clinic and administering COVID-19 vaccines today. The clients will be age 12 and older. The clinic is open from 9 am to 4 pm daily. The staff is preparing the vaccines for the first group this morning. What relevant information should the staff recognize prior to administration of the COVID-19 vaccine? Select all that apply.

   a. The route will be IM.
   b. The vaccine must be kept in the freezer.
   c. If the vial is not empty after the first day, it can be used until empty the next day.
   d. The medication will not be reconstituted.
   e. The dose will be determined by age.
   f. The medication is in a multidose vial.

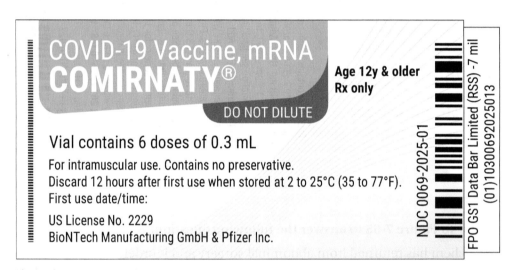

▲ **Figure 7-56**

Answers to Critical Thinking Questions

1. b. The ordered route is wrong, therefore the drug would not be prepared or administered.
2. c. The medication is expired and pharmacy should be notified. According to the label, the medication would not be placed in a syringe, it should be refrigerated, not in the freezer and the lot number would not be a consideration for this medication which is expired.
3. b. 40 mg/1 mL
4. b. Read the package insert.
5. d. Subcutaneous route is on the label.
6. a, d, f (b is incorrect because the temperature does not require a freezer; c is incorrect because the vial must be discarded after 12 hours; e is incorrect because the dose is indicated on the vial).

Ratio and Proportion

Objectives

The learner will:

1. explain the difference between the terms ratio and proportion.

2. set up calculations using ratio and proportion.

3. use ratio and proportion to solve calculations.

Prerequisites

Chapters 1 through 7

A **ratio** consists of two different numbers or quantities that have a significant relationship to each other. There are many examples of ratios in everyday life, as well as health care. For example, if you need 2.5 cups of flour for one cake, the ratio would be 2.5 cups per 1 cake. Recall that dosages can be expressed as a ratio on drug labels, including a certain weight (strength) of drug in a tablet (tab), capsule (cap), or a certain volume of solution, most commonly mL; for example, 50 mg per mL, 100 mcg in 1 tablet, 1,000 units per mL. A proportion is used to show the relationship between two ratios.

Clinical Relevance: Chapters 8 through 10 will introduce three methods of calculation. It is important to choose a method of calculation that you can consistently use to perform calculations in the clinical setting. Consistent use of a method will enable you to become comfortable with its use to calculate dosages and apply it to other calculations in the clinical setting. Whichever method of calculation you use, it is important to clearly label your numbers with the unit of measure so that you are certain about what your end result represents. For example, will your result be tablets, capsules, milliliters, milligrams, or another unit of measure? This attention to detail will serve you well in the prevention of calculation errors.

Common Ways to Express Ratio and Proportion

There are two ways to express, or write, a ratio. The numbers can be written as a common fraction or separated by a colon.

Note: Ratios are typically written without spaces between the number and the colon. However, when solving dosage problems that include the units of measure in the ratio expression, we are adding spaces to clearly separate the two pieces of information in the ratio.

As a common fraction		Separated by a colon
$\dfrac{\frac{1}{3} \text{ cup bleach}}{1 \text{ gallon water}}$	or	$\frac{1}{3}$ cup : 1 gallon
$\dfrac{50 \text{ mg}}{1 \text{ mL}}$	or	50 mg : 1 mL
$\dfrac{100 \text{ mcg}}{1 \text{ tab}}$	or	100 mcg : 1 tab
$\dfrac{1{,}000 \text{ units}}{1 \text{ mL}}$	or	1,000 units : 1 mL

Keypoint: A ratio consists of two numbers that have a significant relationship to each other. It can be expressed as a common fraction or with the numbers separated by a colon.

While a ratio is an expression of a significant relationship between two numbers, a **proportion** is used to show the relationship between two ratios. In a proportion, the ratios are separated by an **equal sign (=)**. Again, a proportion can be shown using fractions or colons.

Example 1 ■ $\dfrac{50}{1} = \dfrac{100}{2}$ or $50{:}1 = 100{:}2$

These expressions are true proportions.

Keypoint: A **true proportion** contains two ratios that are equal. This is a simple comparison, but by using drug strength examples, we can verify that the ratios are equal and that the proportion is true.

Example 2 ■ $\dfrac{50 \text{ mg}}{1 \text{ tab}} = \dfrac{100 \text{ mg}}{2 \text{ tab}}$ or   50 mg : 1 tab = 100 mg : 2 tab

If 1 tablet contains 50 mg, 2 tablets will contain 100 mg.

Example 3 ■ $\dfrac{50 \text{ mg}}{1 \text{ mL}} = \dfrac{100 \text{ mg}}{2 \text{ mL}}$ or   50 mg : 1 mL = 100 mg : 2 mL

If 1 mL contains 50 mg, 2 mL will contain 100 mg.

You can also prove mathematically that these ratios are equal and that the proportion is true. When working with proportions that are set up using colons, it is important to understand the structure and terminology. The **means** are the middle part of the equation and the **extremes** are the ends of the equation. To remember this distinction and prevent errors, notice that the means, or middle of a proportion, both begin with the letter "**m**" (**m**eans, **m**iddle). The extremes, or ends of a proportion, both begin with the letter "**e**" (**e**xtremes, **e**nds). It is critical in all math involving proportions that the means and extremes are not mixed up or an incorrect answer will be obtained.

> **Key**point: In a true proportion set up using fractions, the cross-multiplied products will be identical. To prove that a proportion is true, cross multiply. The products (answers) you obtain will be identical. If using colons to separate the ratios, multiply the extremes and also the means. In a true proportion using colons, the products of the means and the extremes will be equal.

Example 4 ▪

$$\frac{50 \text{ mg}}{1 \text{ tab}} = \frac{100 \text{ mg}}{2 \text{ tab}}$$

$$\frac{50}{1} \diagdown \frac{100}{2}$$ You may eliminate the measurement units.

$$50 \times 2 = 100 \times 1$$ Cross multiply.

$$100 = 100$$

The products of cross multiplying in this proportion, 100, are the same. If using colons to separate your ratio, the setup would be as follows:

$$50 \text{ mg} : 1 \text{ tab} = 100 \text{ mg} : 2 \text{ tab}$$

$$50 \times 2 = 1 \times 100$$ Multiply the extremes and the means.
                                     You may eliminate the measurement units.

$$100 = 100$$

The extremes are equal to the means.

   Regardless of the method used, we have now proved mathematically that the ratios are equal and the proportion is true.

Example 5 ▪

$$\frac{500 \text{ mg}}{2 \text{ mL}} \diagdown \frac{250 \text{ mg}}{1 \text{ mL}}$$

$$250 \times 2 = 500 \times 1$$ Eliminate the measurement units, then
                                     cross multiply.

$$500 = 500$$

The products of cross multiplying, 500, are identical. This is a true proportion; the ratios are equal.

Example 6 ▪

$$\frac{10 \text{ units}}{1 \text{ mL}} = \frac{20 \text{ units}}{2 \text{ mL}}$$

$$10 \times 2 = 20 \times 1$$

$$20 = 20$$

This is a true proportion. The products of cross multiplying, 20, are equal.

Problems 8.1

Express the following using the ratio format you prefer (fraction format or colon format).

Note: If you do not include the units of measure, your answers are incorrect.

1. An injectable solution that contains 100 mg in each 1.5 mL   _____

2. An injectable solution that contains 250 mg in each 0.7 mL   _____

3. A tablet that contains 0.4 mg of drug   _____

4. Two tablets that contain 450 mg of drug   _____

5. A cup of soup has 240 calories   _____

6. A train goes 45 miles over 2 hours   _____

Answers **1.** $\frac{100 \text{ mg}}{1.5 \text{ mL}}$; 100 mg : 1.5 mL **2.** $\frac{250 \text{ mg}}{0.7 \text{ mL}}$; 250 mg : 0.7 mL; **3.** $\frac{0.4 \text{ mg}}{1 \text{ tab}}$; 0.4 mg : 1 tab
4. $\frac{450 \text{ mg}}{2 \text{ tab}}$; 450 mg : 2 tab **5.** $\frac{240 \text{ calories}}{1 \text{ cup}}$; 240 calories : 1 cup **6.** $\frac{45 \text{ miles}}{2 \text{ hours}}$; 45 miles : 2 hours

Problems 8.2

Determine mathematically if these proportions are true.

1. $\dfrac{34 \text{ mg}}{2 \text{ mL}} = \dfrac{51 \text{ mg}}{3 \text{ mL}}$ _____

2. $\dfrac{15 \text{ mg}}{4 \text{ mL}} = \dfrac{45 \text{ mg}}{12 \text{ mL}}$ _____

3. $\dfrac{46 \text{ mg}}{1.3 \text{ mL}} = \dfrac{23 \text{ mg}}{0.65 \text{ mL}}$ _____

4. $\dfrac{150 \text{ units}}{2.3 \text{ mL}} = \dfrac{130 \text{ units}}{1.9 \text{ mL}}$ _____

5. $\dfrac{40 \text{ mg}}{1.1 \text{ mL}} = \dfrac{80 \text{ mg}}{2.2 \text{ mL}}$ _____

Answers **1.** true (2 × 51 = 102 and 34 × 3 = 102) **2.** true (4 × 45 = 180 and 15 × 12 = 180)
3. true (46 × 0.65 = 29.9 and 23 × 1.3 = 29.9) **4.** not true (150 × 1.9 = 285 and 130 × 2.3 = 299)
5. true (40 × 2.2 = 88 and 1.1 × 80 = 88)

Problems 8.3

Determine mathematically if these proportions are true.

1. 24 mg : 2 mL = 36 mg : 3 mL   _____

2. 0.5 mg : 2 mL = 3 mg : 12 mL   _____

3. 48 mg : 1.5 mL = 16 mg : 0.5 mL   _____

4. 250 units : 3 mL = 125 units : 5 mL   _____

5. 8 mcg : 1.6 mL = 4 mcg : 0.8 mL   _____

Relating Ratio and Proportion to Calculations

Ratios and proportions are important in calculations because they can be used when only **one ratio is known**, or **complete**, and **the second is incomplete**. For example, if you know that you can travel by car going 55 miles in 1 hour and you want to know how many hours it will take to go to a town 220 miles away, you can calculate this using ratio and proportion.

Example 1 ▣

$$\frac{55 \text{ miles}}{1 \text{ hour}} = \frac{220 \text{ miles}}{x \text{ hours}} \quad \text{or} \quad 55 \text{ miles} : 1 \text{ hour} = 220 \text{ miles} : x \text{ hours}$$

$$\frac{55 \text{ miles}}{1 \text{ hour}} \diagdown \diagup \frac{220 \text{ miles}}{x \text{ hours}} \qquad \text{Cross multiply.}$$

$$55x = 220 \times 1$$

$$\frac{55x}{55} = \frac{220}{55}$$

$$x = 4 \text{ hours}$$

You can apply this concept to various calculations in health care. You will encounter situations where the ordered dose is in the same system and same unit of measurement as the supply.

Example 2 ▣

The morphine solution strength is 8 mg per mL and will be used to prepare a dosage order of 10 mg. Refer to the label in Figure 8-1 for additional information.

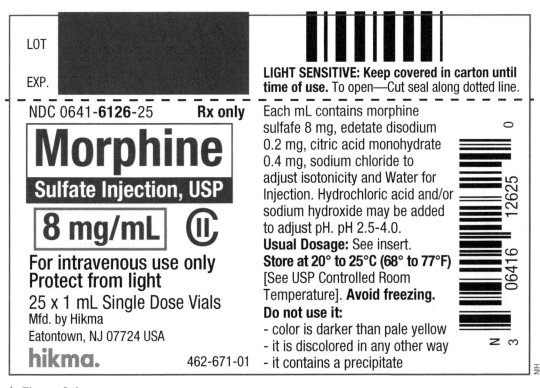

LOT

EXP.

LIGHT SENSITIVE: Keep covered in carton until time of use. To open—Cut seal along dotted line.

NDC 0641-**6126**-25   **Rx only**

Morphine

Sulfate Injection, USP

8 mg/mL   ℗

For intravenous use only
Protect from light
25 x 1 mL Single Dose Vials
Mfd. by Hikma
Eatontown, NJ 07724 USA

hikma.   462-671-01

Each mL contains morphine sulfafe 8 mg, edetate disodium 0.2 mg, citric acid monohydrate 0.4 mg, sodium chloride to adjust isotonicity and Water for Injection. Hydrochloric acid and/or sodium hydroxide may be added to adjust pH. pH 2.5-4.0.
Usual Dosage: See insert.
Store at 20° to 25°C (68° to 77°F) [See USP Controlled Room Temperature]. **Avoid freezing.**
Do not use it:
- color is darker than pale yellow
- it is discolored in any other way
- it contains a precipitate

0

12625

06416

N   3

▲ **Figure 8-1**

The known ratio is provided by the solution strength available, 8 mg per mL. The incomplete ratio is the dosage to be given, 10 mg, and x is used to represent the mL which will contain 10 mg.

$$\frac{8 \text{ mg}}{1 \text{ mL}} = \frac{10 \text{ mg}}{x \text{ mL}}$$

$$\begin{pmatrix} \text{Complete ratio:} \\ \text{Drug strength} \end{pmatrix} \qquad \begin{pmatrix} \text{Incomplete ratio:} \\ \text{Dosage to give} \end{pmatrix}$$

Below is the same example using colons.

$$8 \text{ mg} : 1 \text{ mL} = 10 \text{ mg} : x \text{ mL}$$

$$\begin{pmatrix} \text{Complete ratio:} \\ \text{Drug strength} \end{pmatrix} \qquad \begin{pmatrix} \text{Incomplete ratio:} \\ \text{Dosage to give} \end{pmatrix}$$

 Keypoint: The ratios in a proportion are written in the same sequence of measurement units.

To determine the value of the unknown x mL, follow these steps.

Option 1: Calculation Using Fractions

$\dfrac{8 \text{ mg}}{1 \text{ mL}} = \dfrac{10 \text{ mg}}{x \text{ mL}}$

Set up the proportion to include the measurement units; make sure they are in the same sequence.

$\dfrac{8 \text{ mg}}{1 \text{ mL}} \diagdown\!\!\!\diagup \dfrac{10 \text{ mg}}{x \text{ mL}}$

Drop the measurement units as you cross multiply.

$8x = 10$

Keep x on the left of the equation.

$x = \dfrac{\cancel{10}^{\,5}}{\cancel{8}_{\,4}}$

Divide 10 by the number in front of x; reduce by the highest common denominator (2).

$x = \dfrac{5}{4}$

Divide the final fraction to obtain a decimal fraction.

$x = 1.25 \text{ mL}$

The x in the original proportion was mL, so the answer is 1.25 mL.

Answer: The ordered dosage of 10 mg is contained in 1.25 mL.

In practice, this will be rounded to 1.3 mL. As you will learn in later chapters there are no syringes that allow measurement of 1.25 mL. Remember, it is routine to check your math three times in dosage calculations.

Option 2: Calculation Using Colons

$8 \text{ mg} : 1 \text{ mL} = 10 \text{ mg} : x \text{ mL}$

Set up the proportion to include the measurement units; make sure they are in the same sequence.

$8x = 10$

Eliminate the units of measurement. Multiply the extremes and multiply the means.

$$x = \frac{\cancel{10}^{\,5}}{\cancel{8}_{\,4}}$$

Divide 10 by the number in front of x; reduce by the highest common denominator (2).

$$x = \frac{5}{4}$$

Divide the final fraction to obtain a decimal fraction.

$$x = 1.25 \text{ mL}$$

The x in the original proportion was mL, so the answer is 1.25 mL.

Answer: The ordered dosage of 10 mg is contained in 1.25 mL.

Example 3 ■   The lisinopril tablet strength is 2.5 mg per tablet and will be used to prepare a dosage order of 5 mg. Refer to the label in Figure 8-2 for additional information used in this example.

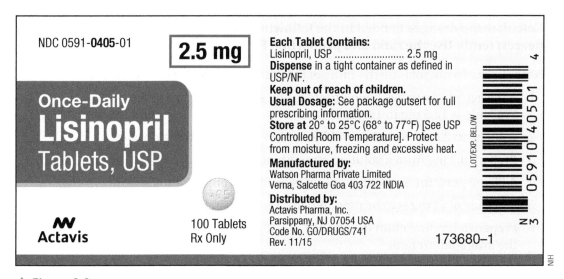

▲ **Figure 8-2**

The strength available is 2.5 mg in 1 tablet. A dosage of 5 mg has been ordered.

Option 1: Calculation Using Fractions

$$\frac{2.5 \text{ mg}}{1 \text{ tab}} = \frac{5 \text{ mg}}{x \text{ tab}}$$

Set up the proportion to include the measurement units; make sure they are in the same sequence.

$$\frac{2.5 \text{ mg}}{1 \text{ tab}} \diagdown\diagup \frac{5 \text{ mg}}{x \text{ tab}}$$

Drop the measurement units as you cross multiply.

$$2.5x = 5$$

Keep x on the left of the equation.

$$x = \frac{5}{2.5}$$

Divide 5 by the number in front of x.

$$x = 2 \text{ tab}$$

The x in the original proportion was tab, so the answer is 2 tab.

Answer: The dosage would be 2 tab.

Option 2: Calculation Using Colons

$2.5 \text{ mg} : 1 \text{ tab} = 5 \text{ mg} : x \text{ tab}$	Set up the proportion to include the measurement units; make sure they are in the same sequence.
$2.5x = 5$	Eliminate the units of measurement. Multiply the extremes and multiply the means.
$x = \dfrac{5}{2.5}$	Divide 5 by the number in front of x.
$x = 2 \text{ tab}$	The x in the original proportion was tab, so the answer is 2 tab.

Answer: The dosage would be 2 tab.

Problems 8.4

Calculate the dosages needed in the following questions. Express answers to the nearest tenth. Use the ratio and proportion format of your choice.

Note: If you do not include the units of measure, your answers are incorrect.

1. A dosage of 24 mg has been ordered. The solution strength available is 12.5 mg in 1.5 mL. _____

2. A 40 mg in 2.5 mL solution will be used to prepare a 30 mg dosage. _____

3. Prepare 0.3 mg from a solution strength of 0.6 mg in 0.8 mL. _____

4. A 36 mg per 2 mL strength solution is used to prepare 24 mg. _____

5. A dosage of 52 mg is to be prepared from a 78 mg in 0.9 mL solution. _____

6. Prepare a levetiracetam dosage of 1,500 mg. Refer to Figure 8-3 for the available strength. _____

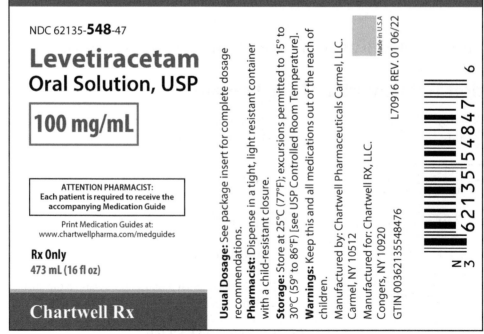

▲ **Figure 8-3**

7. A strength of 3 mL containing 750 mcg is available to prepare 600 mcg. _____

8. If the strength available is 1.5 g per mL, how many mL will a 4 g dosage require? _____

9. Prepare a 0.5 mg dosage of digoxin. Refer to Figure 8-4 for the available strength. _____

10. Prepare a 3 g dosage from a 4 g in 2.7 mL strength solution. _____

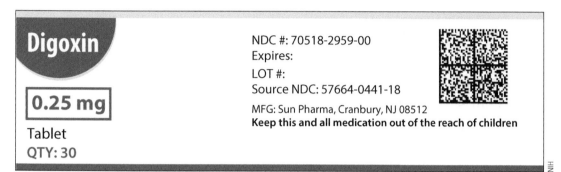

Digoxin

0.25 mg

Tablet

QTY: 30

NDC #: 70518-2959-00
Expires:
LOT #:
Source NDC: 57664-0441-18

MFG: Sun Pharma, Cranbury, NJ 08512
Keep this and all medication out of the reach of children

▲ **Figure 8-4**

Answers   1. 2.9 mL **2.** 1.9 mL **3.** 0.4 mL **4.** 1.3 mL **5.** 0.6 mL **6.** 15 mL **7.** 2.4 mL **8.** 2.7 mL
9. 2 tab **10.** 2 mL

There will be times when the order for a medication and the supply are not in the same system and same unit of measurement. Consider the following calculations. We will show these examples using both formats of ratio and proportion, however you are encouraged to use the ratio and proportion format you chose earlier.

Example 4 ■   The order is to give Neupogen® 0.15 mg of medication. Refer to Figure 8-5 for the available strength.

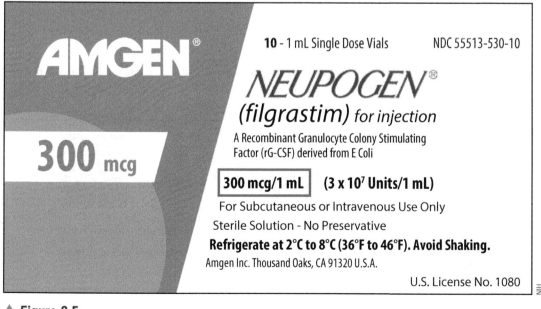

AMGEN®

300 mcg

10 - 1 mL Single Dose Vials   NDC 55513-530-10

NEUPOGEN®

(filgrastim) for injection

A Recombinant Granulocyte Colony Stimulating
Factor (rG-CSF) derived from E Coli

300 mcg/1 mL   (3 x 10⁷ Units/1 mL)

For Subcutaneous or Intravenous Use Only

Sterile Solution - No Preservative

Refrigerate at 2°C to 8°C (36°F to 46°F). Avoid Shaking.

Amgen Inc. Thousand Oaks, CA 91320 U.S.A.

U.S. License No. 1080

▲ **Figure 8-5**

This problem cannot be solved as it is currently written because **the dosages are in different units of measure: mg and mcg**. Recall that it may be safer to convert from larger to smaller units of measure to eliminate/avoid decimal points. Convert the mg to mcg.

Option 1: Calculation Using Fractions

$$\frac{1 \text{ mg}}{1{,}000 \text{ mcg}} = \frac{0.15 \text{ mg}}{x \text{ mcg}}$$

First change the milligrams to micrograms.

$$x = 1{,}000 \times 0.15 = 150$$

$$\frac{300 \text{ mcg}}{1 \text{ mL}} = \frac{150 \text{ mcg}}{x \text{ mL}}$$

Then proceed with your calculation using 150 mcg in place of 0.15 mg.

$$\frac{300 \text{ mcg}}{1 \text{ mL}} \diagdown \diagup \frac{150 \text{ mcg}}{x \text{ mL}}$$

$$300x = 150$$

$$x = \frac{150}{300}$$

$$x = 0.5 \text{ mL}$$

Option 2: Calculation Using Colons

$$1 \text{ mg} : 1{,}000 \text{ mcg} = 0.15 \text{ mg} : x \text{ mcg}$$

First change the milligrams to micrograms.

$$x = 1{,}000 \times 0.15 = 150$$

$$x = 150 \text{ mcg}$$

$$300 \text{ mcg} : 1 \text{ mL} = 150 \text{ mcg} : x \text{ mL}$$

Then proceed with your calculation using 150 mcg in place of 0.15 mg.

$$300x = 1 \times 150$$

$$x = \frac{150}{300}$$

$$x = 0.5 \text{ mL}$$

Example 5 ■   The order is to give amiodarone 0.075 g. Refer to Figure 8-6 for your supply.

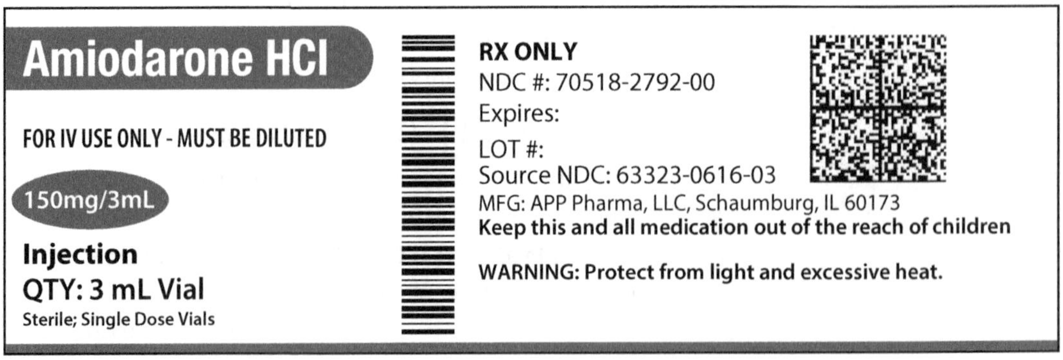

Amiodarone HCl

FOR IV USE ONLY - MUST BE DILUTED

150mg/3mL

Injection
QTY: 3 mL Vial
Sterile; Single Dose Vials

RX ONLY
NDC #: 70518-2792-00
Expires:
LOT #:
Source NDC: 63323-0616-03
MFG: APP Pharma, LLC, Schaumburg, IL 60173
Keep this and all medication out of the reach of children

WARNING: Protect from light and excessive heat.

NIH

▲ **Figure 8-6**

Option 1: Calculation Using Fractions

$$\frac{1 \text{ g}}{1,000 \text{ mg}} = \frac{0.075 \text{ g}}{x \text{ mg}}$$

First change the grams to milligrams.

$$x = 75 \text{ mg}$$

$$\frac{150 \text{ mg}}{3 \text{ mL}} = \frac{75 \text{ mg}}{x \text{ mL}}$$

Then proceed with your calculation using 75 mg in place of 0.075 g.

$$\frac{150 \text{ mg}}{3 \text{ mL}} \diagdown \diagup \frac{75 \text{ mg}}{x \text{ mL}}$$

$$150x = 225$$

$$x = 1.5 \text{ mL}$$

Option 2: Calculation Using Colons

$$1 \text{ g} : 1,000 \text{ mg} = 0.075 \text{ g} : x \text{ mg}$$

First change the grams to milligrams.

$$x = 75 \text{ mg}$$

$$150 \text{ mg} : 3 \text{ mL} = 75 \text{ mg} : x \text{ mL}$$

Then proceed with your calculation using 75 mg in place of 0.075 g.

$$150x = 225$$

$$x = \frac{225}{150}$$

$$x = 1.5 \text{ mL}$$

Ratio and proportion are also used to solve calculations for unit and mEq dosages.

Example 6 ■   The order is to give 1,200 units. The available dosage strength is 1,000 units per 1.5 mL.

Using Fractions

$$\frac{1,000 \text{ units}}{1.5 \text{ mL}} = \frac{1,200 \text{ units}}{x \text{ mL}}$$

or

Using Colons

$$1,000 \text{ units} : 1.5 \text{ mL} = 1,200 \text{ units} : x \text{ mL}$$

$$1,000x = 1.5 \times 1,200$$

$$1,000x = 1.5 \times 1,200$$

$$x = \frac{1.5 \times 1,200}{1,000}$$

$$x = \frac{1.5 \times 1,200}{1,000}$$

$$x = 1.8 \text{ mL}$$

$$x = 1.8 \text{ mL}$$

Example 7 ■   A drug has a dosage strength of 2 mEq per mL. You are to give 10 mEq.

Using Fractions

$$\frac{2\text{ mEq}}{1\text{ mL}} = \frac{10\text{ mEq}}{x\text{ mL}}$$

or

$$2x = 10$$

$$x = 5\text{ mL}$$

Using Colons

$$2\text{ mEq} : 1\text{ mL} = 10\text{ mEq} : x\text{ mL}$$

$$2x = 10$$

$$x = 5\text{ mL}$$

Problems 8.5

Solve these dosage problems. Express answers to the nearest tenth. Use the ratio and proportion format of your choice.

Note: If you do not include the units of measure, your answers are incorrect.

1. The drug label reads 1,000 mcg in 2 mL. The order is 0.4 mg.   _____

2. The ordered dosage is 275 mg. The available drug is labeled 0.5 g per 2 mL.   _____

3. A dosage strength of 0.2 mg in 1.5 mL is available. Give 0.15 mg.   _____

4. The strength available is 1 g in 3.6 mL. Prepare a 600 mg dosage.   _____

5. A dosage of 8,000 units of heparin has been ordered. Refer to Figure 8-7 for the supply.   _____

Rx only   NDC 0409-2721-30

1 mL Single-dose Vial

HEPARIN
Sodium Injection, USP

10,000 USP Units/**mL**

NOT for LOCK FLUSH

For Intravenous or Subcutaneous Use From Porcine Intestines

Contains Preservative

AP/DRUGS/08/2013
M.L.No. 08/VP/AP/2013/F/G

Dist. by Hospira, Inc. *Hospira*
Lake Forest, IL 60045 USA

▲ **Figure 8-7**

6. The dosage available is 20 mEq per 20 mL. You are to prepare 15 mEq.   _____

7. The order is for 200,000 units of nystatin oral suspension. Refer to Figure 8-8 for the supply.   _____

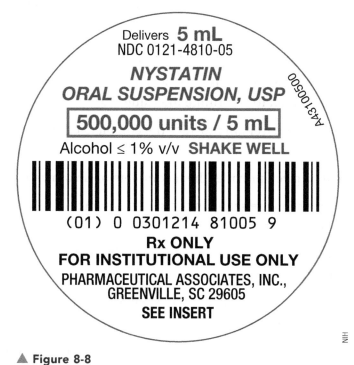

▲ **Figure 8-8**

8. The order is for a 5 mg dose of prednisone. Refer to Figure 8-9 for the supply.   _____

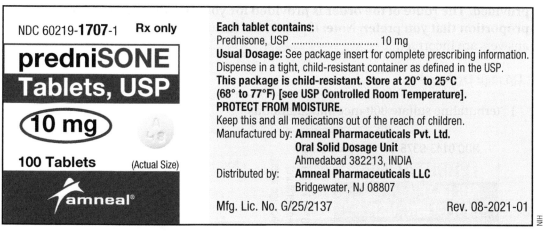

▲ **Figure 8-9**

Answers   **1.** 0.8 mL   **2.** 1.1 mL   **3.** 1.1 mL   **4.** 2.2 mL   **5.** 0.8 mL   **6.** 15 mL   **7.** 2 mL   **8.** 0.5 tab

Summary

This concludes the chapter on ratio and proportion and its uses in calculations in health care. The important points to remember from this chapter are:

▓   A ratio is composed of two numbers that have a significant relationship to each other.

▓   A proportion consists of two ratios with a significant relationship to each other.

▓   If one number in a proportion is missing, it can be determined mathematically by solving an equation to determine the value of x.

▓   The available dosage strength provides the complete or known ratio for calculations.

▓   The dosage to be given provides the incomplete or unknown ratio.

▓   Ratios in a proportion are set up in the same sequence of measurement units; for example, mg : mL = mg : mL.

▓   If the measurement units in a calculation are different—for example, mg and g—one of these must be converted before the problem can be solved.

▓   It may be safer to convert from larger to smaller metric units of measure to eliminate decimal points.

▓   The math of calculations is triple-checked to determine accuracy of the answer.

Summary Self-Test

Calculate these dosages using ratio and proportion. Express mL answers to the nearest tenth (or hundredth where indicated) using the medication labels provided. The route of the order is provided for you. Use the format of ratio and proportion that you prefer. Note: If you do not include the units of measure, your answers are incorrect.

Dosage Ordered   **Answer**

1. terbutaline sulfate 800 mcg subcutaneous   _____

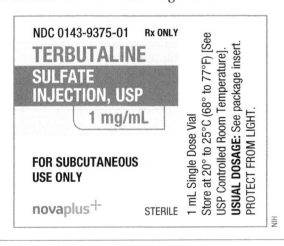

Dosage Ordered   **Answer**

2. furosemide 15 mg IV   _____

NDC 70121-**1163**-1

Furosemide
Injection, USP

20 mg/2 mL

(10 mg/mL)

FOR IV OR IM USE

2 mL SINGLE-DOSE VIAL
Rx only

WARNING: USE ONLY IF SOLUTION IS
CLEAR AND COLORLESS. PROTECT
FROM LIGHT. Store at 20° to 25°C
(68° to 77°F); excursions permitted
between 15° to 30°C (59° to 86°F)
[see USP Controlled Room Temperature].
Directions for Use: See Package Insert.
Mfg. Lic. No. G/28/1539
Distributed by:
Amneal Pharmaceuticals LLC
Bridgewater, NJ 08807

NIH

3. dexamethasone 15 mg IV   _____

NDC 63323-506-41   PRX500601

Dexamethasone
Sodium Phosphate
Injection, USP

10 mg per mL

For IM or IV use only.
Preservative free.
Discard unused portion.
Protect from light.
1 mL Single Dose Vial   Rx only

PREMIERProRx®

Mfd. by: Fresenius Kabi

NIH

4. fentanyl citrate 0.15 mg IV   _____

NDC 17478-030-02   **2 mL Ampule**

Fentanyl Citrate
Injection, USP (II)

100 mcg/2 mL (50 mcg/mL)*

FOR INTRAVENOUS OR
INTRAMUSCULAR USE   Rx only

*Each mL contains: 0.0785 mg fentanyl
citrate equivalent to 50 mcg fentanyl base.
Mfd. by: **Akorn**, Lake Forest, IL 60045

(01)00317478030027

LOT
EXP.

AFCADL Rev.09/21

NIH

Dosage Ordered   Answer

5. naloxone 350 mcg subcutaneous (Round to the hundredth.)   _____

17478-**041**-01

Naloxone HCl Injection, USP

0.4 mg/mL

For I.V., I.M. or S.C. use
1 mL Single-dose Vial

Rx only

Protect from light.

○AKORN

Mfd. by: Akorn Inc.
Lake Forest, IL 60045

NLAAL   Rev. 10/17

NIH

6. clindamycin 225 mg IM   _____

NDC 25021-115-02   1030283

Clindamycin

Injection, USP

300 mg per **2** mL
(150 mg per mL)

SAGENT

Lot:

Rx only

For IM or IV Use
Dilute Before IV Use
2 mL Single-Dose Vial

Exp.:

**Sterile, Nonpyrogenic.
Each mL contains:** clindamycin phosphate equivalent to clindamycin 150 mg. Also contains 0.5 mg disodium edetate and 9.45 mg benzyl alcohol as a preservative. **Usual Dosage:** See insert. Store at 20° to 25°C (68° to 77°F). [See Insert.]

Mfd. for: SAGENT Pharmaceuticals, Inc. Schaumburg, IL 60195 (USA) Made in India ©2011 Sagent Pharmaceuticals, Inc. Code No.: KR/DRUGS/KTK/28/384/2009

NIH

7. Robinul® 75 mcg IV (Round to the nearest hundredth.)   _____

NDC 0641-6104-01

Robinul Injection

(glycopyrrolate injection, USP)

0.2 mg/mL   Rx only

CONTAINS BENZYL ALCOHOL
FOR IM OR IV USE
1 mL Single Dose Vial

Manufactured by:
 WEST-WARD

462-176-02

(01)00306416104012

Lot:

Exp.:

NIH

Dosage Ordered   **Answer**

8. bumetanide 1.5 mg IV   _____

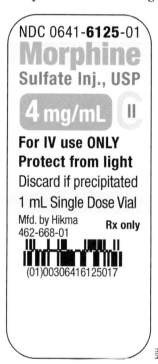

NDC 65219-**570**-01   **Rx only**

Bumetanide
Injection, USP

1 mg/4 mL (0.25 mg/mL)

For Intravenous or
Intramuscular Use
Contains Benzyl Alcohol
4 mL Single-Dose Vial
Discard unused portion.

Each mL contains bumetanide
0.25 mg, sodium chloride 8.5 mg
and ammonium acetate 4 mg as
buffers, edetate disodium dihydrate
0.1 mg and benzyl alcohol 10 mg
as preservative: pH adjusted to
6.8-7.8 with sodium hydroxide.
This container closure is not made
with natural rubber latex.
Usual Dosage: See package insert.
Store at 20°C to 25°C (68°F to
77°F). Protect from light.

Code No.: TS/DRUGS/2/2015

NIH

9. morphine sulfate 2.5 mg IV (Round to the nearest hundredth.)   _____

NDC 0641-**6125**-01

Morphine
Sulfate Inj., USP

4 mg/mL   II

For IV use ONLY
Protect from light
Discard if precipitated
1 mL Single Dose Vial
Mfd. by Hikma   **Rx only**
462-668-01

(01)00306416125017

NIH

10. heparin sodium 2,500 units subcutaneous (Calculate to the   _____
    hundredth.)

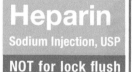

Heparin
Sodium Injection, USP
NOT for lock flush

5,000
USP units
per 0.5 mL

For Intravenous or Subcutaneous Use.
Derived from Porcine Intestinal Mucosa
Do NOT place syringe on a Sterile Field.

24 x 0.5 mL Prefilled Single-Dose Syringes
Discard unused portion.

Simplist®   FRESENIUS KABI

NIH

Dosage Ordered   **Answer**

11. phenytoin 0.1 g PO   _____

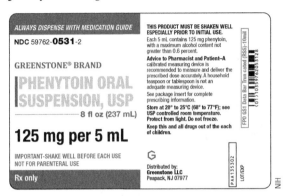

12. medroxyprogesterone 200 mg IM   _____

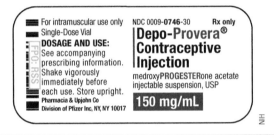

13. lorazepam 2.5 mg PO   _____

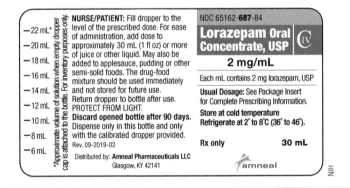

14. atropine sulfate 150 mcg IM (Round to the nearest hundredth.)   _____

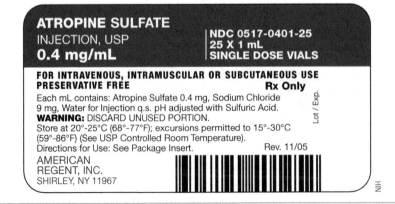

Dosage Ordered   **Answer**

15. cefaclor 75 mg PO   _____

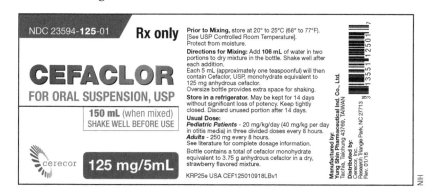

16. phenytoin 0.15 g PO   _____

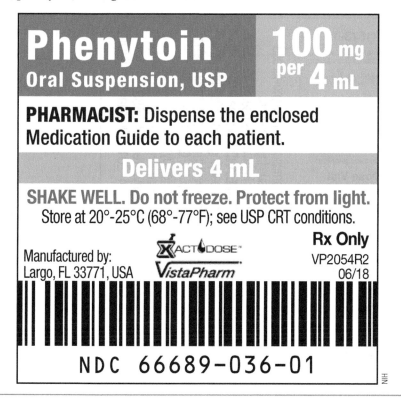

17. methotrexate 40 mg IV   _____

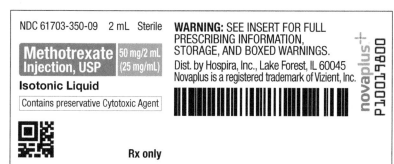

Dosage Ordered   *   **Answer**

18. ondansetron 3 mg IV   _____

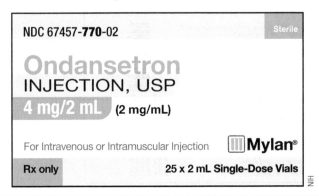

19. methylprednisolone 25 mg IM (Round to the nearest hundredth).   _____

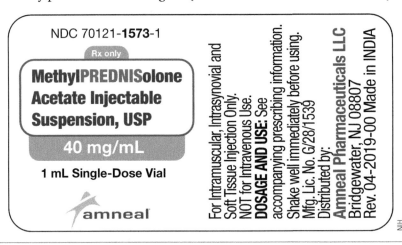

20. ketorolac tromethamine 20 mg IV   _____

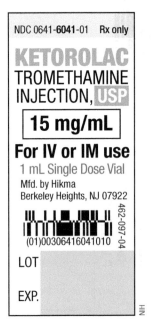

Dosage Ordered   **Answer**

21. nalbuphine 15 mg subcutaneous (Round to the nearest   _____
    hundredth.)

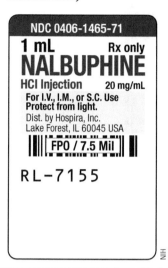

22. hydromorphone 1.5 mg IV (Round to the nearest hundredth.)   _____

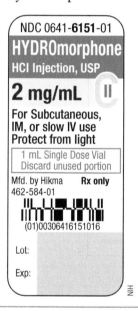

23. ondansetron 6 mg PO   _____

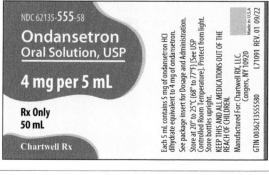

Dosage Ordered   **Answer**

24. prednisone 7.5 mg PO   _____

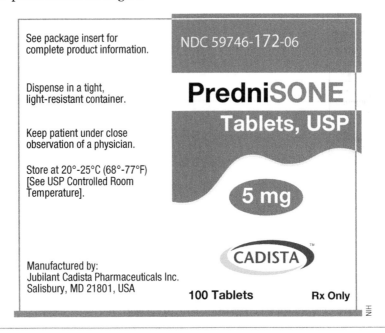

See package insert for complete product information.

NDC 59746-**172**-06

Dispense in a tight, light-resistant container.

Keep patient under close observation of a physician.

Store at 20°-25°C (68°-77°F) [See USP Controlled Room Temperature].

PredniSONE

Tablets, USP

5 mg

CADISTA™

Manufactured by:
Jubilant Cadista Pharmaceuticals Inc.
Salisbury, MD 21801, USA

100 Tablets   **Rx Only**

25. digoxin 0.25 mg PO   _____

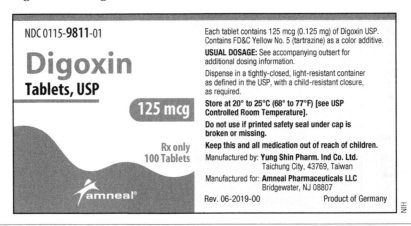

NDC 0115-**9811**-01

Digoxin

Tablets, USP

125 mcg

Rx only
100 Tablets

amneal®

Each tablet contains 125 mcg (0.125 mg) of Digoxin USP. Contains FD&C Yellow No. 5 (tartrazine) as a color additive.

USUAL DOSAGE: See accompanying outsert for additional dosing information.

Dispense in a tightly-closed, light-resistant container as defined in the USP, with a child-resistant closure, as required.

Store at 20° to 25°C (68° to 77°F) [see USP Controlled Room Temperature].

Do not use if printed safety seal under cap is broken or missing.

Keep this and all medication out of reach of children.

Manufactured by: **Yung Shin Pharm. Ind Co. Ltd.**
                Taichung City, 43769, Taiwan

Manufactured for: **Amneal Pharmaceuticals LLC**
                 Bridgewater, NJ 08807

Rev. 06-2019-00   Product of Germany

Answers to Summary Self-Test

1. 0.8 mL	**6.** 1.5 mL	**11.** 4 mL	**16.** 6 mL	**21.** 0.75 mL
2. 1.5 mL	**7.** 0.38 mL	**12.** 1.3 mL	**17.** 1.6 mL	**22.** 0.75 mL
3. 1.5 mL	**8.** 6 mL	**13.** 1.3 mL	**18.** 1.5 mL	**23.** 7.5 mL
4. 3 mL	**9.** 0.63 mL	**14.** 0.38 mL	**19.** 0.63 mL	**24.** 1.5 tab
5. 0.88 mL	**10.** 0.25 mL	**15.** 3 mL	**20.** 1.3 mL	**25.** 2 tab

Dimensional Analysis

You may already be familiar with **dimensional analysis (DA)**, also known as factor label method or unit analysis. This calculation method is used in chemistry, physics, and for other scientific calculations. DA was first introduced.for dosage calculations in the 1950s, but it has had several other names since then, including the label factor and factor label methods. The strength of dimensional analysis is that it reduces multiple-step calculations to a single equation.

Clinical Relevance: Chapters 8 through 10 will introduce three methods of calculation. It is important to choose a method of calculation that you can consistently use to perform calculations in the clinical setting. Consistent use of a method will enable you to become comfortable with its use to calculate dosages and apply it to other calculations in the clinical setting. Whichever method of calculation you use, it is important to clearly label your numbers with the unit of measure so that you are certain about what your end result represents. For example, will your result be tablets, capsules, milliliters, milligrams, or another unit of measure? This attention to detail will serve you well in the prevention of calculation errors.

The Basic Dimensional Analysis Equation

Relationships between units of measurement provide the components for all the calculations you have already learned and will be learning in the remainder of this text. Some examples of these relationships

Objectives

The learner will:

1. set up equations using dimensional analysis.

2. use dimensional analysis for calculations.

Prerequisites

Chapters 1 through 7

include the following, which may be found on labels of different medications and when utilizing various conversions:

oral medications: 1 tab = 250 mg; 5 mL = 125 mg

IM and subcutaneous medications: 2 g = 1.5 mL; 10 units = 1 mL; 20 mEq = 10 mL

metric conversions: 1,000 mcg = 1 mg; 1 g = 1,000 mg

In addition, you will be using relationships between units of measurement in more advanced dosage calculations. Later chapters will provide further information.

We use relationships between units of measurement in our daily life, and it may be easier initially to apply dimensional analysis to everyday situations. Practicing with familiar situations will help when applying DA to clinical situations and dosage calculations.

The first step in setting up a DA equation is to write the unit of measure being calculated. A situation that requires calculations in our daily life is adapting recipes. For example, if we are baking a cake and we want to triple the recipe, we can use DA to calculate the amount needed to make three cakes. Notice that color is used in the first DA examples to help you learn the sequence of entry.

Example 1 ■   The cake you are baking requires 2.5 cups of flour. To calculate how much flour is needed to make a total of 3 cakes, write the unit of measure being calculated – cups – followed by an equal sign.

$$\text{cups} =$$

There are two important reasons for identifying the unit of measure being calculated first: It eliminates any confusion over exactly which measure is being calculated, and it dictates how the first or "starting" relationship is entered in the equation.

Keypoint: In a DA equation, the unit of measure being calculated is written first, followed by an equal sign.

Next, identify the information that contains cups. This information is provided in the cake recipe. For one cake, 2.5 cups of flour are needed. Enter this as a common fraction so that the 2.5 cups *numerator* matches the cups unit of measure being calculated; 1 cake becomes the *denominator*.

$$\text{cups} = \frac{2.5 \text{ cups}}{1 \text{ cake}}$$

Keypoint: In a DA equation, the unit of measure being calculated is matched in the numerator of the first fraction entered.

All additional fractions are entered so that each *denominator* is matched in its successive *numerator*. The denominator in the first ratio is cake, so the next numerator must be cake. Review the problem to identify three cakes are needed. Enter this information as the next numerator to complete this single-step equation.

$$\text{cups} = \frac{2.5 \text{ cups}}{1 \text{ cake}} \times \frac{3 \text{ cakes}}{}$$

Keypoint: The unit of measure in each denominator of a DA equation is matched in the successive numerator entered.

All the pertinent fractional relationships have now been entered in this one-step DA equation. The next step is to cancel the alternate denominator/numerator measurement units (but not their quantities) to be sure they match. This ensures that the fractional relationships were entered correctly. **After cancellation, only the unit of measure being calculated may remain in the equation**. Cake in the first denominator will be canceled along with cake in the numerator of the subsequent fraction.

$$\text{cups} = \frac{2.5 \text{ cups}}{1 \text{ cake}} \times \frac{3 \text{ cakes}}{}$$

Keypoint: Only the unit of measure being calculated will remain in the equation after the denominator/numerator units of measure are canceled.

Only the cups being calculated remains in the equation. The math can now be completed.

$$\text{cups} = 2.5 \text{ cups} \times 3 = 7.5 \text{ cups}$$

Answer: To make three cakes, you need 7.5 cups of flour.

Keypoint: It is very important to label your numbers with the unit of measure and methodically strike through the unit of measure in the numerator that matches the unit of measure in the denominator. This is the best way to maintain an understanding of what you are calculating.

There are no complicated rules to memorize; DA works the same way for every calculation regardless of the number of fractions entered. With these simple steps, you can use DA for all types of calculations. It is important to set the calculation up and follow through with the calculations correctly.

When there are multiple fractions in the calculation, it is important to multiply first and then divide for consistency. This means you should multiply all the numerators, multiply all the denominators, and then finally divide the product of the numerators by the product of the denominators. Performing the calculation in this manner will prevent multiple episodes of rounding, which may lead to inaccuracies in your final answer.

Problems 9.1

Set up the following using DA. Do not solve. Refer to the conversions in Chapters 4 and 5 and Appendix A. Be sure to label your units of measure.

1. Convert 50 mg to g
2. Convert 3 oz to mL
3. Convert 220 lb to kg
4. Convert 60 kg to lb
5. Convert 5 g to mg

6. Convert 0.25 mg to mcg
7. Convert 75 mL to oz
8. Convert 20 mL to tsp
9. Convert 30 mcg to mg
10. Convert 0.75 g to mg

Answers

1. 1,000 mg = 1 gram (required conversion)

$$g = \frac{1\text{ g}}{1{,}000\text{ mg}} \times \frac{50\text{ mg}}{}$$

2. 30 mL = 1 ounce (required conversion)

$$mL = \frac{30\text{ mL}}{1\text{ oz}} \times \frac{3\text{ oz}}{}$$

3. 2.2 lb = 1 kg (required conversion)

$$kg = \frac{1\text{ kg}}{2.2\text{ lb}} \times \frac{220\text{ lb}}{}$$

4. 2.2 lb = 1 kg (required conversion)

$$lb = \frac{2.2\text{ lb}}{1\text{ kg}} \times \frac{60\text{ kg}}{}$$

5. 1 g = 1,000 mg (required conversion)

$$mg = \frac{1{,}000\text{ mg}}{1\text{ g}} \times \frac{5\text{ g}}{}$$

6. 1 mg = 1,000 mcg (required conversion)

$$mcg = \frac{1{,}000\text{ mcg}}{1\text{ mg}} \times \frac{0.25\text{ mg}}{}$$

7. 30 mL = 1 oz (required conversion)

$$oz = \frac{1\text{ oz}}{30\text{ mL}} \times \frac{75\text{ mL}}{}$$

8. 5 mL = 1 tsp (required conversion)

$$tsp = \frac{1\text{ tsp}}{5\text{ mL}} \times \frac{20\text{ mL}}{}$$

9. 1,000 mcg = 1 mg (required conversion)

$$mg = \frac{1\text{ mg}}{1{,}000\text{ mcg}} \times \frac{30\text{ mcg}}{}$$

10. 1 g = 1,000 mg (required conversion)

$$mg = \frac{1{,}000\text{ mg}}{1\text{ g}} \times \frac{0.75\text{ g}}{}$$

Relating Dimensional Analysis to Calculations

For clinical calculations, follow the principles and don't focus on the type of calculation being completed. We have reviewed the basics of setting up a dimensional analysis equation. Let's now apply this to common calculations in health care. A calculation that you may commonly perform will be conversions within a system of measurement or between systems of measurement. If we have a patient's weight in pounds and must document the weight in kilograms, we will need to convert. The conversion for pounds and kilograms is 2.2 pounds is equal to 1 kilogram. Let's now use this conversion in a DA equation to convert pounds to kilograms.

Example 1 ■   The client weighs 110 pounds. For treatment purposes, we must calculate their weight in kilograms. We know the conversion for pounds to kilograms is 2.2 pounds per kilogram. Let's set this conversion up using DA.

$$kg = \frac{1\text{ kg}}{2.2\text{ lb}} \times \frac{110\text{ lb}}{}$$

$$kg = \frac{110}{2.2}$$

$$kg = 50$$

Answer: 110 pounds is equal to 50 kg.

Clinical calculations may require conversion of milliliters to teaspoons for purposes of giving information to a client who must take medication at home. We know that 5 mL is equal to 1 teaspoon. If we have a physician order to give 30 mL of a medication to a client, the client may voice confusion about the amount. We could convert the amount to teaspoons to give the client a measure that is more familiar.

Example 2 ■   To convert 30 mL to teaspoons, the first step is to place teaspoon to the left of the equal sign. Then proceed to set up the calculation as explained in the previous examples.

$$tsp = \frac{1 \text{ tsp}}{5 \text{ mL}} \times \frac{30 \text{ mL}}{}$$

$$tsp = \frac{30}{5}$$

$$tsp = 6$$

Answer: 30 mL is equivalent to 6 teaspoons. The client would be more familiar with this measurement.

Now we will look at a clinical calculation that involves calculating the volume of medication, which is equivalent to the dosage ordered by the physician. While this may seem challenging at first, remember the principles of dimensional analysis and set the problem up as discussed previously.

Example 3 ■   A dosage of 50,000 units is ordered to be administered. The strength available is 10,000 units in 1.5 mL. Calculate how many mL will contain this dosage. First, since mL is what we desire to know, write the mL being calculated to the left of the equation followed by an equal sign.

$$mL =$$

Locate the information in the problem which contains mL. This would be the available dosage strength of 10,000 units in 1.5 mL. Enter this now, with 1.5 mL as the numerator to match the mL being calculated; 10,000 units becomes the denominator.

$$mL = \frac{1.5 \text{ mL}}{10,000 \text{ units}}$$

The units denominator must be matched in the next numerator. This is provided by the 50,000 units ordered. Enter this now to complete this one-step equation.

$$mL = \frac{1.5 \text{ mL}}{10,000 \text{ units}} \times 50,000 \text{ units}$$

Cancel the alternate denominator and numerator term of units. Canceling these units of measure will help you double-check for the correct entry of your numbers and units of measure. Therefore, it is so important to include the units of measure with the numbers when entering them into the DA equation. In this equation, then, only the mL being calculated remains in the equation. Finally, do the math.

$$mL = \frac{1.5 \text{ mL}}{10,000 \text{ units}} \times \frac{50,000 \text{ units}}{}$$

You can reduce 50,000 and 10,000 by dividing 10,000 into both the numerator and the denominator.

$$mL = 1.5 \times 5$$

$$mL = 7.5 \text{ mL}$$

Answer: It will require a 7.5 mL volume of the 10,000 units in 1.5 mL solution to prepare the 50,000 units ordered.

Just as the example of the recipe calculation gave us the total number of cups of flour that would be needed for 3 cakes; this equation gives us the total number of mL required to prepare the 50,000 units of medication ordered.

Tablet calculations are not common but would be done the same way using DA.

Example 4 ■   Alprazolam 1.25 mg is ordered for your client. Refer to Figure 9-1 for your supply. Note the tablets are scored (breakable). How many tablets must you give the client?

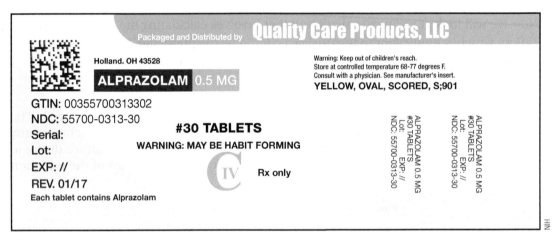

▲ **Figure 9-1**

Enter the tab being calculated to the left of the equation followed by an equal sign.

$$\text{tab} =$$

The tab unit being calculated is matched by the tab strength available, 0.5 mg in 1 tab. Enter this as the first ratio with 1 tab as the numerator and 0.5 mg as the denominator.

$$\text{tab} = \frac{1 \text{ tab}}{0.5 \text{ mg}}$$

The mg denominator must be matched in the next numerator. This is provided by the 1.25 mg ordered. Enter this to complete the equation.

$$\text{tab} = \frac{1 \text{ tab}}{0.5 \text{ mg}} \times \frac{1.25 \text{ mg}}{}$$

Cancel the alternate denominator/numerator mg units of measure to check that you have entered the information correctly. Only the tab being calculated remains in the equation. Complete the math.

$$\text{tab} = \frac{1 \text{ tab}}{0.5 \text{ mg}} \times \frac{1.25 \text{ mg}}{}$$

$$\text{tab} = \frac{1.25}{0.5} = 2.5 \text{ tab}$$

Answer: To obtain the 1.25 mg dosage ordered, 2.5 tab must be given.

Example 5 ■   How many mL will you draw up to prepare a 1.2 g dosage if you are using the medication in Figure 9-2?

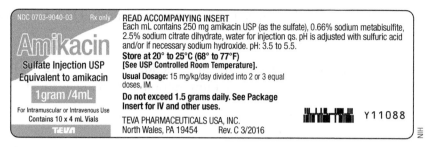

▲ Figure 9-2

Write the mL unit being calculated to the left of the equation followed by an equal sign. Enter the starting fraction, 1 g in 4 mL, with 4 mL as the numerator to match the mL being calculated and 1 g as the denominator.

$$mL = \frac{4 \text{ mL}}{1 \text{ g}}$$

Match the g denominator in the next numerator with the 1.2 g ordered to complete the equation.

$$mL = \frac{4 \text{ mL}}{1 \text{ g}} \times \frac{1.2 \text{ g}}{}$$

Cancel the alternate denominator/numerator g units of measure to double-check that the entries are correct. Only the mL being calculated remains.

$$mL = \frac{4 \text{ mL}}{1 \text{ g}} \times \frac{1.2 \text{ g}}{}$$

Do the math, expressing fractional answers to the nearest tenth.

$$mL = \frac{4.8}{1} = 4.8 \text{ mL}$$

Answer: The 1.2 g dosage ordered is contained in 4.8 mL of the 1 g in 4 mL solution available.

Example 6 ◼   A client will be taking 3 mg of dulaglutide as a weekly dose. Based on the label in Figure 9-3, how many mL will this client be receiving?

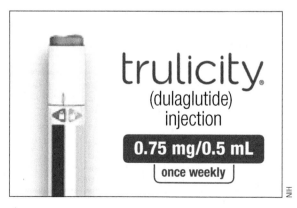

▲ Figure 9-3

Write the mL being calculated to the left of the equation followed by an equal sign.

$$mL =$$

The mL being calculated is provided for the first fraction by the 0.75 mg per 0.5 mL dosage strength available. Enter 0.5 mL as the numerator and 0.75 mg as the denominator.

$$mL = \frac{0.5 \text{ mL}}{0.75 \text{ mg}}$$

The mg denominator must now be matched. This is provided by the 3 mg dosage ordered. Enter this now to complete this one-step equation.

$$mL = \frac{0.5 \text{ mL}}{0.75 \text{ mg}} \times \frac{3 \text{ mg}}{}$$

Cancel the alternate denominator/numerator mg units of measure to check for correct fraction entry, then do the math. Remember to multiply first and then divide.

$$mL = \frac{0.5 \text{ mL}}{0.75 \cancel{\text{ mg}}} \times \frac{3 \cancel{\text{ mg}}}{} = 2 \text{ mL}$$

Answer: The client will receive 2 mL of the 0.75 mg in 0.5 mL dosage available.

These are the basics of using DA in calculations. The key points are summarized below:

- The unit being calculated in the equation is identified to the left of the equal sign.
- The starting fraction is entered so that its numerator matches the unit of measure being calculated.
- The unit of measure in each denominator is matched in each successively entered numerator.
- The only unit of measure that remains after cancellation of like terms is the same as the unit of measure being calculated.
- Triple check that quantities have been entered correctly.
- Triple check the math to ensure accuracy.

A major advantage of DA is that it allows multiple fractions to be entered in a single equation. This is especially useful when a drug is ordered in one unit of measure—for example, mg—but is labeled in another—for example, g or mcg.

There are two ways to handle a conversion. Sometimes, it will be easier to do the conversion before setting up the equation. In other instances, you may elect to incorporate the conversion into an equation. For practice purposes, let's review how we would incorporate the conversion into the DA equation.

Example 7 ■   The IM dosage ordered is 0.8 mg. Refer to Figure 9-4 for the supply. How many mL must you give?

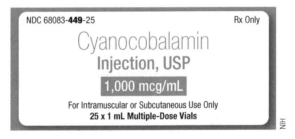

▲ **Figure 9-4**

Enter the mL to be calculated to the left of the equation. Locate the fraction containing mL, the 1,000 mcg per mL dosage strength, and enter it, with 1 mL as the numerator; 1,000 mcg becomes the denominator.

$$mL = \frac{1\ mL}{1,000\ mcg}$$

When you refer back to the problem, you will not find a mcg measure to match the mcg in the starting fraction denominator. The dosage to be given is in mg. So, a conversion fraction between mcg and mg is needed: 1 mg = 1,000 mcg. Enter this now, with 1,000 mcg as the numerator to match the mcg of the previous denominator; 1 mg becomes the new denominator.

$$mL = \frac{1\ mL}{1,000\ mcg} \times \frac{1,000\ mcg}{1\ mg}$$

The final entry, the 0.8 mg dosage to be given, will automatically fall into its correct position as it is entered as the final numerator to match the mg of the previous denominator. The equation is now complete.

$$mL = \frac{1\ mL}{1,000\ mcg} \times \frac{1,000\ mcg}{1\ mg} \times \frac{0.8\ mg}{}$$

Cancel the alternate denominator/numerator mcg/mcg and mg/mg units of measure to double-check the fraction entry. Only the mL being calculated remains. Complete the math.

$$mL = \frac{1\ mL}{1,000\ mcg} \times \frac{1,000\ mcg}{1\ mg} \times \frac{0.8\ mg}{} = 0.8\ mL$$

Answer: To give a dosage of 0.8 mg, you must prepare 0.8 mL of the 1,000 mcg in 1 mL strength solution.

Example 8 ■ The IM dosage ordered is 0.6 mg. The drug available is labeled 800 mcg in 1.5 mL. Enter the mL to be calculated followed by an equal sign to the left of the equation. Locate the fraction containing mL, 800 mcg in 1.5 mL. Enter 1.5 mL as the numerator to match the mL being calculated; 800 mcg becomes the denominator.

$$mL = \frac{1.5\ mL}{800\ mcg}$$

There is no mcg measure in the problem, which is your clue to the necessity for a conversion fraction. Enter the 1,000 mcg = 1 mg conversion, with 1,000 mcg as the numerator to match the mcg of the previous denominator; 1 mg becomes the denominator.

$$mL = \frac{1.5\ mL}{800\ mcg} \times \frac{1,000\ mcg}{1\ mg}$$

The mg denominator is now matched by the 0.6 mg dosage to be given and completes the equation.

$$mL = \frac{1.5\ mL}{800\ mcg} \times \frac{1,000\ mcg}{1\ mg} \times \frac{0.6\ mg}{}$$

Cancel the alternate denominator/numerator mcg/mcg and mg/mg units of measure to check for correct fraction entry. Only the mL being calculated should remain in the equation. Do the math.

$$\text{mL} = \frac{1.5\text{ mL}}{800\text{ mcg}} \times \frac{1,000\text{ mcg}}{1\text{ mg}} \times \frac{0.6\text{ mg}}{} = 1.12 = 1.1\text{ mL}$$

Answer: To give a dosage of 0.6 mg from the available 1.5 mL per 800 mcg strength, you must prepare 1.1 mL.

Problems 9.2

Calculate the following using DA. Express mL answers to the nearest tenth, unless instructed to round to the hundredth. Be sure to label your units of measure.

1. A dosage of 30 mg of diphenhydramine has been ordered. Refer to Figure 9-5 for the strength available.   _____

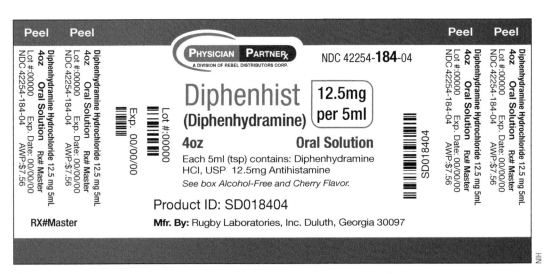

▲ **Figure 9-5**

2. A dosage strength of 0.8 mg in 2 mL is to be used to prepare a 0.5 mg dosage.   _____

3. Prepare a 1.8 mg dosage from a solution labeled 2 mg in 3 mL.   _____

4. The order is for 1,500 mg. You have available a 1,200 mg per mL solution.   _____

5. A dosage strength of 0.2 mg in 1.5 mL is available. Give 0.15 mg.   _____

6. The strength available is 1,000 mg in 3.6 mL. Prepare a 600 mg dosage.   _____

7. A dosage of 7.5 mg oxycodone is to be prepared. Refer to Figure 9-6 for the supply. _____

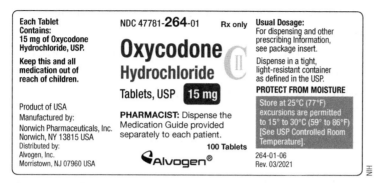

▲ **Figure 9-6**

8. You are to prepare a dose of 2 tsp, but your equipment only measures milliliters. Convert 2 tsp to milliliters. _____

9. An order is for 1.2 g. Convert 1.2 g to mg. _____

10. Convert 400 mcg to mg. _____

Answers 1. 12 mL **2.** 1.3 mL **3.** 2.7 mL **4.** 1.3 mL **5.** 1.1 mL **6.** 2.2 mL **7.** 1/2 tab **8.** 10 mL **9.** 1,200 mg **10.** 0.4 mg

Problems 9.3

Calculate these dosages which require conversion using DA. Express mL answers to the nearest tenth. Be sure to label your units of measure.

1. Prepare 0.1 g of an IM medication from a strength of 200 mg per mL. _____

2. A drug label reads 0.1 g in 2 mL. Prepare a 130 mg dosage. _____

3. Prepare an oral dose of 160 mg of Vancomycin. Refer to Figure 9-7 for the supply. _____

4. Prepare a 0.75 g dosage from a 250 mg per mL strength solution. _____

5. Prepare 500 mg for IM injection from an available strength of 1 g per 3 mL. _____

6. A dosage of 0.065 g of gentamicin is ordered. See Figure 9-8 for the supply. _____

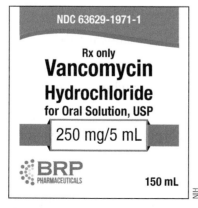

▲ **Figure 9-7**

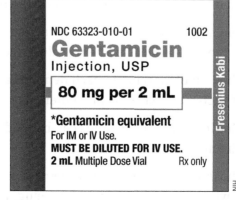

▲ **Figure 9-8**

7. The strength available is 500 mcg in 1.5 mL. Prepare a 0.75 mg dosage.   _____

8. A dosage of 1,500 mg has been ordered. The solution available is 0.5 g per mL.   _____

9. The dosage strength available is 200 mcg per mL. A 0.5 mg dosage has been ordered.   _____

10. The dosage ordered is 350 mcg of levothyroxine. Refer to Figure 9-9 for the supply.   _____

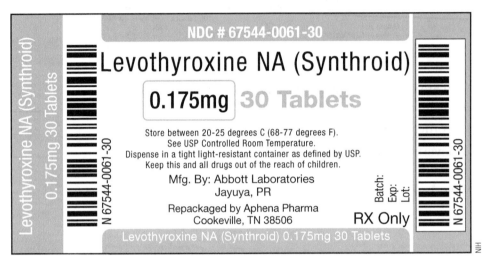

NDC # 67544-0061-30

Levothyroxine NA (Synthroid)

0.175mg 30 Tablets

Store between 20-25 degrees C (68-77 degrees F).
See USP Controlled Room Temperature.
Dispense in a tight light-resistant container as defined by USP.
Keep this and all drugs out of the reach of children.

Mfg. By: Abbott Laboratories
Jayuya, PR

Repackaged by Aphena Pharma
Cookeville, TN 38506

Batch:
Exp:
Lot:

RX Only

Levothyroxine NA (Synthroid) 0.175mg 30 Tablets

N 67544-0061-30

N 67544-0061-30

Levothyroxine NA (Synthroid)
0.175mg 30 Tablets

▲ **Figure 9-9**

Answers   **1.** 0.5 mL   **2.** 2.6 mL   **3.** 3.2 mL   **4.** 3 mL   **5.** 1.5 mL   **6.** 1.6 mL   **7.** 2.3 mL   **8.** 3 mL   **9.** 2.5 mL
10. 2 tab

Summary

This ends your introduction to clinical calculations using dimensional analysis. The important points to remember from this chapter are:

- The unit of measure being calculated is written first to the left of the equation, followed by an equal sign.

- All fractions entered must include the quantity and the unit of measure.

- The numerator in the starting fraction must be in the same measurement unit as the unit of measure being calculated.

- The unit of measure in each denominator must be matched in the numerator of each successive fraction entered.

- Metric system conversions can be made by incorporating a conversion fraction directly into the DA equation.

- The unit of measure in each alternate denominator and numerator must cancel, leaving only the unit of measure being calculated remaining in the equation.

■ The numerator of the starting fraction is never canceled.

■ Remember to multiply numerators first, then multiply denominators and finally divide the product of the numerators by the product of the denominators.

Summary Self-Test

Calculate these dosages using DA. Express mL answers to the nearest tenth (or hundredth where indicated) using the medication labels provided. The route of the order is provided for you.

Dosage Ordered   **Answer**

1. terbutaline sulfate 800 mcg subcutaneous   _____

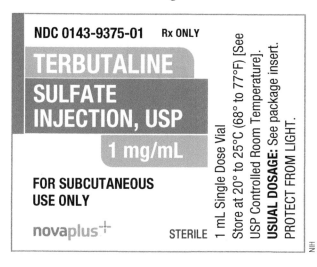

NDC 0143-9375-01   Rx ONLY

TERBUTALINE
SULFATE
INJECTION, USP
1 mg/mL

FOR SUBCUTANEOUS
USE ONLY

novaplus⁺   STERILE

1 mL Single Dose Vial
Store at 20° to 25°C (68° to 77°F) [See USP Controlled Room Temperature].
USUAL DOSAGE: See package insert.
PROTECT FROM LIGHT.

---

2. furosemide 15 mg IV   _____

NDC 70121-**1163**-1

Furosemide
Injection, USP

20 mg/2 mL
(10 mg/mL)
FOR IV OR IM USE

2 mL SINGLE-DOSE VIAL
Rx only

WARNING: USE ONLY IF SOLUTION IS CLEAR AND COLORLESS. PROTECT FROM LIGHT. Store at 20° to 25°C (68° to 77°F); excursions permitted between 15° to 30°C (59° to 86°F) [see USP Controlled Room Temperature]. Directions for Use: See Package Insert.

Dosage Ordered   **Answer**

3. dexamethasone 15 mg IV   _____

NDC 63323-506-41   PRX500601

**Dexamethasone
Sodium Phosphate**
Injection, USP

10 mg per mL

For IM or IV use only.
Preservative free.
Discard unused portion.
Protect from light.
1 mL Single Dose Vial   Rx only

PREMIER ProRx®

Mfd. by: Fresenius Kabi

NIH

---

4. fentanyl citrate 0.15 mg IV   _____

NDC 17478-030-02   **2 mL Ampule**

**Fentanyl Citrate
Injection, USP** Ⓒ

100 mcg/2 mL (50 mcg/mL)*

**FOR INTRAVENOUS OR
INTRAMUSCULAR USE**   Rx only

Each mL contains: 0.0785 mg fentanyl
citrate equivalent to 50 mcg fentanyl base.
Mfd. by: **Akorn,** Lake Forest, IL 60045

(01)00317478030027

AFCADL   Rev.09/21

LOT
EXP.

NIH

Dosage Ordered   **Answer**

5. naloxone 350 mcg subcutaneous (Round to the hundredth.)   _____

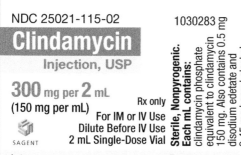

6. clindamycin 225 mg IM   _____

7. Robinul® (glycopyrrolate) 75 mcg IV (Round to the nearest   _____
   hundredth.)

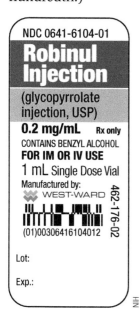

Dosage Ordered   **Answer**

8. bumetanide 1.5 mg IV   _____

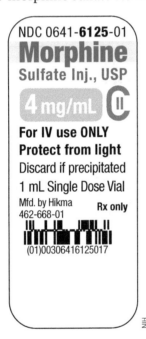

NDC 65219-**570**-01   **Rx only**

Bumetanide
Injection, USP

1 mg/4 mL (0.25 mg/mL)

**For Intravenous or
Intramuscular Use
Contains Benzyl Alcohol**

4 mL Single-Dose Vial
Discard unused portion.

Each mL contains bumetanide
0.25 mg, sodium chloride 8.5 mg
and ammonium acetate 4 mg as
buffers, edetate disodium dihydrate
0.1 mg and benzyl alcohol 10 mg
as preservative; pH adjusted to
6.8-7.8 with sodium hydroxide.
This container closure is not made
with natural rubber latex.

Usual Dosage: See package insert.
**Store at 20°C to 25°C (68°F to
77°F). Protect from light.**

Code No.: TS/DRUGS/2/2015

9. morphine sulfate 2.5 mg IV (Round to the nearest hundredth.)   _____

NDC 0641-**6125**-01

Morphine
Sulfate Inj., USP

4 mg/mL C II

**For IV use ONLY
Protect from light**

Discard if precipitated

1 mL Single Dose Vial

Mfd. by Hikma
462-668-01   **Rx only**

(01)00306416125017

10. heparin sodium 2,500 units subcutaneous (Calculate to the   _____
    hundredth.)

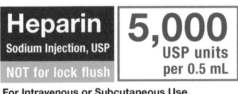

Heparin
Sodium Injection, USP

NOT for lock flush

5,000
**USP units
per 0.5 mL**

**For Intravenous or Subcutaneous Use.
Derived from Porcine Intestinal Mucosa**
Do NOT place syringe on a Sterile Field.

24 x 0.5 mL Prefilled Single-Dose Syringes
Discard unused portion.

Simplist®   FRESENIUS KABI

Dosage Ordered   **Answer**

11. phenytoin 0.1 g po   _____

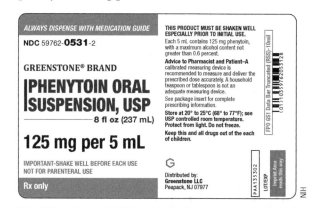

12. medroxyprogesterone 200 mg IM   _____

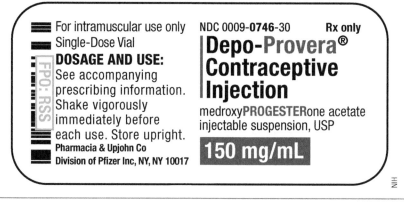

13. lorazepam 2.5 mg po   _____

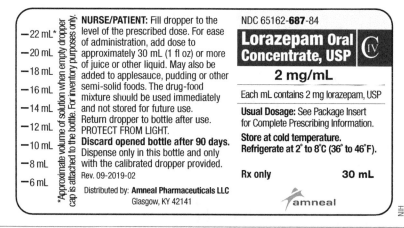

Dosage Ordered   **Answer**

14. atropine sulfate 150 mcg IM (Round to the nearest hundredth.)   _____

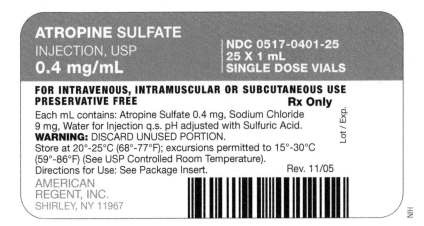

15. cefaclor 75 mg po   _____

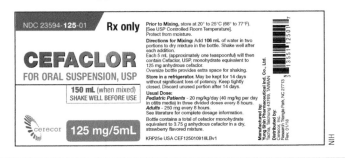

16. phenytoin 0.15 g po   _____

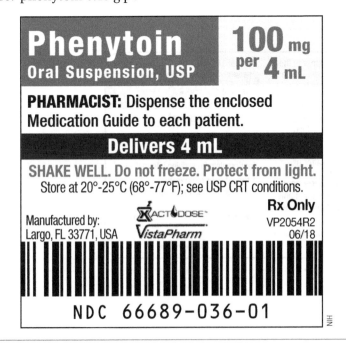

Dosage Ordered **Answer**

17. methotrexate 40 mg IV _____

18. ondansetron 3 mg IV _____

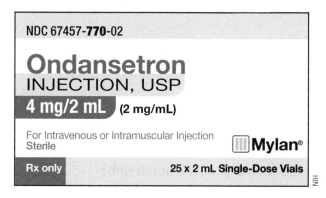

19. methylprednisolone 25 mg IM (Round to the nearest hundredth.) _____

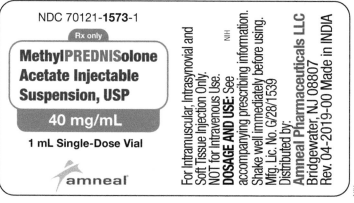

Dosage Ordered   **Answer**

20. ketorolac tromethamine 20 mg IV   _____

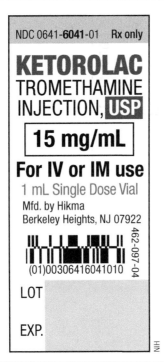

21. nalbuphine 15 mg subcutaneous (Calculate to the hundredth)   _____

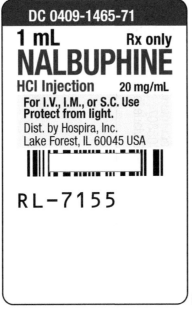

Dosage Ordered   **Answer**

22. hydromorphone 1.5 mg IV (Calculate to the hundredth.)   _____

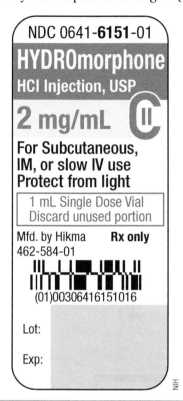

23. ondansetron 6 mg po   _____

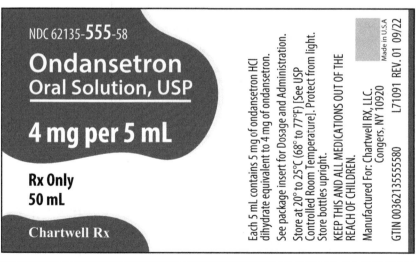

Dosage Ordered   **Answer**

24. prednisone 7.5 mg po   _____

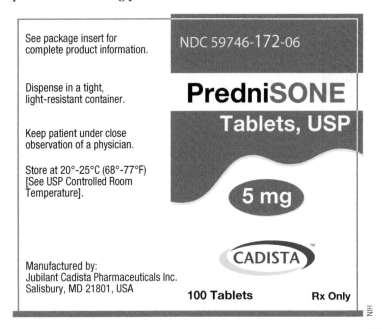

25. digoxin 0.25 mg po   _____

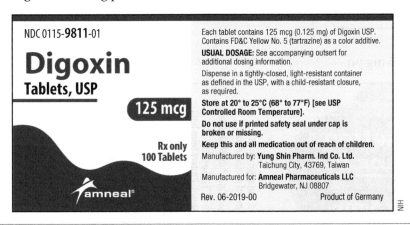

Answers to Summary Self-Test

1. 0.8 mL	**6.** 1.5 mL	**11.** 4 mL	**16.** 6 mL	**21.** 0.75 mL
2. 1.5 mL	**7.** 0.38 mL	**12.** 1.3 mL	**17.** 1.6 mL	**22.** 0.75 mL
3. 1.5 mL	**8.** 6 mL	**13.** 1.3 mL	**18.** 1.5 mL	**23.** 7.5 mL
4. 3 mL	**9.** 0.63 mL	**14.** 0.38 mL	**19.** 0.63 mL	**24.** 1.5 tab
5. 0.88 mL	**10.** 0.25 mL	**15.** 3 mL	**20.** 1.3 mL	**25.** 2 tab

Formula Method

The formula method presents a systematic method for calculation within the health care setting. As the formula involves a fraction, it is important to remember to multiply first and then divide, as this will allow greater consistency and accuracy in your answers. The letters D, H, and Q will represent the variables used in the formula method. Consistent application of the formula in calculations in the health care setting is paramount for accuracy.

Clinical Relevance: Chapters 8 through 10 will introduce three methods of calculation. It is important to choose a method of calculation that you can consistently use to perform calculations in the clinical setting. Consistent use of a method will enable you to become comfortable with its use to calculate dosages and apply it to other calculations in the clinical setting. Whichever method of calculation you use, it is important to clearly label your numbers with the unit of measure so that you are certain about what your end result represents. For example, will your result be tablets, capsules, milliliters, milligrams, or another unit of measure? This attention to detail will serve you well in the prevention of calculation errors.

Objectives

The learner will:

1. explain the letters D, H, and Q used in the basic formula method.

2. set up calculations using the formula method.

3. use the formula method to solve calculations.

Prerequisites

Chapters 1 through 7

The Basic Formula

It is necessary to memorize the following formula for calculating dosages:

$$\frac{D \times Q}{H} = x$$

The letters in the formula mean the following:

D is the **desired dosage** ordered in mg, g, etc.

H is the dosage strength you **have available** in mg, g, etc.

Q is the **quantity** or volume the dosage strength available is contained in.

x is the **unknown** value of the **liquid volume**, **number of tables**, or **capsules** the desired dosage will be contained in.

Notice the *H*, have available, and *Q*, quantity, values are closely related. Both are located on the label of the supplied medication. It is also important to note that *D*, desired dosage, and *H*, have available, must be in the same system and unit of measurement. Remember to triple check the numbers you enter in the formula to ensure proper placement and accurate results.

Just as with dimensional analysis (DA), we must be able to eliminate all the units of measurement except for the measurement unit that we are solving for.

Example 1 ■   Consider the following equation.

$$\frac{0.25 \text{ mg} \times 5 \text{ mL}}{500 \text{ mcg}} = x \text{ mL}$$

This cannot be solved as written since we cannot eliminate the units of measurement, mg and mcg, to leave only mL in the formula. You will need to convert mg to mcg or mcg to mg.

 Keypoint: The *D*, desired dosage, and *H*, have available, values must be in the same system and same unit of measure so the units of measurement can be eliminated. This will leave only the units of measurement of *Q*, the quantity, which should be the same as the units of measurement needed for the answer.

This example also shows how important it is to label your entries in the formula with the units of measurement. This will clearly show you whether the calculation can be completed.

Example 2 ■   Compare Example 1 to the following equation.

$$\frac{250 \text{ mcg} \times 5 \text{ mL}}{500 \text{ mcg}} = x \text{ mL}$$

After converting mg to mcg, this calculation can now be solved. Since we can eliminate mcg in the numerator and denominator, we will be left with mL, which is the unit of measurement for our answer.

 Keypoint: The unknown, X, will always be expressed in the same units of measure as Q.

Let's consider a calculation where the unit of measurement for *x*, the unknown, is different from the unit of measure *Q*, the quantity entered.

Example 3 ▣
$$\frac{250 \text{ mcg} \times 1 \text{ tsp}}{500 \text{ mcg}} = x \text{ mL}$$

In this equation, although the units of measure in the numerator (mcg) and denominator (mcg) can be eliminated, the units of measure that remain are not the same. Again, conversion will be needed. In this example, tsp will be converted to mL to provide the final answer.

If you label your entries with the unit of measure, you can be assured that you are calculating accurately. It is important for you to be confident in your setup of calculations using the formula method.

When using the formula method for conversions, *D* will be the unit of measure we want to convert, and *H* and *Q* will come from the conversion factor. *H* will need to be the part of the conversion that matches the unit of measurement in *D*, and *Q* will be the other piece of the conversion factor.

Recall that *D*, desired dosage, and *H*, have available, must be in the same system and same unit of measure, and *Q*, quantity, and *x*, unknown answer, must be in the same unit of measure.

Example 4 ▣   Consider the following information and set up a conversion using the formula method.

- We must convert 0.25 mg to mcg (*D*).
- We know that 1,000 mcg (*Q*) is equal to 1 mg (*H*).

Using the formula method, we will set this conversion up as:

$$\frac{0.25 \text{ mg} \times 1,000 \text{ mcg}}{1 \text{ mg}} = x \text{ mcg}$$

Answer: Completing the calculation will result in 250 mcg.

Example 5 ▣   We must convert 1 tsp to mL. We know the conversion is 5 mL is equal to 1 tsp. Using the formula method, we will set this conversion up as:

$$\frac{1 \text{ tsp} \times 5 \text{ mL}}{1 \text{ tsp}} = x \text{ mL}$$

Answer: Completing the calculation will result in 5 mL.

Problems 10.1

Set up the following using the formula method. Do not solve. Refer to the conversions in Chapters 4 and 5 and Appendix A. Be sure to label your units of measure.

1. Convert 50 mg to g
2. Convert 3 oz to mL
3. Convert 220 lb to kg
4. Convert 60 kg to lb
5. Convert 5 g to mg
6. Convert 0.25 mg to mcg
7. Convert 75 mL to oz
8. Convert 20 mL to tsp
9. Convert 30 mcg to mg
10. Convert 0.75 g to mg

Answers

1. 1,000 mg = 1 gram (required conversion)
$$\frac{50 \text{ mg} \times 1 \text{ g}}{1,000 \text{ mg}} = x \text{ g}$$

2. 30 mL = 1 ounce (required conversion)
$$\frac{3 \text{ oz} \times 30 \text{ mL}}{1 \text{ oz}} = x \text{ mL}$$

3. 2.2 lb = 1 kg (required conversion)
$$\frac{220 \text{ lb} \times 1 \text{ kg}}{2.2 \text{ lb}} = x \text{ kg}$$

4. 2.2 lb = 1 kg (required conversion)
$$\frac{60 \text{ kg} \times 2.2 \text{ lb}}{1 \text{ kg}} = x \text{ lb}$$

5. 1 g = 1,000 mg (required conversion)
$$\frac{5 \text{ g} \times 1,000 \text{ mg}}{1 \text{ g}} = x \text{ mg}$$

6. 1 mg = 1,000 mcg (required conversion)
$$\frac{0.25 \text{ mg} \times 1,000 \text{ mcg}}{1 \text{ mg}} = x \text{ mcg}$$

7. 30 mL = 1 oz (required conversion)
$$\frac{75 \text{ mL} \times 1 \text{ oz}}{30 \text{ mL}} = x \text{ oz}$$

8. 5 mL = 1 tsp (required conversion)
$$\frac{20 \text{ mL} \times 1 \text{ tsp}}{5 \text{ mL}} = x \text{ tsp}$$

9. 1,000 mcg = 1 mg (required conversion)
$$\frac{30 \text{ mcg} \times 1 \text{ mg}}{1,000 \text{ mcg}} = x \text{ mg}$$

10. 1g = 1,000 mg (required conversion)
$$\frac{0.75 \text{ g} \times 1,000 \text{ mg}}{1 \text{ g}} = x \text{ mg}$$

Relating the Formula Method to Calculations

When using the formula for clinical calculations, follow the principles and don't focus on the type of calculation being completed. Common calculations you will perform in health care will be conversions within a system of measurement or between systems of measurement. We have reviewed the key components of setting up the formula for the calculation of conversions.

If we have a patient's weight in pounds and must document the weight in kilograms, we will need to convert. The conversion for pounds and kilograms is 2.2 pounds is equal to 1 kilogram. Let's now use this conversion in the formula to convert pounds to kilograms.

Example 1 ■ The client weighs 220 pounds and for treatment purposes, we must calculate their weight in kilograms. Recall that 2.2 pounds is equal to 1 kilogram. Recall that, for conversions, *D* will be the unit of measure we want to convert. In this example, we are given the information of 220 pounds. Use the formula method to set up this conversion.

$$\frac{220 \text{ lb} \times 1 \text{ kg}}{2.2 \text{ lb}} = x \text{ kg}$$

Next, eliminate lb in the numerator and denominator.

$$\frac{220 \text{ lb} \times 1 \text{ kg}}{2.2 \text{ lb}} = x \text{ kg}$$

$$100 \text{ kg} = x$$

Answer: After completing the calculation, 220 pounds is equal to 100 kg.

The formula method can also be used for calculations of medication dosages.

Example 2 ■ A dosage of 80 mg is ordered. Refer to Figure 10-1 for the available supply. How many mL are needed to administer this dosage? How do we know where to place these numbers in the formula?

Keypoint: The desired dosage (*D*) will be the doctor's order.

You can remember this by the *D* in **D**esire and in **d**octor's order. The *H*, have, and *Q*, quantity, values will be found on the supply of the medication.

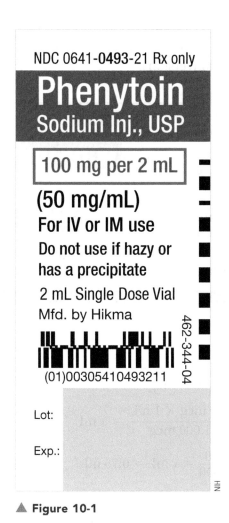

▲ **Figure 10-1**

The desired dosage (*D*) is 80 mg. In Figure 10-1, you have (*H*) 100 mg in (*Q*) 2 mL available. Recall that *x* will always be expressed in the same units of measure as *Q*, which is mL in this example. **Always include units of measure when setting up the formula.**

$$\frac{80 \text{ mg} \times 2 \text{ mL}}{100 \text{ mg}} = x \text{ mL}$$

Next, eliminate the units of measure in the numerator and denominator.

$$\frac{80 \text{ m\!\!\!/g} \times 2 \text{ mL}}{100 \text{ m\!\!\!/g}} = x \text{ mL}$$

$$\frac{80 \times 2 \text{ mL}}{100} = x \text{ mL}$$

$$\frac{160}{100} = 1.6 \text{ mL}$$

Answer: To give a dosage of 80 mg, you must administer 1.6 mL.

Example 3 ■   A dosage of 750 mcg has been ordered by the physician. Refer to Figure 10-2 for the supply that is available and set up the formula for conversions.

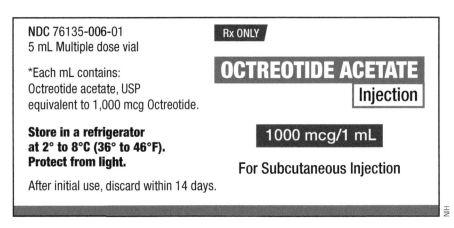

NDC 76135-006-01
5 mL Multiple dose vial

*Each mL contains:
Octreotide acetate, USP
equivalent to 1,000 mcg Octreotide.

**Store in a refrigerator
at 2° to 8°C (36° to 46°F).
Protect from light.**

After initial use, discard within 14 days.

Rx ONLY

OCTREOTIDE ACETATE
Injection

1000 mcg/1 mL

For Subcutaneous Injection

▲ **Figure 10-2**

$$\frac{750 \text{ mcg} \times 1 \text{ mL}}{1,000 \text{ mcg}} = x \text{ mL}$$

$$\frac{750 \text{ m\cancel{c}g} \times 1 \text{ mL}}{1,000 \text{ m\cancel{c}g}} = x \text{ mL}$$

$$\frac{750}{1,000} = x \text{ mL} = 0.75 \text{ mL}$$

Answer: The amount of 0.75 mL will be the most accurate since the answer is less than 1 mL.

In later chapters, we discuss measuring devices that will measure to the hundredth if the volume is less than 1 mL.

The doctor's order and the supply are not always in the same system and same unit of measurement. When this happens, conversion will be needed as the first step.

Example 4 ■   A dosage of 0.125 mg is ordered. Refer to Figure 10-3 for the available supply.

This problem cannot be solved with the information given because the drug strengths, *D* and *H*, are in different units of measure. One of them must be changed before the problem can be solved.

$$\frac{0.125 \text{ mg} \times 1 \text{ tab}}{250 \text{ mcg}} = x \text{ tab}$$

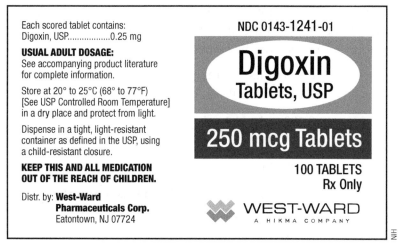

▲ **Figure 10-3**

First, convert mg to mcg to eliminate the decimal point. Use the conversion factor of 1 mg = 1,000 mcg and move the decimal point three places to the right.

$$0.125 \text{ mg} = 125 \text{ mcg}$$

To use the formula to perform the conversion, 0.125 mg would be *D*, desire, 1 mg would be *H*, have, and *Q*, quantity, would be 1,000 mcg.

$$\frac{0.125 \text{ mg} \times 1,000 \text{ mcg}}{1 \text{ mg}} = 125 \text{ mcg}$$

Next, use the formula to complete the calculation.

$$\frac{125 \text{ mcg} \times 1 \text{ tab}}{250 \text{ mcg}} = x \text{ tab}$$

$$\frac{125 \times 1 \text{ tab}}{250} = \frac{1}{2} \text{ tab}$$

Answer: To give 125 mcg, you must administer ½ tablet.

Example 5 ■   A dosage of 8,500 units has been ordered. Refer to Figure 10-4 for the available supply.

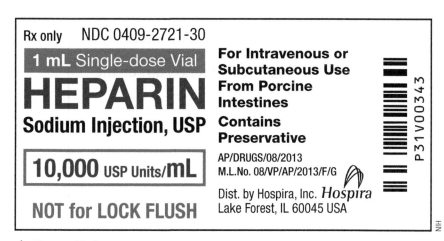

▲ **Figure 10-4**

When calculating this dosage, note that both the ordered dose (D) and the available strength (H) are already in the same unit of measurement so no conversion is needed. Using the formula method, set up the calculation.

$$\frac{8{,}500 \text{ units} \times 1 \text{ mL}}{10{,}000 \text{ units}} = x \text{ mL}$$

$$\frac{8{,}500 \text{ units} \times 1 \text{ mL}}{10{,}000 \text{ units}} = x \text{ mL}$$

$$x = 0.85 \text{ mL}$$

Answer: For accuracy, keep this amount at 0.85 mL.

In later chapters, we will discuss measuring devices that measure to the hundredth if the volume is less than 1 mL.

Example 6 ■   You are to prepare a dose of 30 mEq. Refer to Figure 10-5 for the available supply.

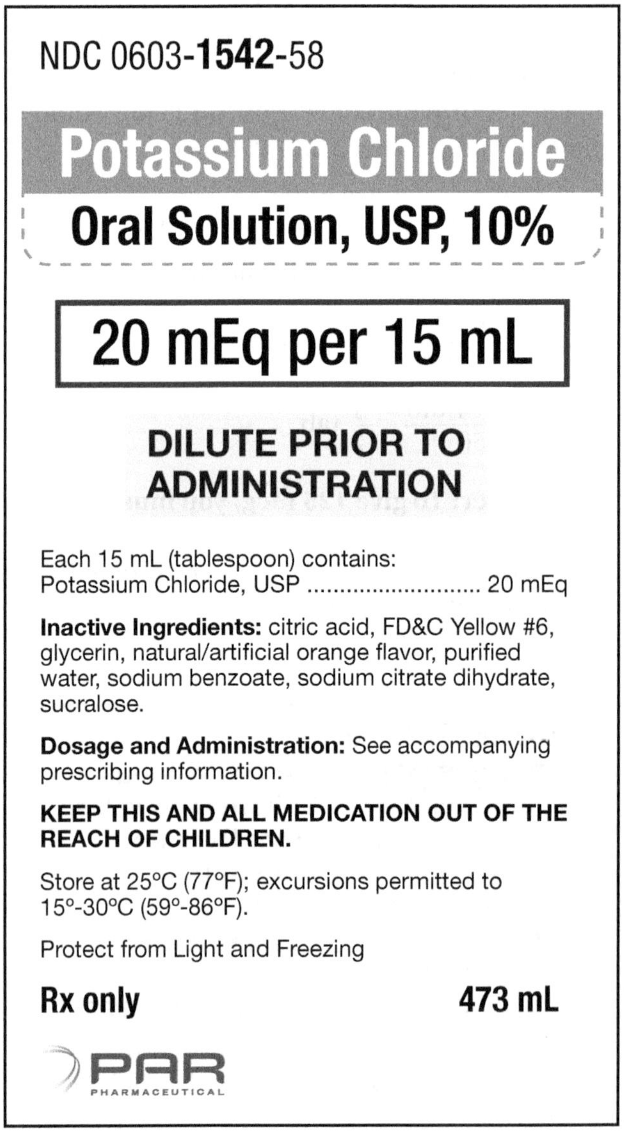

NDC 0603-**1542**-58

Potassium Chloride
Oral Solution, USP, 10%

20 mEq per 15 mL

DILUTE PRIOR TO ADMINISTRATION

Each 15 mL (tablespoon) contains:
Potassium Chloride, USP .... 20 mEq

Inactive Ingredients: citric acid, FD&C Yellow #6, glycerin, natural/artificial orange flavor, purified water, sodium benzoate, sodium citrate dihydrate, sucralose.

Dosage and Administration: See accompanying prescribing information.

KEEP THIS AND ALL MEDICATION OUT OF THE REACH OF CHILDREN.

Store at 25°C (77°F); excursions permitted to 15°-30°C (59°-86°F).

Protect from Light and Freezing

Rx only   **473 mL**

PAR
PHARMACEUTICAL

▲ **Figure 10-5**

When calculating this dosage, note that *D*, desire, and *H*, have, are in the same unit of measure, milliequivalents. Therefore, the calculation will be completed as follows:

$$\frac{30 \text{ mEq} \times 15 \text{ mL}}{20 \text{ mEq}} = x \text{ mL}$$

$$\frac{30 \cancel{\text{ mEq}} \times 15 \text{ mL}}{20 \cancel{\text{ mEq}}} = x \text{ mL}$$

$$\frac{30 \times 15 \text{ mL}}{20} = x \text{ mL}$$

$$\frac{450 \text{ mL}}{20} = 22.5 \text{ mL}$$

Answer: A dosage of 30 mEq would be supplied in 22.5 mL.

Problems 10.2

Calculate the dosages. Express answers to the nearest tenth, unless otherwise instructed.

1. The dosage ordered is 780 mcg. The strength available is 1 mg per mL. Round to the nearest hundredth.   _____

2. The available dosage strength is 0.1 g per mL. The dosage ordered is 250 mg.   _____

3. Prepare a dosage of 0.6 mg from an available strength of 1,000 mcg per 2 mL.   _____

4. A dosage of 0.4 g has been ordered. The strength available is 500 mg per 1.3 mL.   _____

5. The dosage ordered is 400 mg of amoxicillin. Refer to Figure 10-6 for the available strength.   _____

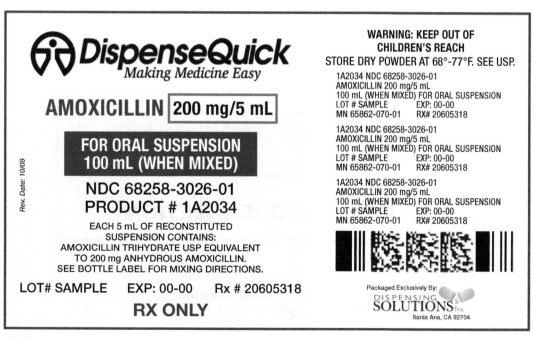

▲ **Figure 10-6**

6. A dosage of 6,000 units of heparin has been ordered. Refer to Figure 10-7 for the available supply. _____

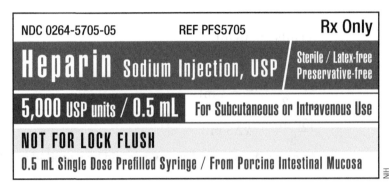

NDC 0264-5705-05   REF PFS5705   **Rx Only**

Heparin Sodium Injection, USP / Sterile / Latex-free Preservative-free

5,000 USP units / **0.5 mL**   For Subcutaneous or Intravenous Use

NOT FOR LOCK FLUSH

0.5 mL Single Dose Prefilled Syringe / From Porcine Intestinal Mucosa

▲ **Figure 10-7**

7. A dosage of 45 units has been ordered. The strength available is 80 units per mL. Round to the nearest hundredth. _____

8. The supply available has a strength of 200 mEq per 20 mL. Prepare a 50 mEq dosage. _____

9. A dosage of 30 mg of enoxaparin has been ordered. Refer to Figure 10-8 for the available supply. _____

ENOXAPARIN SODIUM INJECTION

40 mg/0.4 mL

NDC 0548-5632-00

Rx ONLY ///

10 x 40 mg Single Dose Syringes with Automatic Safety Device

FOR SUBCUTANEOUS INJECTION

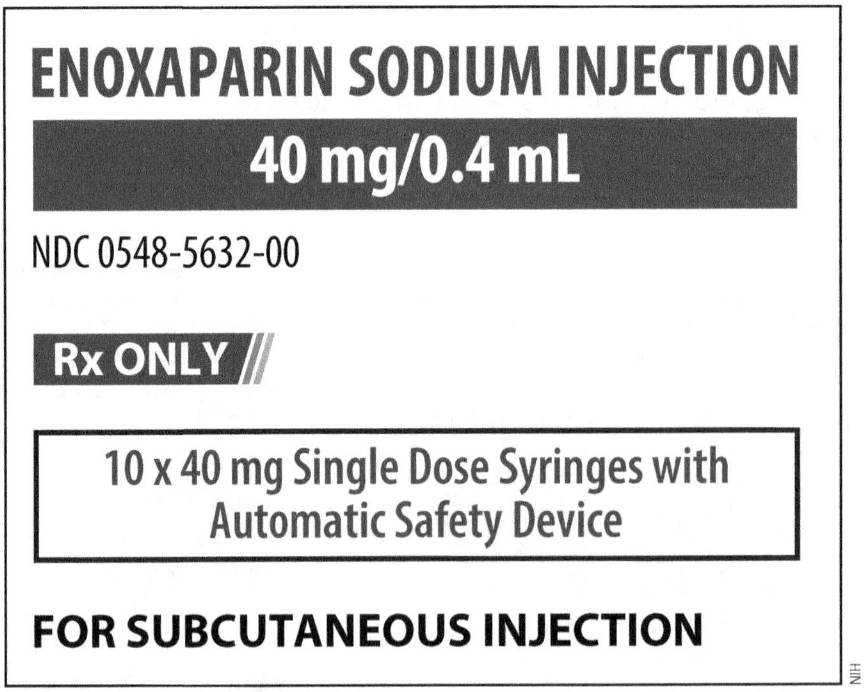

▲ **Figure 10-8**

10. The dosage ordered is 600 mcg of Nitrostat. Refer to Figure 10-9 for the available strength. _____

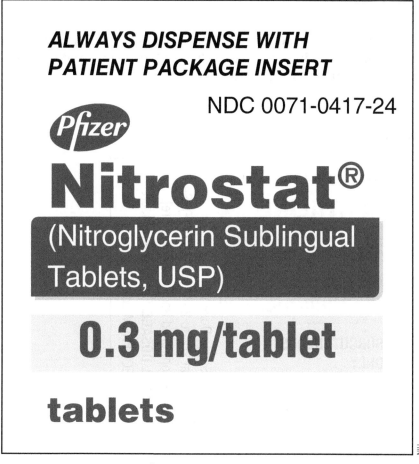

ALWAYS DISPENSE WITH
PATIENT PACKAGE INSERT

NDC 0071-0417-24

Pfizer

Nitrostat®

(Nitroglycerin Sublingual Tablets, USP)

0.3 mg/tablet

tablets

NIH

▲ **Figure 10-9**

Answers **1.** 0.78 mL **2.** 2.5 mL **3.** 1.2 mL **4.** 1 mL **5.** 10 mL **6.** 0.6 mL **7.** 0.56 mL
8. 5 mL **9.** 0.3 mL **10.** 2 tab

Summary

This concludes the chapter on using the formula method to solve dosage calculations. The important points to remember from this chapter are:

- The formula utilizes the letters *D* for desired dosage, *H* for have available, *Q* for quantity, and *x* for the unknown.

- When using the formula method, *D* and *H* must be expressed in the same units of measure.

- The answer obtained, *x*, will always be in the same unit of measure as *Q*, the quantity.

- Always multiply the numbers in the numerator first and then divide the product by the denominator.

- Routinely triple-check the math for all calculations.

Summary Self-Test

Calculate the following dosages using the formula method. Express mL answers to the nearest tenth (or hundredth where indicated) using the medication labels provided. The route of the order is provided for you.

Dosage Ordered   **Answer**

1. terbutaline sulfate 800 mcg subcutaneous   _____

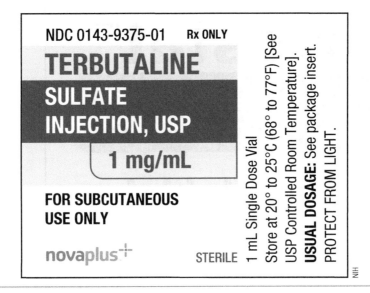

2. furosemide 15 mg IV   _____

Dosage Ordered   **Answer**

3. dexamethasone 15 mg IV   _____

NDC 63323-506-41   PRX500601

Dexamethasone Sodium Phosphate
Injection, USP

10 mg per mL

For IM or IV use only.
Preservative free.
Discard unused portion.
Protect from light.
1 mL Single Dose Vial   Rx only

PREMIER ProRx®

Mfd. by: Fresenius Kabi

NIH

4. fentanyl citrate 0.15 mg IV   _____

NDC 17478-030-02   **2 mL Ampule**

Fentanyl Citrate Injection, USP Ⓒⓛ

100 mcg/2 mL (50 mcg/mL)*

FOR INTRAVENOUS OR INTRAMUSCULAR USE

Rx only

*Each mL contains:** 0.0785 mg fentanyl
citrate equivalent to 50 mcg fentanyl base.
Mfd. by: **Akorn,** Lake Forest, IL 60045

AFCADL Rev.09/21

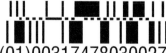

(01)00317478030027

LOT
EXP.

Dosage Ordered   **Answer**

5. naloxone 350 mcg subcutaneous (Round to the nearest   _____
   hundredth.)

17478-**041**-01

Naloxone HCl Injection, USP

0.4 mg/mL

For I.V., I.M. or S.C. use
1 mL Single-dose Vial

Rx only

Protect from light.

○AKORN

Mfd. by: **Akorn Inc.**
Lake Forest, IL 60045

NLAAL   Rev. 10/17

NIH

6. clindamycin 225 mg IM   _____

NDC 25021-115-02   1030283

Clindamycin

Injection, USP

300 mg per **2** mL
(150 mg per mL)

SAGENT

Rx only
For IM or IV Use
Dilute Before IV Use
2 mL Single-Dose Vial

Lot: Exp.:

**Sterile, Nonpyrogenic.
Each mL contains:** clindamycin phosphate equivalent to clindamycin 150 mg. Also contains 0.5 mg disodium edetate and 9.45 mg benzyl alcohol as a preservative. **Usual Dosage:** See insert. Store at 20° to 25°C (68° to 77°F). [See Insert.]

Mfd. for:
SAGENT Pharmaceuticals
Schaumburg, IL 60195 (USA)
Made in India
©2011 Sagent Pharmaceuticals, Inc.
Code No.: KR/DRUGS/KTK/28/384/2009

NIH

Dosage Ordered   **Answer**

7. Robinul® 75 mcg IV (Round to the nearest hundredth.)   _____

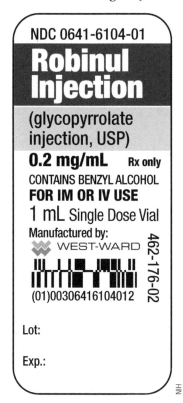

---

8. bumetanide 1.5 mg IV   _____

NDC 65219-**570**-01   **Rx only**

Bumetanide
Injection, USP

1 mg/4 mL (0.25 mg/mL)

**For Intravenous or
Intramuscular Use
Contains Benzyl Alcohol**

4 mL Single-Dose Vial
Discard unused portion.

Each mL contains bumetanide
0.25 mg, sodium chloride 8.5 mg
and ammonium acetate 4 mg as
buffers, edetate disodium dihydrate
0.1 mg and benzyl alcohol 10 mg
as preservative; pH adjusted to
6.8-7.8 with sodium hydroxide.
This container closure is not made
with natural rubber latex.

Usual Dosage: See package insert.
**Store at 20°C to 25°C (68°F to
77°F). Protect from light.**

Dosage Ordered   **Answer**

9. morphine sulfate 2.5 mg IV (Round to the nearest   _____
   hundredth.)

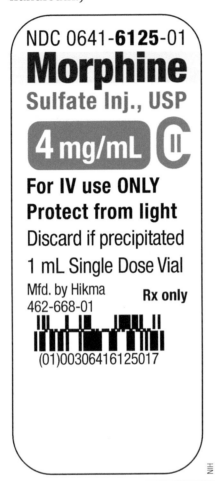

NDC 0641-**6125**-01

Morphine

Sulfate Inj., USP

4 mg/mL ⒈Ⅱ

For IV use ONLY
Protect from light
Discard if precipitated
1 mL Single Dose Vial

Mfd. by Hikma   **Rx only**
462-668-01

(01)00306416125017

10. heparin sodium 2,500 units subcutaneous (Round to   _____
    the nearest hundredth.)

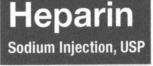

Heparin   **5,000**
Sodium Injection, USP   **USP units**
NOT for lock flush   **per 0.5 mL**

For Intravenous or Subcutaneous Use.
Derived from Porcine Intestinal Mucosa
Do NOT place syringe on a Sterile Field.

24 x 0.5 mL Prefilled Single-Dose Syringes
Discard unused portion.

Simplist®   FRESENIUS KABI

Dosage Ordered   **Answer**

11. phenytoin 0.1 g po   _____

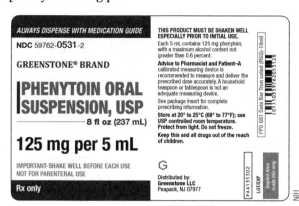

12. medroxyprogesterone 200 mg IM   _____

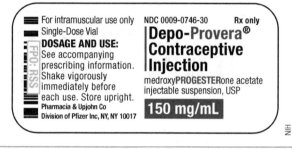

13. lorazepam 2.5 mg po   _____

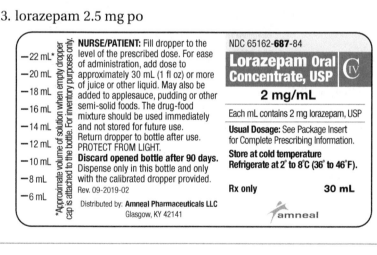

Dosage Ordered	**Answer**

14. atropine sulfate 150 mcg IM (Round to the nearest hundredth.) _____

ATROPINE SULFATE
INJECTION, USP
0.4 mg/mL

NDC 0517-0401-25
25 X 1 mL
SINGLE DOSE VIALS

FOR INTRAVENOUS, INTRAMUSCULAR OR SUBCUTANEOUS USE
PRESERVATIVE FREE
Rx Only

Each mL contains: Atropine Sulfate 0.4 mg, Sodium Chloride 9 mg, Water for Injection q.s. pH adjusted with Sulfuric Acid.
WARNING: DISCARD UNUSED PORTION.
Store at 20°-25°C (68°-77°F); excursions permitted to 15°-30°C (59°-86°F) (See USP Controlled Room Temperature).
Directions for Use: See Package Insert.

Rev. 11/05

Lot / Exp.

AMERICAN
REGENT, INC.
SHIRLEY, NY 11967

NIH

15. cefaclor 75 mg po _____

NDC 23594-125-01

Rx only

CEFACLOR
FOR ORAL SUSPENSION, USP

150 mL (when mixed)
SHAKE WELL BEFORE USE

cerecor

125 mg/5mL

Prior to Mixing, store at 20° to 25°C (68° to 77°F). [See USP Controlled Room Temperature]. Protect from moisture.
Directions for Mixing: Add 106 mL of water in two portions to dry mixture in the bottle. Shake well after each addition.
Each 5 mL (approximately one teaspoonful) will then contain Cefaclor, USP, monohydrate equivalent to 125 mg anhydrous cefaclor.
Oversize bottle provides extra space for shaking.
Store in a refrigerator. May be kept for 14 days without significant loss of potency. Keep tightly closed. Discard unused portion after 14 days.
Usual Dose:
Pediatric Patients - 20 mg/kg/day (40 mg/kg per day in otitis media) in three divided doses every 8 hours.
Adults - 250 mg every 8 hours.
See literature for complete dosage information.
Bottle contains a total of cefaclor monohydrate equivalent to 3.75 g anhydrous cefaclor in a dry, strawberry flavored mixture.

KRP25e USA CEF125010918LBv1

Manufactured by:
Yung Shin Pharmaceutical Ind. Co., Ltd.
Tachia, Taichung 43769, TAIWAN
Distributed by:
Cerecor, Inc.
Research Triangle Park, NC 27713
Rev. 01/18

3 13551 12501 7

NIH

Dosage Ordered   **Answer**

16. phenytoin 0.15 g po   _____

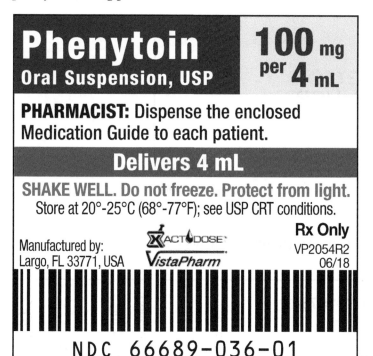

17. methotrexate 40 mg IV   _____

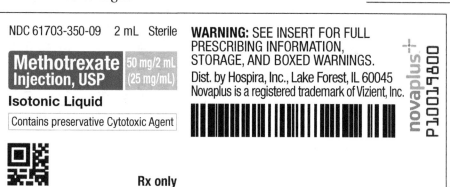

Dosage Ordered   **Answer**

18. ondansetron 3 mg IV   _____

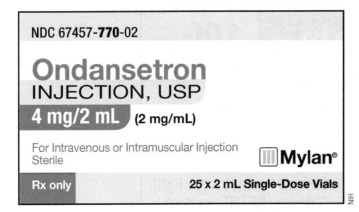

19. methylprednisolone 25 mg IM (Round to the nearest   _____
    hundredth.)

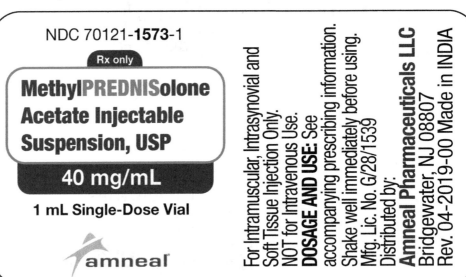

Dosage Ordered   **Answer**

20. ketorolac tromethamine 20 mg IV   _____

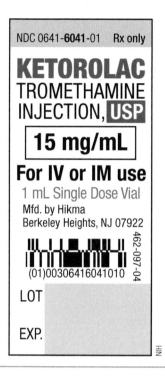

---

21. nalbuphine 15 mg subcutaneous (Round to the nearest   _____
    hundredth.)

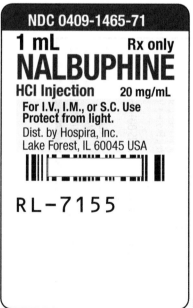

Dosage Ordered   **Answer**

22. hydromorphone 1.5 mg IV (Round to the nearest   _____
    hundredth.)

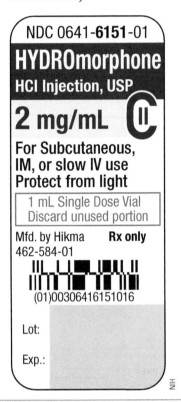

23. ondansetron 6 mg po   _____

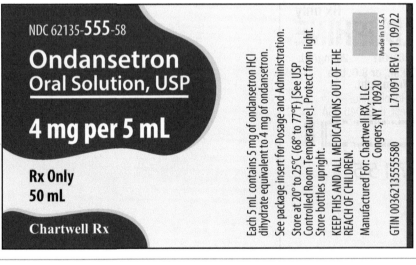

Dosage Ordered   **Answer**

24. prednisone 7.5 mg po   _____

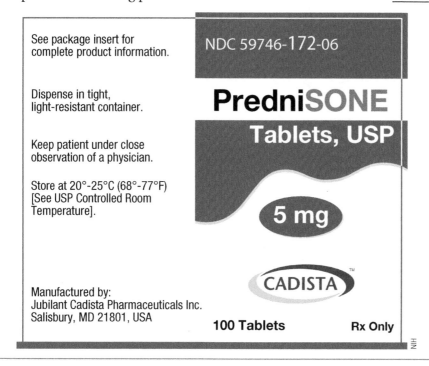

See package insert for
complete product information.

NDC 59746-172-06

PredniSONE

Tablets, USP

Dispense in tight,
light-resistant container.

Keep patient under close
observation of a physician.

5 mg

Store at 20°-25°C (68°-77°F)
[See USP Controlled Room
Temperature].

CADISTA™

Manufactured by:
Jubilant Cadista Pharmaceuticals Inc.
Salisbury, MD 21801, USA

100 Tablets   **Rx Only**

25. digoxin 0.25 mg po   _____

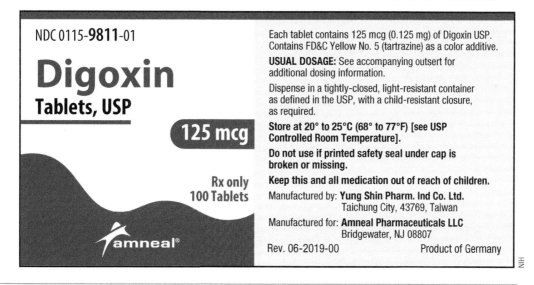

NDC 0115-9811-01

Digoxin

Tablets, USP

125 mcg

Rx only
100 Tablets

amneal®

Each tablet contains 125 mcg (0.125 mg) of Digoxin USP.
Contains FD&C Yellow No. 5 (tartrazine) as a color additive.

USUAL DOSAGE: See accompanying outsert for
additional dosing information.

Dispense in a tightly-closed, light-resistant container
as defined in the USP, with a child-resistant closure,
as required.

**Store at 20° to 25°C (68° to 77°F) [see USP
Controlled Room Temperature].**

**Do not use if printed safety seal under cap is
broken or missing.**

Keep this and all medication out of reach of children.

Manufactured by: **Yung Shin Pharm. Ind Co. Ltd.**
                  Taichung City, 43769, Taiwan

Manufactured for: **Amneal Pharmaceuticals LLC**
                  Bridgewater, NJ 08807

Rev. 06-2019-00   Product of Germany

Answers to Summary Self-Test

1. 0.8 mL	**6.** 1.5 mL	**11.** 4 mL	**16.** 6 mL	**21.** 0.75 mL
2. 1.5 mL	**7.** 0.38 mL	**12.** 1.3 mL	**17.** 1.6 mL	**22.** 0.75 mL
3. 1.5 mL	**8.** 6 mL	**13.** 1.3 mL	**18.** 1.5 mL	**23.** 7.5 mL
4. 3 mL	**9.** 0.63 mL	**14.** 0.38 mL	**19.** 0.63 mL	**24.** 1.5 tab
5. 0.88 mL	**10.** 0.25 mL	**15.** 3 mL	**20.** 1.3 mL	**25.** 2 tab

Section 4

Calculating Drug Dosages

Chapter

11

Oral Dosage Calculations

Objectives

The learner will:

1. utilize the correct conversion factor to convert when needed.

2. use one of the three calculation methods presented in this book to calculate the equivalent number of tablets, capsules, mL, etc., to administer prescribed medication amounts.

3. evaluate the calculated amount to determine if it is logical.

4. explain the equipment available to measure oral solutions.

In this chapter, you will use medication labels to calculate prescribed oral dosages. Remember, the physician will prescribe medications for administration, but will not provide the number of tablets, capsules, milliliters, etc., that the nurse will need to give the patient. It will be the responsibility of the nurse to calculate how to provide the dosage ordered utilizing the supply provided by the pharmacist. Chapter 7 introduced the information provided on medication labels. Chapters 8 through 10 introduced three methods to calculate dosages so medication orders can be implemented. This chapter will expand on the ability to read and interpret medication labels to prepare to provide the medications to our patients that have been ordered by the physician.

Clinical Relevance: In the past three chapters, you have learned three methods to apply to dosage calculation. While all three methods produce accurate, reliable answers when applied correctly, it is important for you to develop confidence with the method of your choice. To apply this to practice in the clinical setting, you are encouraged to utilize the method that you prefer. This chapter will begin looking at additional examples of calculation of oral dosages. Consistent use of a method of calculation during practice will give you the confidence you need to accurately calculate oral dosages in the clinical setting. Including your units of measure when using these calculation methods is very important. Doing this consistently will help you maintain accuracy and decrease the chances of placing your numbers in the wrong place in the calculation method. When you set up your calculation, review your equations and determine a reasonable, logical answer. To help avoid errors, compare your calculation to what you have determined would be a reasonable answer. Now that we are calculating dosages, we must also be mindful of the equipment available to measure oral liquids. In this chapter, you will be exposed to examples of equipment used to measure oral liquid dosages. The equipment available will require rounding of some dosages. In order to be consistent, we would round to the tenth if the volume calculated is greater than 1 mL and round to the hundredth if the volume calculated is less than 1 mL. Consistency in rounding will promote safety and accuracy in the clinical setting.

Solid Drug Preparations

We will begin with labels and dosage calculations for solid drug preparations. These include tablets, scored tablets (which contain an indented marking to make breakage for partial dosages possible), enteric-coated tablets (which delay absorption until the drug reaches the small intestine), capsules (powdered or oily drugs in a gelatin cover), and sustained or controlled-release capsules (action spread over a prolonged period of time; for example, 12 hours). When reading the drug label of solid forms of medications, it is important to understand that the dosage strength is usually associated with a quantity of one (1) tablet, capsule, enteric-coated tablet, and so on.

The physician will prescribe the medication for the patient. In the clinical setting, this order will be on the Medication Administration Record (MAR). In an outpatient setting, the order will be on a prescription form. The order or prescription will tell you the name and amount of drug to be given, but it will not tell you how many tablets or capsules contain this dosage. You will need to calculate this.

Most orders will involve giving $\frac{1}{2}$ to 3 tablets (or 1–3 capsules, because capsules cannot be broken in half). You should consider questioning orders that require administration of more than 3 tablets or capsules; however, it is more important to use your critical reasoning abilities. Although some drugs require multiple tablets, it is important to consider what makes sense and is reasonable. For example, if you were receiving medication, you would most likely question if you were given 6 tablets of the same medication at the same time.

There are limited exceptions where a large number of tablets may be given—for example, initial doses of steroids, such as prednisone and dexamethasone. In these cases, there may be 60 mg ordered and you have available 10 mg tablets. This would require administration of 6 tablets. Although we may question this, we would see in our drug references that a dose of this amount would be appropriate. In most instances we do not expect to take more than 1 or 2 tablets of the same medication at the same time. While it is true that some clinical pharmacies only carry a limited quantity of a particular medication as a cost-saving factor, typically enough variation of doses are available so that unreasonable numbers of tablets are not required. Always triple-check your calculations to ensure that your calculations are accurate.

> **Key**point: Most oral dosages consist of no more than 3 tablets or capsules. An unusual number of tablets or capsules could be a warning of an error in prescribing, transcribing, or calculating. Consider the reason the medication is being given. For example, we would not expect to give a patient 3 tablets of the same heart medication at the same time. We need to remember to check our drug references and use our critical-thinking abilities.

Since the dosage strength of a solid form of oral medication is associated with a quantity of 1, it is important to recognize the advantage of continuing to set up the dosage problem and always include both parts of the supply—the dosage strength and the quantity. This is especially important as you are learning and practicing calculation of dosages to bolster your confidence. Do not fall into the pitfall of taking shortcuts and sacrificing safety. Let's look at a few examples of calculations for medication administration.

Example 1 ▧   The physician has ordered glipizide 5 mg po bid. Refer to Figure 11-1 for the supply.

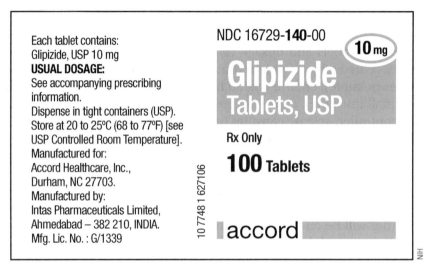

Each tablet contains:
Glipizide, USP 10 mg
USUAL DOSAGE:
See accompanying prescribing information.
Dispense in tight containers (USP).
Store at 20 to 25°C (68 to 77°F) [see USP Controlled Room Temperature].
Manufactured for:
Accord Healthcare, Inc.,
Durham, NC 27703.
Manufactured by:
Intas Pharmaceuticals Limited,
Ahmedabad – 382 210, INDIA.
Mfg. Lic. No. : G/1339

NDC 16729-**140**-00   **10 mg**

Glipizide
Tablets, USP

Rx Only

100 Tablets

10 7748 1 627106

❚accord

▲ **Figure 11-1**

The doctor's order is 5 mg. The supply is 10 mg per tablet. Notice the label indicates there are a total of 100 tablets in this bottle, but we want to use the quantity that is associated with 10 mg, and that is 1 tablet.

Calculate how many tablets we will need to administer to ensure the patient receives 5 mg. We will assume all tablets are scored. In all these examples, we will show all three methods of calculation to determine how many tablets to administer to your patient. You are encouraged to use the format of your choice.

Method 1: Ratio and Proportion

In Colon Format

$10 \text{ mg} : 1 \text{ tab} = 5 \text{ mg} : x \text{ tab}$

$10x = 5$

$x = 0.5 \text{ or } \frac{1}{2} \text{ tab}$

In Fraction Format

$$\frac{10 \text{ mg}}{1 \text{ tab}} = \frac{5 \text{ mg}}{x \text{ tab}}$$

$10x = 5$

$x = \frac{5}{10} = 0.5 \text{ or } \frac{1}{2} \text{ tab}$

Method 2: Dimensional Analysis

$$\text{tab} = \frac{1 \text{ tab}}{10 \text{ mg}} \times \frac{5 \text{ mg}}{}$$

$$\text{tab} = \frac{1 \text{ tab}}{10 \text{ mg}} \times \frac{5 \text{ mg}}{}$$

$$\text{tab} = \frac{5}{10} = 0.5 \text{ or } \frac{1}{2} \text{ tab}$$

Method 3: Formula Method

$$\frac{5 \text{ mg (D)} \times 1 \text{ tab (Q)}}{10 \text{ mg (H)}} = x \text{ tab}$$

$$\frac{5 \cancel{\text{mg}} \times 1 \text{ tab}}{10 \cancel{\text{mg}}} = x \text{ tab}$$

$$\frac{5 \times 1}{10} = 0.5 \text{ or } \tfrac{1}{2} \text{ tab}$$

These three methods of calculation arrive at the same answer. This answer is logical based on the information we have. We know the doctor's order is for 5 mg and the supply we have is 10 mg per tablet. We can determine that we will give less than 1 tablet—precisely, $\tfrac{1}{2}$ tablet of this medication.

Example 2 ▪   The physician orders diltiazem 90 mg PO every 8 hours. Refer to Figure 11-2 for the supply provided for this order.

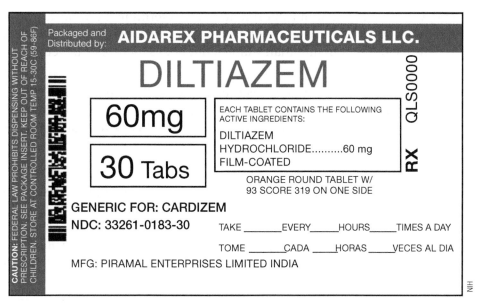

▲ **Figure 11-2**

We recognize that the doctor's order is 90 mg for each dose. The supply is 60 mg per tablet. Let's calculate how many tablets we will need to administer to ensure the patient receives 90 mg.

Method 1: Ratio and Proportion

In Colon Format

60 mg : 1 tab = 90 mg : x tab

$60x = 90$

$x = 1.5$ or $1\tfrac{1}{2}$ tab

In Fraction Format

$$\frac{60 \text{ mg}}{1 \text{ tab}} = \frac{90 \text{ mg}}{x \text{ tab}}$$

$60x = 90$

$x = \dfrac{90}{60} = 1.5$ or $1\tfrac{1}{2}$ tab

Method 2: Dimensional Analysis

$$\text{tab} = \frac{1 \text{ tab}}{60 \text{ mg}} \times \frac{90 \text{ mg}}{}$$

$$\text{tab} = \frac{1 \text{ tab}}{60 \text{ mg}} \times \frac{90 \text{ mg}}{}$$

$$\text{tab} = \frac{90}{60} = 1.5 \text{ or } 1\tfrac{1}{2} \text{ tab}$$

Method 3: Formula Method

$$\frac{90 \text{ mg (D)} \times 1 \text{ tab (Q)}}{60 \text{ mg (H)}} = x \text{ tab}$$

$$\frac{90 \text{ mg} \times 1 \text{ tab}}{60 \text{ mg}} = x \text{ tab}$$

$$\frac{90 \times 1}{60} = 1.5 \text{ or } 1\tfrac{1}{2} \text{ tab}$$

Again, we should look at our information and determine if our answer is logical. The order was for 90 mg and the supply had 60 mg per tablet. We can logically determine that the answer should be greater than 1 tablet, but not as many as 2 tablets.

Keypoint: Only tablets that are scored can be split. They must be broken along the score line. If a tablet is not scored, it cannot be broken. In addition, capsules cannot be split and therefore, $\frac{1}{2}$ capsule would not be appropriate.

Let's look now at an example where the order and the supply are not in the same system and same unit of measure.

Example 3 ■ The physician orders ciprofloxacin 0.5 g PO every 8 hours. Refer to Figure 11-3 for the supply provided for this order. Calculate one dose.

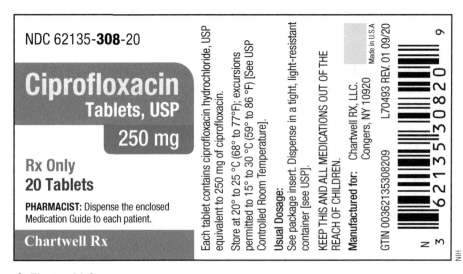

▲ **Figure 11-3**

We see that the doctor's order and the supply are not in the same unit of measure. The order is 0.5 g and the supply 250 mg per tablet. Our first consideration will be to convert so that both the order and the supply are in the same unit of measure. We know that our conversion factor will be 1,000 mg equal to 1 g. It will be best to convert to mg so we can eliminate the decimal point.

Method 1: Ratio and Proportion

In Colon Format   *In Fraction Format*

$$1 \text{ g} : 1{,}000 \text{ mg} = 0.5 \text{ g} : x \text{ mg}$$

$$\frac{1 \text{ g}}{1{,}000 \text{ mg}} = \frac{0.5 \text{ g}}{x \text{ mg}}$$

$$x = 500 \text{ mg} \qquad\qquad x = 500 \text{ mg}$$

Now we can substitute 500 mg for 0.5 g and continue with the calculation. As you can see from your labels, we have not calculated the number of tablets to administer.

$$250 \text{ mg} : 1 \text{ tab} = 500 \text{ mg} : x \text{ tab} \qquad \frac{250 \text{ mg}}{1 \text{ tab}} = \frac{500 \text{ mg}}{x \text{ tab}}$$

$$250x = 500 \qquad\qquad\qquad 250x = 500$$

$$x = 2 \text{ tab} \qquad\qquad\qquad x = 2 \text{ tab}$$

Method 2: Dimensional Analysis

$$\text{tab} = \frac{1 \text{ tab}}{250 \text{ mg}} \times \frac{1{,}000 \text{ mg}}{1 \text{ g}} \times \frac{0.5 \text{ g}}{}$$

$$\text{tab} = \frac{1 \text{ tab}}{250 \ \cancel{\text{mg}}} \times \frac{1{,}000 \ \cancel{\text{mg}}}{1 \ \cancel{\text{g}}} \times \frac{0.5 \ \cancel{\text{g}}}{}$$

$$\text{tab} = \frac{500}{250} = 2 \text{ tab}$$

Method 3: Formula Method

First, we need to convert 0.5 g to mg.

$$\frac{0.5 \text{ g} \times 1{,}000 \text{ mg}}{1 \text{ g}} = 500 \text{ mg}$$

Next, substitute 500 mg for the doctor's order, or the desire. Our have and quantity will come from the label and will be 250 mg per tablet.

$$\frac{500 \text{ mg} \times 1 \text{ tab}}{250 \text{ mg}} = x \text{ tab}$$

$$\frac{500 \ \cancel{\text{mg}} \times 1 \text{ tab}}{250 \ \cancel{\text{mg}}} = 2 \text{ tab}$$

In this example, we are better able to logically determine an answer after we have converted to the same unit of measure. Once we realize the doctor's order of 0.5 g is equivalent to 500 mg, it is easier to look at our supply and logically determine that our answer should be 2 tablets. This allows us to recognize that the answer we calculated is reasonable.

Problems 11.1

Calculate the number of tablets, capsules, or milligrams to administer in each question. Assume all tablets are scored and can be broken in half. Calculate one dose unless otherwise instructed. Answers must be labeled to be correct.

1. The order is verapamil PO 0.12 g TID. Refer to Figure 11-4.

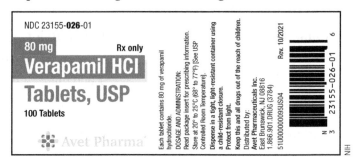

▲ **Figure 11-4**

2. Chlordiazepoxide 50 mg has been ordered PO once today. Refer to Figure 11-5.

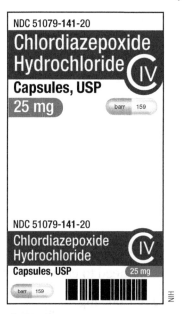

▲ **Figure 11-5**

3. The order is for levothyroxine 0.2 mg PO once daily. Refer to Figure 11-6.

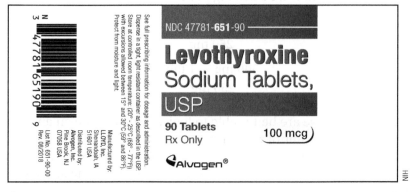

▲ **Figure 11-6**

4. Nitrostat 0.6 mg has been ordered SL route once today. Refer to Figure 11-7.

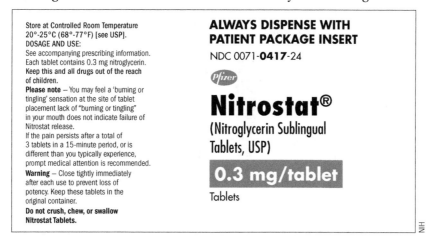

▲ **Figure 11-7**

5. The order is for sulfasalazine 1 g PO BID. How many total tablets will the patient receive daily? Refer to Figure 11-8.

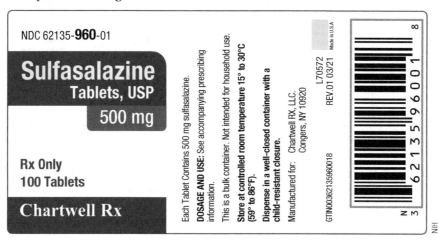

▲ **Figure 11-8**

6. The order is for isosorbide dinitrate 15 mg BID PO. Refer to Figure 11-9.

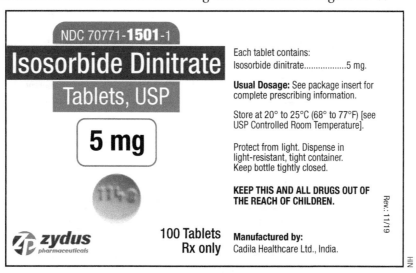

▲ **Figure 11-9**

7. Halcion® 125 mcg PO has been ordered at bedtime. Refer to Figure 11-10.

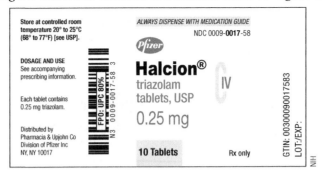

▲ **Figure 11-10**

8. Gabapentin 300 mg PO has been ordered TID. Refer to Figure 11-11.

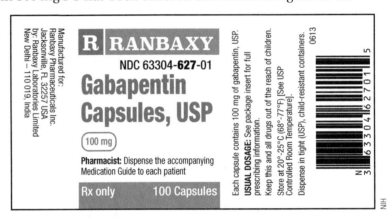

▲ **Figure 11-11**

9. The order is for 16 mEq of potassium chloride PO daily. How many total mgs will the patient receive daily? Please be sure to read this question carefully! Refer to Figure 11-12.

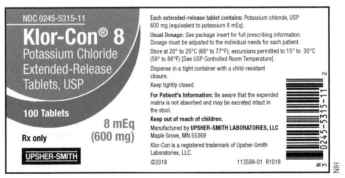

▲ **Figure 11-12**

10. Prednisone 60 mg has been ordered PO for 2 days. Refer to Figure 11-13.

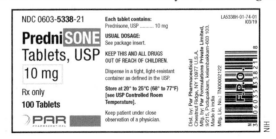

▲ **Figure 11-13**

11. The order is for penicillin V 800,000 units PO q 6 hours. Refer to Figure 11-14.

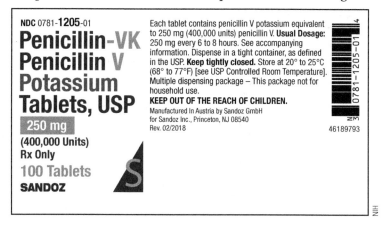

▲ **Figure 11-14**

12. The order is for digoxin 500 mcg PO daily. Refer to Figure 11-15.

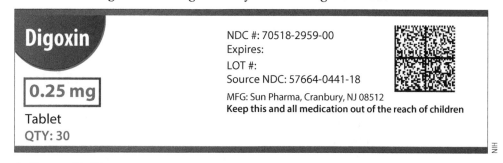

▲ **Figure 11-15**

13. Terbutaline 3.75 mg has been ordered PO TID. Refer to Figure 11-16.

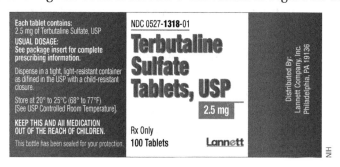

▲ **Figure 11-16**

14. The order is for methotrexate 10 mg PO weekly. Refer to Figure 11-17.

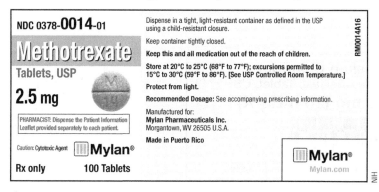

▲ **Figure 11-17**

15. The order is for alprazolam extended release tab 1 mg PO daily in the morning. Refer to Figure 11-18.

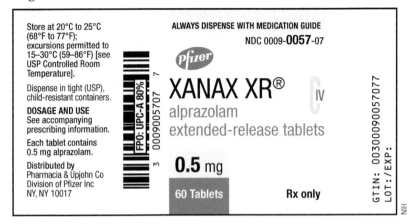

Store at 20°C to 25°C (68°F to 77°F); excursions permitted to 15–30°C (59–86°F) [see USP Controlled Room Temperature].

Dispense in tight (USP), child-resistant containers.

DOSAGE AND USE See accompanying prescribing information.

Each tablet contains 0.5 mg alprazolam.

Distributed by Pharmacia & Upjohn Co Division of Pfizer Inc NY, NY 10017

ALWAYS DISPENSE WITH MEDICATION GUIDE
NDC 0009-**0057**-07

Pfizer

XANAX XR® ℂ IV
alprazolam
extended-release tablets

0.5 mg

60 Tablets   Rx only

▲ **Figure 11-18**

Answers 1. 1.5 tab **2.** 2 cap **3.** 2 tab **4.** 2 tab **5.** 4 tab **6.** 3 tab **7.** $\frac{1}{2}$ tab **8.** 3 cap **9.** 1,200 mg
10. 6 tab **11.** 2 tab **12.** 2 tab **13.** 1.5 tab **14.** 4 tab **15.** 2 tab

Liquid Drug Preparations for Oral Medications

In liquid drug preparations, the dosage is contained in a certain volume of solution. Some of the drug preparations will come as a powder and will need to be diluted. The instructions will be on the label, and we will discuss this process further in Chapter 13, which looks at reconstitution. Let's review dosages in some solid and liquid drug preparations to illustrate the difference.

Example 1 ▪   **Solid:** 250 mg in 1 tablet   **Liquid:** 250 mg in 5 mL

Example 2 ▪   **Solid:** 100 mg in 1 capsule   **Liquid:** 100 mg in 10 mL

Example 3 ▪   **Solid:** 20 mEq in 1 tablet   **Liquid:** 20 mEq in 15 mL

Refer to Figures 11-19A and 11-19B for examples of labels from an oral solid preparation and an oral liquid. These are both unit dose labels.

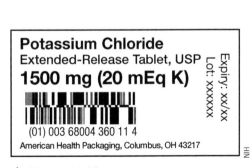

Potassium Chloride
Extended-Release Tablet, USP
1500 mg (20 mEq K)

(01) 003 68004 360 11 4
American Health Packaging, Columbus, OH 43217

Expiry: xx/xx
Lot: xxxxxx

NDC 43598-891-16
Potassium Chloride
Oral Solution, USP 10%

20 mEq/15 mL
DILUTE PRIOR TO ADMINISTRATION

0 43598 89116 2

15 mL
Lot #:   Exp. Date:
FOR INSTITUTIONAL USE ONLY
Manufactured for:
Dr.Reddy's Laboratories, Inc.
Princeton, NJ 08540

▲ **Figure 11-19a**   ▲ **Figure 11-19b**

In Figure 11-19a, although the number of tablets is not listed on the label, it is understood that it is 20 mEq per 1 tablet, as there is only 1 tablet in this unit dose package. In the unit dose of the oral solution in Figure 11-19b, it is identified on the label that there are 20 mEq in 15 mL. It is the same medication but in two different forms for oral administration.

When putting this information into the dosage calculation equations that have been presented in this book, it is very important to include all aspects required in the equation, even if the quantity is 1. This practice will help you calculate safely and accurately, and you will not miss key pieces of the calculation information. As with solid drugs, the Medication Administration Record (MAR) will tell you the dosage of the drug to be administered, but it will not specify the volume that contains this dosage.

Let's look at a few examples of dosage calculations involving oral solutions.

Example 4 ▨   The doctor has ordered metoclopramide 7.5 mg PO every 6 hours. Refer to Figure 11-20 for your supply.

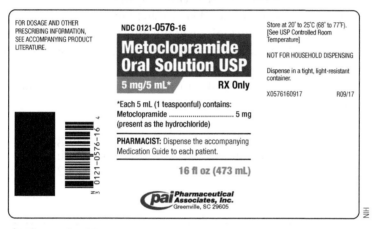

▲ **Figure 11-20**

When you are giving medications to your patient, you will have to calculate to determine the volume you will administer to your patient. From the physician's order you recognize that you are to administer 7.5 mg po for each dose every 6 hours. Let's utilize the three methods of calculation that were discussed in previous chapters.

Method 1: Ratio and Proportion

In Colon Format

$$5 \text{ mg} : 5 \text{ mL} = 7.5 \text{ mg} : x \text{ mL}$$

$$5x = 37.5$$

$$x = 7.5 \text{ mL}$$

In Fraction Format

$$\frac{5 \text{ mg}}{5 \text{ mL}} = \frac{7.5 \text{ mg}}{x \text{ mL}}$$

$$5x = 37.5$$

$$x = \frac{37.5}{5} = 7.5 \text{ mL}$$

Method 2: Dimensional Analysis

$$mL = \frac{5 \text{ mL}}{5 \text{ mg}} \times \frac{7.5 \text{ mg}}{}$$

$$mL = \frac{5 \text{ mL}}{5 \text{ mg}} \times \frac{7.5 \text{ mg}}{}$$

$$mL = \frac{37.5}{5} = 7.5 \text{ mL}$$

Method 3: Formula Method

$$\frac{7.5 \text{ mg (D)} \times 5 \text{ mL (Q)}}{5 \text{ mg (H)}} = x \text{ mL}$$

$$\frac{7.5 \cancel{\text{ mg}} \times 5 \text{ mL}}{5 \cancel{\text{ mg}}} = x \text{ mL}$$

$$\frac{7.5 \times \cancel{5}}{\cancel{5}} = 7.5 \text{ mL}$$

Regardless of the method of calculation used, the answer remains the same. Consistency and accuracy of answers will depend on insertion of the correct numbers into the equation of your choice. You may choose to reduce numbers in the numerator and denominators, as we discussed in Chapter 2, or you may choose to use the numbers as they are. Multiply numerators first before dividing by the denominators. This prevents the need to round multiple times, which will lead to slight inaccuracies. It is also important to evaluate your calculated answer by looking at the information you are given. In this case, the answer of 7.5 mL is logical, as we know that the order of 7.5 mg will require more than 5 milliliters.

Let's look at another example and apply the equations to calculate the volume of medication to administer.

Example 5 ■   The medication order is the following: "Administer nystatin 450,000 units PO qid." You are to administer one dose during your shift. Using the label in Figure 11-21, calculate how much to administer.

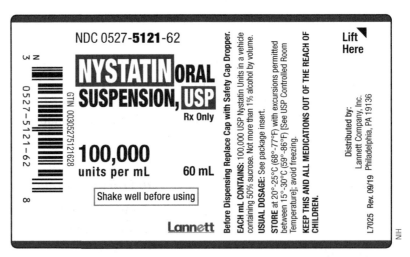

▲ **Figure 11-21**

In this order, you recognize that you must give 450,000 units of the medication to your client for each dose. Although this is not a unit of measure in the metric system, the label supply is also in units. Therefore, you will not need to convert anything. On the label, we recognize that the supply is 100,000 units per mL. Let's use our three methods of dosage calculation to calculate the volume that we must give the client.

Option 1: Ratio and Proportion

In Colon Format

100,000 units : 1 mL = 450,000 units : x mL

$100,000x = 450,000$

$x = 4.5$ mL

In Fraction Format

$$\frac{100,000 \text{ units}}{1 \text{ mL}} = \frac{450,000 \text{ units}}{x \text{ mL}}$$

$100,000x = 450,000$

$$x = \frac{450,000}{100,000} = \frac{45}{10} = 4.5 \text{ mL}$$

Note: Reducing numbers makes them more manageable.

Option 2: Dimensional Analysis

$$mL = \frac{1 \text{ mL}}{100,000 \text{ units}} \times \frac{450,000 \text{ units}}{}$$

$$mL = \frac{1 \text{ mL}}{100,000 \text{ units}} \times \frac{450,000 \text{ units}}{}$$

Eliminate the units of measure and reduce if desired.

$$mL = \frac{45}{10} = 4.5 \text{ mL}$$

Option 3: Formula Method

$$\frac{450,000 \text{ units (D)} \times 1 \text{ mL (Q)}}{100,000 \text{ units (H)}} = x \text{ mL}$$

$$\frac{450,000 \text{ units} \times 1 \text{ mL}}{100,000 \text{ units}} = x \text{ mL}$$

$$\frac{45 \times 1}{10} = 4.5 \text{ mL}$$

On completing the calculations, we recognize that we must give 4.5 mL of the available medication in order for the client to receive 450,000 units in each dose. This calculation result is logical. We know the order was for 450,000 units, which is at least four times the concentration of the solution. Therefore, we know that we must give more than 4 mL of the solution.

Finally, let's look at an example where the order and the supply are not in the same unit of measure.

Example 6 ▣   The physician orders nitrofurantoin 0.1 g po every 6 hours. Refer to Figure 11-22 for the supply.

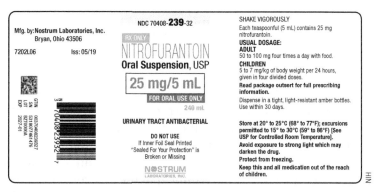

▲ **Figure 11-22**

Let's look at the order and the supply and determine the numbers that will go into the dosage calculation equations. The doctor's order is 0.1 g. The supply is 25 mg in 5 mL. We will have to convert so that the order and the supply are in the same unit of measure. We will convert 0.1 g to mg.

Option 1: Ratio and Proportion

<table>
<tr><td align="center">***In Colon Format***</td><td align="center">***In Fraction Format***</td></tr>
<tr><td align="center">$1\text{ g} : 1{,}000\text{ mg} = 0.1\text{ g} : x\text{ mg}$</td><td align="center">$\dfrac{1\text{ g}}{1{,}000\text{ mg}} = \dfrac{0.1\text{ g}}{x\text{ mg}}$</td></tr>
<tr><td align="center">$x = 100\text{ mg}$</td><td align="center">$x = 100\text{ mg}$</td></tr>
</table>

Now we can substitute 100 mg for 0.1 g and continue with the calculation. As you can see from including the units of measure, we have not yet calculated the volume to administer.

<table>
<tr><td align="center">$25\text{ mg} : 5\text{ mL} = 100\text{ mg} : x\text{ mL}$</td><td align="center">$\dfrac{25\text{ mg}}{5\text{ mL}} = \dfrac{100\text{ mg}}{x\text{ mL}}$</td></tr>
<tr><td align="center">$25x = 500$</td><td align="center">$25x = 500$</td></tr>
<tr><td align="center">$x = 20\text{ mL}$</td><td align="center">$x = 20\text{ mL}$</td></tr>
</table>

Option 2: Dimensional Analysis

$$\text{mL} = \frac{5\text{ mL}}{25\text{ mg}} \times \frac{1{,}000\text{ mg}}{1\text{ g}} \times \frac{0.1\text{ g}}{}$$

$$\text{mL} = \frac{5\text{ mL}}{25\ \cancel{\text{mg}}} \times \frac{1{,}000\ \cancel{\text{mg}}}{1\ \cancel{\text{g}}} \times \frac{0.1\ \cancel{\text{g}}}{}$$

$$\text{mL} = \frac{500}{25} = 20\text{ mL}$$

Option 3: Formula Method

First, convert 0.1 g to mg.

$$\frac{0.1\text{ g} \times 1{,}000\text{ mg}}{1\text{ g}} = 100\text{ mg}$$

Next, substitute 100 mg for the doctor's order, or the desire. Our have and quantity will come from the label and will be 25 mg per 5 mL.

$$\frac{100\ \cancel{\text{mg}} \times 5\text{ mL}}{25\ \cancel{\text{mg}}} = x\text{ mL}$$

$$\frac{100 \times 5}{25} = \frac{500}{25} = 20\text{ mL}$$

When we look at the information we are provided, we realize we cannot determine a logical answer until both the order and the supply are in the same unit of measure.

When the conversion is completed, we can look at our information and realize that the amount we will be giving to our patient will be more than 5 mL and the answer will be more than 5 mL. We can actually determine that the answer should be 20 mL and our calculation is validated.

Problems 11.2

Calculate the number of milliliters, teaspoons, or tablespoons for the following oral solutions/suspensions. Calculate one dose unless otherwise instructed. Answers must be labeled to be correct.

1. A patient has been ordered 8 mg of ondansetron oral solution PO 2 hours prior to radiation therapy. How many milliliters will the nurse administer? Refer to Figure 11-23.

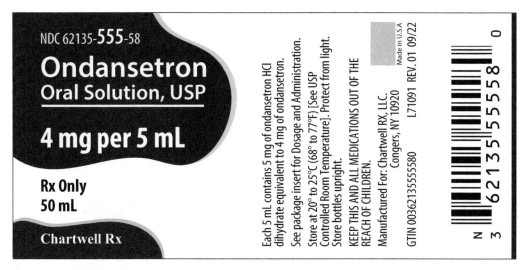

▲ **Figure 11-23**

2. A client is ordered 400 mg of cephalexin oral suspension every 6 hours for a soft tissue infection. How many milliliters will the client receive in each dose? Refer to Figure 11-24.

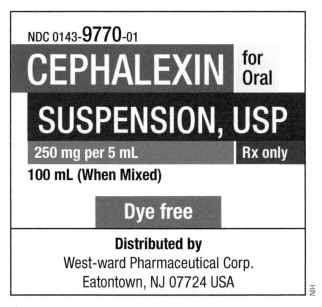

▲ **Figure 11-24**

3. The physician has ordered a patient 350 mg of penicillin V oral suspension PO four times daily. The available supply is penicillin 125 mg per 5 mL. How many mL will the nurse administer?

4. Cefixime 180 mg oral suspension is ordered once daily for a patient with an infection. How many mL will the patient receive? Refer to Figure 11-25.

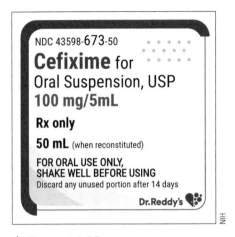

▲ **Figure 11-25**

5. Diphenhydramine 50 mg oral solution has been ordered for a client 20–30 min before bedtime once daily. Calculate the mL dose. Refer to Figure 11-26.

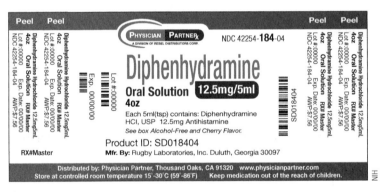

▲ **Figure 11-26**

6. In question 5, if the nurse has equipment that measures teaspoons only, how many tsp of diphenhydramine will be administered?

7. A patient with a urinary tract infection has been ordered nitrofurantoin oral suspension 70 mg every 8 hours. The patient will receive how many mL? Refer to Figure 11-27.

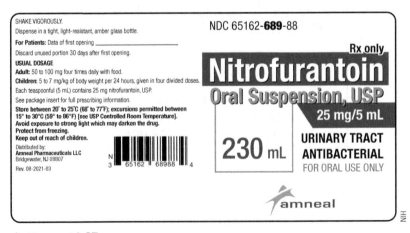

▲ **Figure 11-27**

8. The physician has ordered linezolid 600 mg PO every 12 hr to a client with pneumonia. How many tablespoons will the nurse administer? Refer to Figure 11-28.

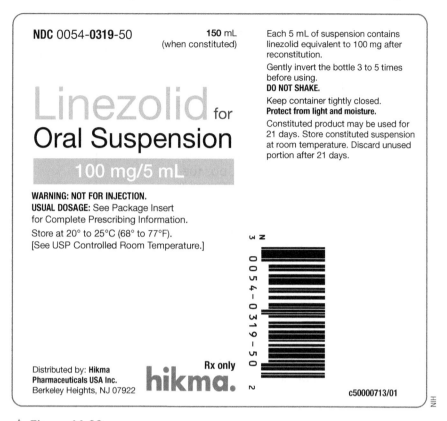

NDC 0054-**0319**-50

150 mL
(when constituted)

Each 5 mL of suspension contains linezolid equivalent to 100 mg after reconstitution.

Gently invert the bottle 3 to 5 times before using.
DO NOT SHAKE.

Keep container tightly closed.
Protect from light and moisture.

Constituted product may be used for 21 days. Store constituted suspension at room temperature. Discard unused portion after 21 days.

Linezolid for
Oral Suspension

100 mg/5 mL

WARNING: NOT FOR INJECTION.
USUAL DOSAGE: See Package Insert for Complete Prescribing Information.
Store at 20° to 25°C (68° to 77°F).
[See USP Controlled Room Temperature.]

Distributed by: **Hikma**
Pharmaceuticals USA Inc.
Berkeley Heights, NJ 07922

hikma.

Rx only

c50000713/01

▲ **Figure 11-28**

9. A client with a low potassium level has been ordered potassium chloride 20 mEq PO once daily. How many mL will the nurse prepare from the medication container? Calculate to the tenth. Refer to Figure 11-29.

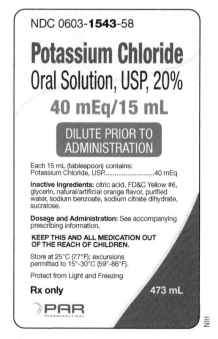

NDC 0603-**1543**-58

Potassium Chloride
Oral Solution, USP, 20%

40 mEq/15 mL

DILUTE PRIOR TO
ADMINISTRATION

Each 15 mL (tablespoon) contains:
Potassium Chloride, USP...........................40 mEq

Inactive Ingredients: citric acid, FD&C Yellow #6, glycerin, natural/artificial orange flavor, purified water, sodium benzoate, sodium citrate dihydrate, sucralose.

Dosage and Administration: See accompanying prescribing information.

KEEP THIS AND ALL MEDICATION OUT OF THE REACH OF CHILDREN.

Store at 25°C (77°F); excursions permitted to 15°-30°C (59°-86°F).

Protect from Light and Freezing

Rx only   473 mL

PAR
PHARMACEUTICAL

▲ **Figure 11-29**

10. A patient has been ordered the anti-inflammatory medication dexamethasone 1.5 mg PO daily for a skin rash. How many mL will the nurse administer? Refer to Figure 11-30.

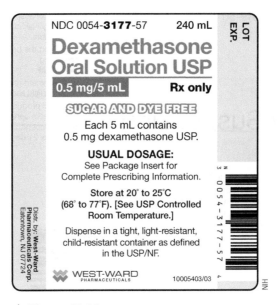

▲ Figure 11-30

11. A young client is ordered 7.5 mg of morphine oral solution every 6 hours for pain. How many mL will be administered? Round to the nearest tenth. Refer to Figure 11-31.

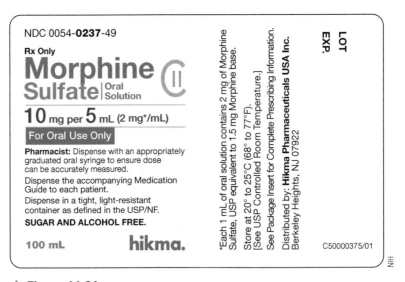

▲ Figure 11-31

12. Spironolactone oral suspension 75 mg has been ordered PO once daily to treat lower extremity edema (swelling/water retention). The available supply is 25 mg in 5 mL. How many mL will the nurse administer?

13. A client is ordered 600 mg amoxicillin every 12 hours PO for an infection. How many mL will the nurse administer? Round to the nearest tenth. Refer to Figure 11-32.

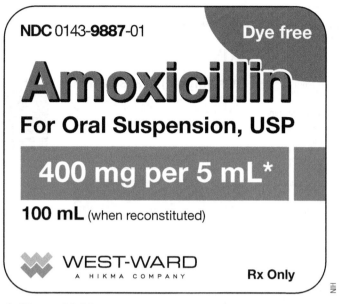

▲ **Figure 11-32**

14. A client is ordered metformin oral solution 850 mg once daily for the management of diabetes. How many mL will the nurse administer? Round to the nearest tenth. Refer to Figure 11-33.

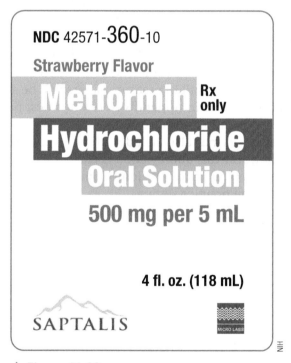

▲ **Figure 11-33**

15. Nimodipine oral solution 30 mg has been ordered PO every 4 hours for a client with liver impairment. How many total mL will the client receive each day? Refer to Figure 11-34.

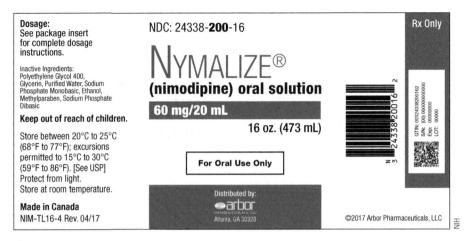

Dosage:
See package insert for complete dosage instructions.

Inactive Ingredients:
Polyethylene Glycol 400, Glycerin, Purified Water, Sodium Phosphate Monobasic, Ethanol, Methylparaben, Sodium Phosphate Dibasic

Keep out of reach of children.

Store between 20°C to 25°C (68°F to 77°F); excursions permitted to 15°C to 30°C (59°F to 86°F). [See USP] Protect from light. Store at room temperature.

Made in Canada
NIM-TL16-4 Rev. 04/17

NDC: 24338-**200**-16

Rx Only

NYMALIZE®
(nimodipine) oral solution

60 mg/20 mL

16 oz. (473 mL)

For Oral Use Only

Distributed by:
arbor
PHARMACEUTICALS, LLC
Atlanta, GA 30328

©2017 Arbor Pharmaceuticals, LLC

▲ **Figure 11-34**

Answers 1. 10 mL **2.** 8 mL **3.** 14 mL **4.** 9 mL **5.** 20 mL **6.** 20 mL = 4 tsp **7.** 14 mL **8.** 30 mL = 2 tbsp **9.** 7.5 mL **10.** 15 mL **11.** 3.75 = 3.8 mL **12.** 15 mL **13.** 7.5 mL **14.** 8.5 mL **15.** 10 mL given q 4 hrs = 60 mL daily total

Measurement Devices for Oral Solutions

Oral solutions are most commonly measured using a disposable calibrated medication cup. Examine the schematic drawing of the medication cup calibrations in Figure 11-35. Many disposable medication cups, like this one, still contain the tsp (teaspoon), tbs (tablespoon), and oz (ounce) calibrations of the household system.

While the apothecary system is obsolete, there may still be calibrated medication cups that include the dram as a unit of measure. There will be some brief information related to the apothecary system in Appendix A, but it is best not to utilize the apothecary system for calculation or for measurement.

Some measuring devices may also include cc (cubic centimeter), which is identical in measure to a mL, however this abbreviation is easily misinterpreted and should be avoided. The abbreviation, cc, is not on the Joint Commission's Do Not Use list and may still be found in use in some practice settings.

Oral solutions are most safely poured at eye level. Because of the number of units of measure on these cups, always read calibrations very carefully, and be clear on the amount being measured.

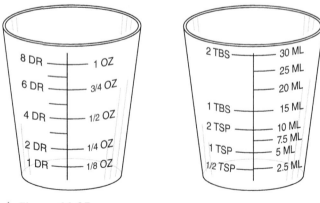

▲ **Figure 11-35**

Small-volume solution dosages can also be measured using specially calibrated oral syringes such as those illustrated in Figures 11-36 and 11-37. Oral syringes have safety features built into their design to prevent their being mistaken for parenteral or hypodermic syringes. A feature of the oral syringe that distinguishes it from a parenteral syringe is the syringe tip. The syringe tip on an oral syringe is usually a different size and shape and is often off center.

Figure 11-36 illustrates an oral syringe with a tip that is off center. The tips of the syringe are also non-luer lock tips, meaning a needle cannot be attached securely on the tip; instead, it is a slip tip, so there is no ability to securely attach a needle. Figure 11-37 shows medication prepared in an oral syringe.

With the availability of oral syringes and other equipment for oral medication administration, parenteral or hypodermic syringes should *not* be used to measure and administer oral dosages. It would be too easy to inadvertently administer the medication by an incorrect route and have a medication error and possibly cause injury to the patient.

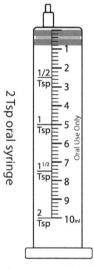

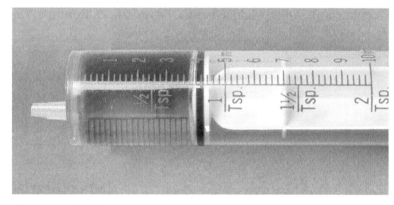

▲ **Figure 11-36**   ▲ **Figure 11-37**

Another consideration with correct syringe identification is that oral syringes are not sterile, and must not be confused and used for parenteral medications, which are sterile. This mistake has been made although hypodermic needles do not fit correctly on oral syringes. The precaution, therefore, does need to be stressed.

Oral solutions may also be ordered as drops (gtt), and when this is the case, the dropper is attached to the bottle stopper. Medicine droppers are often calibrated in mL or by actual dosage, such as 125 mg, and so forth. Chapter 17 will discuss droppers and other medication equipment that may be used with pediatric dosages.

Problems 11.3

Identify the following calculated amounts on the measuring device provided for each question.

1. A patient is ordered penicillin V oral solution 200 mg PO. The supply available is 250 mg in 5 mL. How many mL will be administered? Draw a line to the calculated mL on the device below, Figure 11-38.

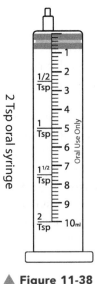

▲ **Figure 11-38**

2. The physician has ordered Vancomycin oral solution 375 mg PO. The supply available is 250 mg in 5 mL. How many mL will be administered? Draw a line to the calculated mL on the device below, Figure 11-39. Round to the nearest tenth.

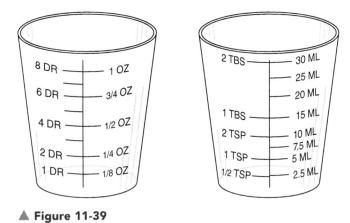

▲ **Figure 11-39**

3. A client is ordered fluconazole oral suspension 20 mg PO. The supply available is 10 mg in 5 mL. Calculate the number of teaspoons and draw a line on the device below, Figure 11-40.

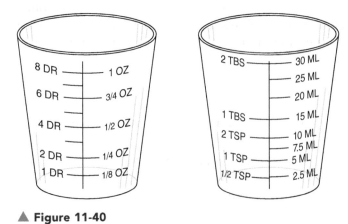

▲ **Figure 11-40**

4. The physician has ordered a patient 0.45 g of penicillin V oral suspension PO. The supply available is 125 mg per 5 mL. Draw a line to the calculated mL on the device below, Figure 11-41.

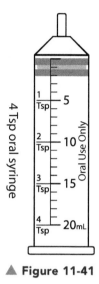

▲ **Figure 11-41**

5. The physician has ordered a client morphine sulfate oral solution 8 mg PO. The supply available is 20 mg in 5 mL. Draw a line to the calculated mL on the device below, Figure 11-42.

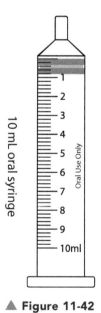

▲ **Figure 11-42**

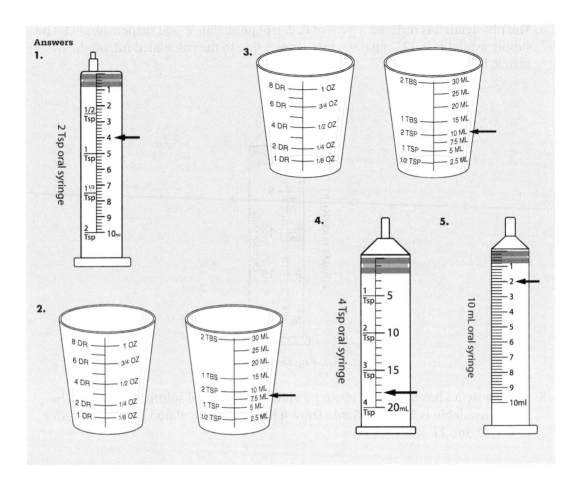

Summary

This concludes the chapter on calculating oral dosages. The important points to remember from this chapter are:

- Most dosages of tablets or capsules consist of $\frac{1}{2}$ to 3 tablets (1–3 capsules, which cannot be broken in half). An unusual number of tablets or capsules may indicate an error.

- Any of the three methods of calculation can be used to calculate dosages. It is recommended that you develop a level of confidence with one of the methods and use it consistently.

- When appropriate, you should always multiply numerators first and then divide that product by the product of the denominators. Using this method will prevent the need to round in the middle of the calculation. Rounding should occur at the end of the calculation.

- The equipment used to measure oral dosages may necessitate rounding of your answer. For purposes of consistency, please use the following guidance: If your end result is greater than 1 mL, round to the tenth. If your end result is less than 1 mL, round to the hundredth.

For accurate measurement, solutions are poured at eye level when a medicine cup is used.

Liquid oral medications may be measured and administered using an oral medication syringe. It is *not* recommended to use a hypodermic syringe without a needle.

Care must be taken not to use oral syringes for hypodermic medication preparation because these are not sterile.

Summary Self-Test

Part I

Locate the appropriate label for each of the following drug orders, and calculate the number of tablets or capsules to be administered. Assume all tablets are scored and can be broken in half. Answers must be labeled to be correct.

1. Glucotrol XL® 7.5 mg _____

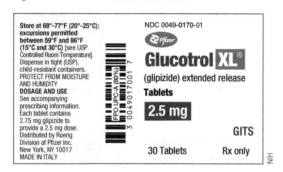

2. dexamethasone 6 mg _____

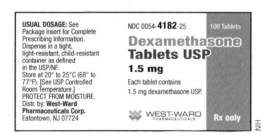

3. triazolam 250 mcg _____

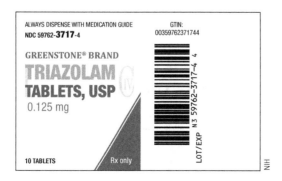

4. alprazolam 500 mcg   _____

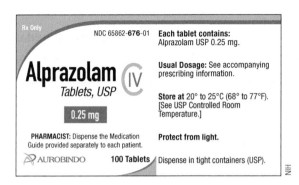

5. gabapentin 0.1 g   _____

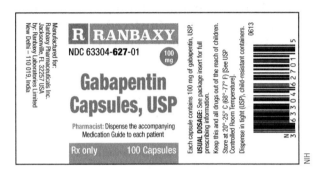

6. clarithromycin 0.5 g   _____

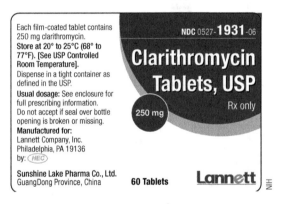

7. codeine 45 mg   _____

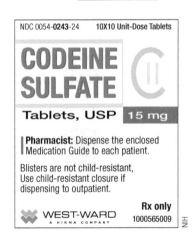

8. levothyroxine 0.225 mg   _____

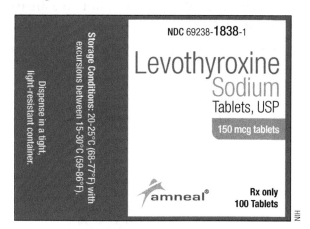

9. nitroglycerin 600 mcg   _____

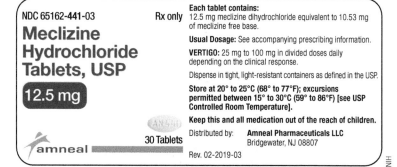

10. meclizine 25 mg   _____

Part II

Calculate answers and locate the calculated amount on a measuring device. Answers must be labeled to be correct.

11. methylphenidate oral solution 12 mg. Calculate the answer in mL. Refer to Figure 11-43.

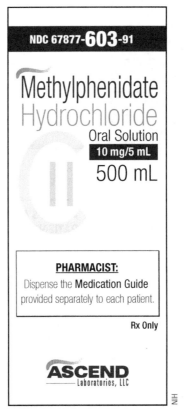

NDC 67877-**603**-91

Methylphenidate
Hydrochloride
Oral Solution
10 mg/5 mL
500 mL

PHARMACIST:
Dispense the **Medication Guide** provided separately to each patient.

Rx Only

ASCEND
Laboratories, LLC

▲ **Figure 11-43**

12. Draw a line on the measuring device below, Figure 11-44, to the calculated mL in the previous question.

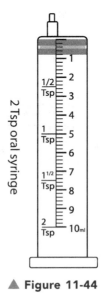

2 Tsp oral syringe

1/2 Tsp
1 Tsp
1 1/2 Tsp
2 Tsp

1
2
3
4
5
6
7
8
9
10 ml

▲ **Figure 11-44**

13. Nystatin oral suspension 300,000 units. Calculate the answer in mL. Refer to Figure 11-45.

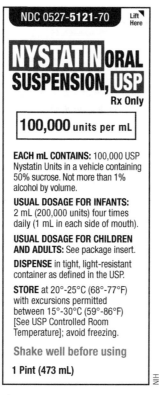

▲ **Figure 11-45**

14. Draw a line on the measuring device below, Figure 11-46, to the calculated mL in the previous question.

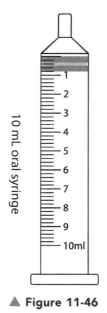

▲ **Figure 11-46**

15. Vibramycin® oral suspension 75 mg. Calculate the answer in tablespoon(s). Refer to Figure 11-47.

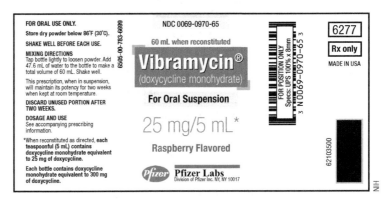

▲ **Figure 11-47**

16. Draw a line on the measuring device below, Figure 11-48, to the calculated tablespoon(s) in the previous question.

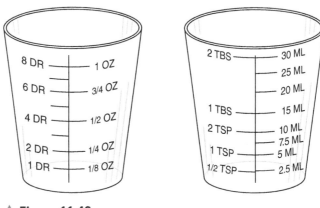

▲ **Figure 11-48**

17. Diphenhydramine oral solution 30 mg. Calculate the answer in mL. Refer to Figure 11-49.

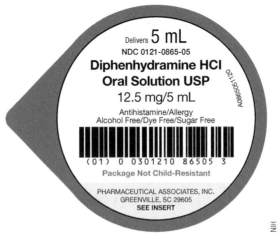

▲ **Figure 11-49**

18. Draw a line on the measuring device below, Figure 11-50, to the calculated mL in the previous question.

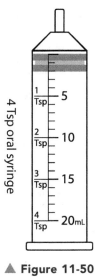

▲ **Figure 11-50**

19. Glycopyrrolate oral solution 600 mcg. Calculate the answer in mL. Refer to Figure 11-51.

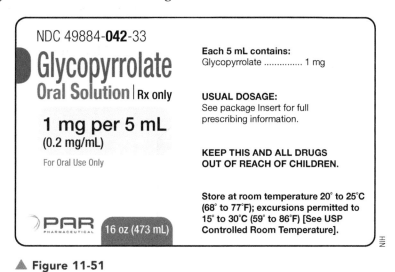

▲ **Figure 11-51**

20. Draw a line on the measuring device below, Figure 11-52, to the calculated mL in the previous question.

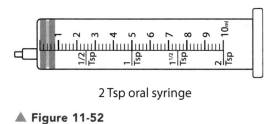

2 Tsp oral syringe

▲ **Figure 11-52**

21. Cimetidine oral solution 525 mg. Calculate the answer in mL, and round to the nearest tenth. Refer to Figure 11-53.

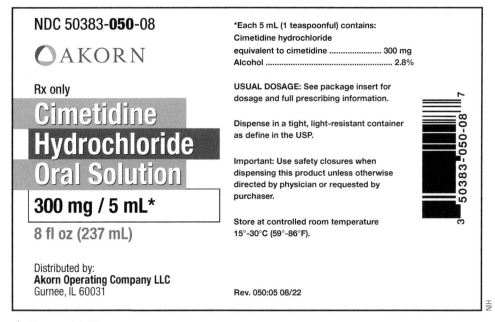

▲ **Figure 11-53**

22. Draw a line on the measuring device below, Figure 11-54, to the calculated mL in the previous question.

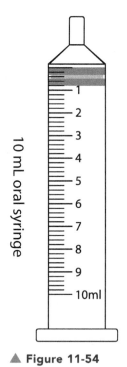

▲ **Figure 11-54**

23. Lactulose solution 20 g. Calculate the answer in mL. Refer to Figure 11-55.

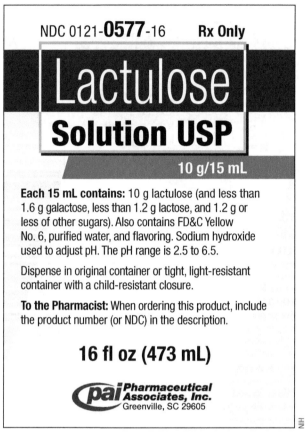

▲ Figure 11-55

24. Draw a line on the measuring device below, Figure 11-56, to the calculated mL in the previous question.

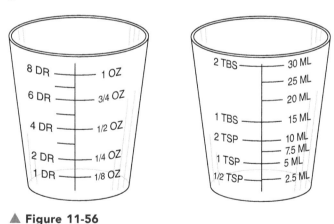

▲ Figure 11-56

25. Propranolol hydrochloride oral solution 20 mg. Calculate the answer in teaspoon(s). Refer to Figure 11-57.

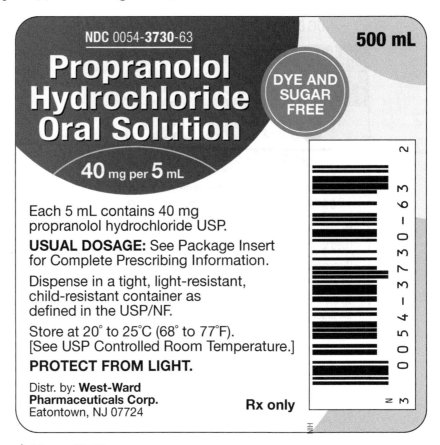

▲ **Figure 11-57**

26. Draw a line on the measuring device below, Figure 11-58, to the calculated teaspoon(s) in the previous question.

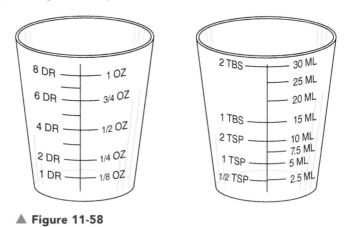

▲ **Figure 11-58**

27. Children's Tylenol® oral suspension 180 mg. Calculate in mL and round to the nearest tenth. Refer to Figure 11-59.

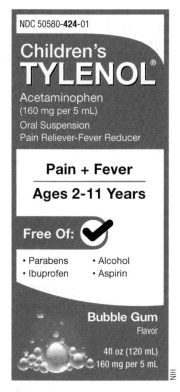

▲ **Figure 11-59**

28. Draw a line on the measuring device below, Figure 11-60, to the calculated mL in the previous question.

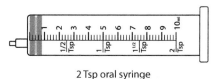

2 Tsp oral syringe

▲ **Figure 11-60**

29. Gabapentin oral solution 500 mg. Calculate the answer in mL. Refer to Figure 11-61.

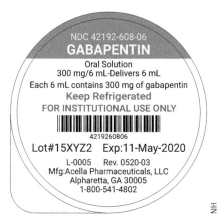

▲ **Figure 11-61**

30. Draw a line on the measuring device below, Figure 11-62, to the calculated mL in the previous question.

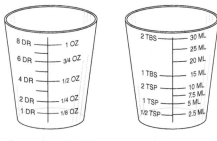

▲ **Figure 11-62**

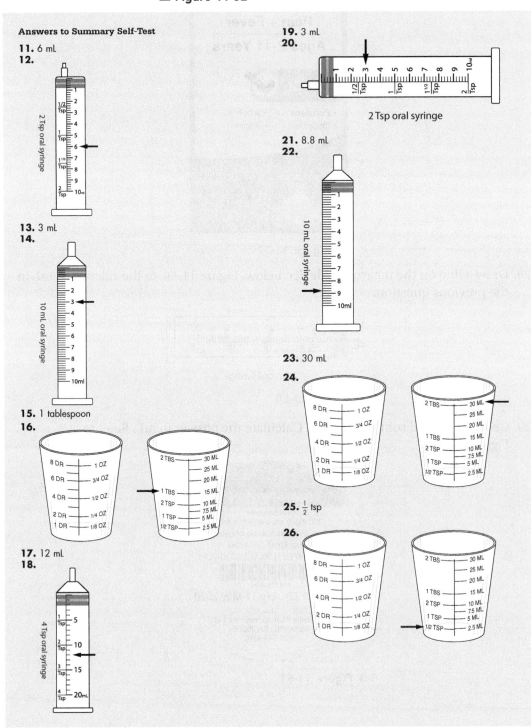

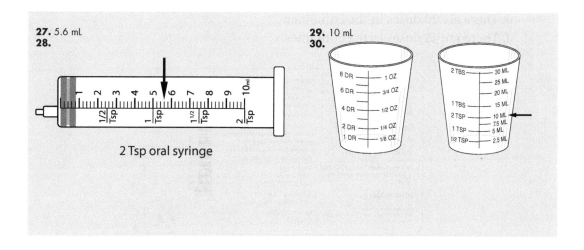

27. 5.6 mL
28.

2 Tsp oral syringe

29. 10 mL
30.

Critical Thinking Questions

1. A client is to receive 5 mL of Carafate QID PO for stomatitis. How many mg is the nurse administering daily? Refer to Figure 11-63.

   a. 2,000
   b. 1,000
   c. 1,500
   d. 500

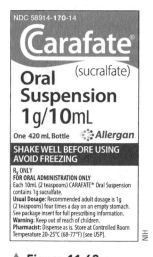

▲ **Figure 11-63**

2. A client is ordered to receive digoxin 0.75 mg oral solution once daily to treat arrhythmias. The nurse reviews the label, Figure 11-64, against the order and is preparing the medication. Of the following choices, which are relevant to this label? Select all that apply.

   a. Administer 3 mL.
   b. Administer 15 mL.
   c. Administer 1.5 mL.
   d. There are 4 doses in the container.

  e. There are 20 doses in the container.

  f. There are 45 doses in the container.

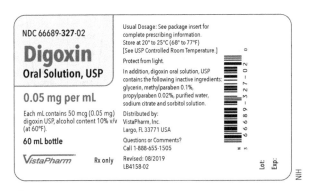

▲ **Figure 11-64**

3. A nurse is preparing propranolol 160 mg oral solution for a client with hypertension. There are two containers of the solutions; refer to Figures 11-65a and 11-65b. The nurse prepares an amount of 20 mL of the medication and pours it in a calibrated medication cup for administration. Based on this information, which of the following would apply? Select all that apply.

  a. The nurse chose the 40 mg to 5 mL drug label option.

  b. The calibrated medication cup does not measure the medication amount.

  c. The nurse chose the correct measuring device.

  d. The nurse chose the 20 mg to 5 mL drug label option.

  e. The nurse prepared the wrong amount for both dosage strengths.

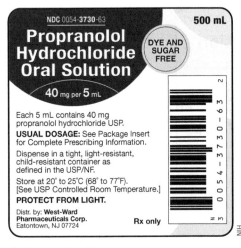

▲ **Figure 11-65a**

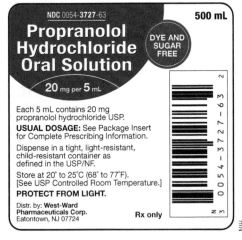

▲ **Figure 11-65b**

4. The physician orders the anticonvulsant drug phenobarbital 60 mg oral solution BID. Refer to Figure 11-66. The nurse is educating the client prior to discharge. How many tsp will the nurse instruct the client to take at home?

  a. 5 tsp

  b. 4 tsp

  c. 6 tsp

  d. 3 tsp

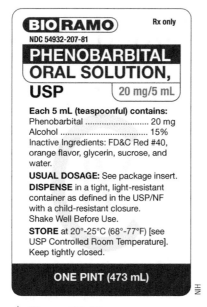

▲ **Figure 11-66**

5. A client is ordered Vancomycin 600 mg oral solution TID for a staph infection. Refer to Figure 11-67. How many milliliters will the nurse prepare?

   a. 2.4
   b. 2
   c. 12
   d. 8

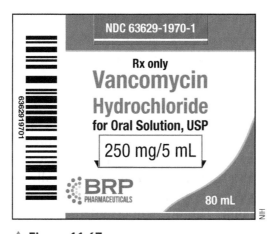

▲ **Figure 11-67**

Answers to Critical Thinking Questions

1. A. 2,000 mg

2. B, D. (A and C are the wrong calculations, B is the correct calculation, E and F are the wrong number of doses in the container, D is the correct number of doses in the container.)

3. A, C. (A is correct because the dosage calculation with this label is 20 mL, B is incorrect because the calibrated oral medication cup does measure 20 mL, C is correct because the correct measuring device was used, D is incorrect because it is the wrong label choice to calculate 20 mL, E is incorrect because the nurse did calculate the medication correctly.)

4. D. 60 mg dose = 15 mL = 3 tsp

5. C. 12 mL

Parenteral Dosages and Syringe Measurements

Objectives

The learner will:

1. utilize the correct conversion factor to convert when needed.

2. calculate parenteral dosages using one of the three calculation methods presented in this book.

3. evaluate the calculated amount to determine if it is logical.

4. measure parenteral dosages using a standard 3 mL syringe.

5. measure parenteral dosages using a tuberculin syringe.

6. measure parenteral solutions using 5, 10, and 20 mL syringes.

Parenteral medications are administered by injection, with intravenous (IV), intramuscular (IM), and subcutaneous being the most frequently used routes. The labels of oral and parenteral solutions are similar, but the size of the average parenteral dosage label is much smaller. Intramuscular solutions are manufactured so that the average adult dosage will be contained in a volume of between 0.5 mL and 3 mL. The safe volume to administer will vary based on the muscle being injected. For example, a volume on the smaller side of that range would be appropriate for a deltoid muscle, which is very small. Some facility protocols may allow up to 4 mL to be injected in a single large muscle, such as the ventrogluteal or vastus lateralis. Subcutaneous injections have a smaller range of volume. They seldom exceed 1 mL. Excessively larger or smaller volumes for IM or subcutaneous injections would need to be questioned and calculations rechecked.

Keypoint: Volumes larger than 3 mL are difficult for a single IM injection site to absorb, and the 0.5 to 3 mL volume can be used as a guideline for accuracy of calculations in IM dosages. Subcutaneous dosages usually have a maximum volume of 1 mL in one site. Calculations that fall outside these ranges should be questioned and rechecked.

Intravenous medication administration is usually a two-step procedure. First, the dosage is prepared, then the dosage may be further diluted in IV fluids before administration. In this chapter, we will focus on the first step of IV drug preparation, which is accurate calculation and measurement of the prescribed dosage. Volume guidelines will be different for intravenous medications, as the injection is being given into the circulating blood, so the ranges of volume are much broader.

To administer parenteral medications, syringes are needed. This chapter will review the equipment necessary for intramuscular, subcutaneous, and intradermal administration. This equipment would also be used to perform the first step of IV drug administration. A variety of hypodermic syringes are in clinical use. It is necessary to learn the similarities and differences of all syringes in use. Regardless of a syringe's volume or capacity, all syringes are calibrated in mL, except specialized insulin syringes. Most syringes will display the measurements and label them as milliliters; however, you may encounter the term cubic centimeter (cc) used when referring to volume. The abbreviation, cc, can be easily misread so it's use is discouraged. Measures in mL and cc are essentially identical. They will be correctly referred to throughout this text as mL. Recognizing the difference in syringe calibrations is one of the key concepts in this chapter.

 Keypoint: The calibrations on different volume syringes differ from each other, requiring particular care in dosage measurement.

When preparing and giving parenteral medications, it will be your responsibility to choose the most appropriate syringe. This chapter will help us integrate the ability to read and interpret parenteral labels to ensure dosages are calculated accurately. With these calculations, we will also need to determine the most appropriate syringe to use to prepare and administer the dosage required.

Clinical Relevance: Parenteral medications are medications that are given intravenously, intramuscularly, subcutaneously, or intradermally. It is important to identify the equipment that would be appropriate for giving parenteral medications. The equipment used for giving parenteral medications must be labeled for parenteral use and sterility must be maintained.

It is also important to maintain safety of the patient and the health care provider when administering parenteral injections, as well as be familiar with the protocol in your practice setting. You must use critical thinking and clinical judgment when calculating parenteral dosages. Knowledge of appropriate volumes to administer via the various routes will be very important as you logically assess each amount that you calculate. For example, if you calculate an intramuscular dosage of 20 mL, you should recognize that something is wrong—either the numbers were not placed appropriately in the dosage equation or perhaps a decimal was misplaced. The important thing to realize is that 20 mL is not an appropriate amount to administer intramuscularly. This realization will stop you from giving an incorrect dose.

With parenteral dosages, it is also critical to be familiar with your equipment and the calibrations on the equipment to administer parenteral dosages safely and accurately. Calibrations on the syringe will help you determine if a dosage amount needs to be rounded. Again, we will use the consistent approach to round to the tenth if our calculation is greater than 1 mL and to round to the hundredth if our calculation is less than 1 mL.

It is important to carefully check the medication order for the route of administration and administer the medication by the ordered route. Parenteral routes are not interchangeable, and the medication orders must be followed accurately.

Parenteral Drug Preparations and Calculations

Parenteral medications are packaged in a variety of single-use glass ampules, single- and multiple-use rubber-stoppered vials, and premeasured syringes and cartridges. Refer to Figure 12-1 for examples of vials and ampules.

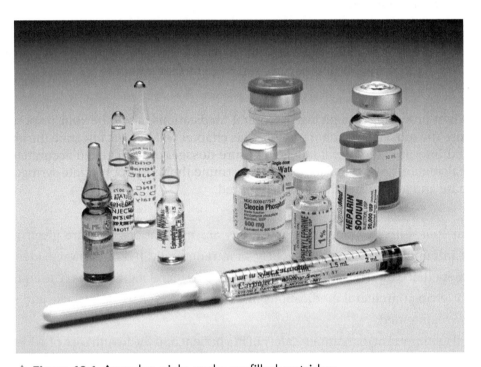

▲ **Figure 12-1** Ampules, vials, and a prefilled cartridge

Notice that the labels on the vials and ampules are smaller than some of the labels on oral medications. The same information must be present on the label, so the print is very small in some cases. Be aware of this and read your labels very carefully.

Ampules will always be for single use. To access the medication in an ampule, the top will need to be snapped off. Once it is open, it cannot be closed again, so any medication that is not used for the medication order must be discarded. Vials may be single use or multiple use. There is a rubber stopper on the vial that can preserve the sterility of the solution as long as strict sterile technique is used when preparing dosages. In addition, if the manufacturer intends for it to be a multiple-use vial, an antimicrobial or preservative agent will be added to the solution to maintain sterility of the medication. Prefilled cartridges are for single-use only. They would be placed in a cartridge holder for use or would be used as a vial and the medication would be withdrawn.

Reading and interpreting the medication label on an ampule or vial will follow the guidelines that were introduced in Chapter 7. To calculate parenteral dosages, follow the guidelines presented when we introduced the three methods of dosage calculation. Review the label to determine what is available; the order will provide the information for what the client is to receive.

Let's look at some examples of dosage calculation using all three methods presented earlier in this book. Each example will include a parenteral label so you can practice identifying the relevant information for your calculation equations.

Example 1 ■   Phenobarbital 100 mg IM has been ordered as a one-time dose prior to surgery. Refer to Figure 12-2 for your supply. How many milliliters will you administer?

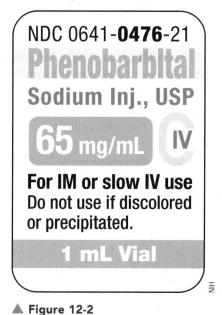

▲ **Figure 12-2**

According to this label, our supply is 65 mg in 1 mL. This vial contains a total of 1 mL, so at this point we can look at our order for 100 mg and compare it to the supply. Doing this, we can logically identify that we will need more than 1 vial since we need more than 65 mg. Let's calculate this now using the three methods of calculation shown in this book.

Method 1: Ratio and Proportion

In Colon Format

65 mg : 1 mL = 100 mg : x mL

$65x = 100$

$x = 1.53$ mL = 1.5 mL

In Fraction Format

$$\frac{65 \text{ mg}}{1 \text{ mL}} = \frac{100 \text{ mg}}{x \text{ mL}}$$

$65x = 100$

$x = \frac{100}{65} = 1.53$ mL = 1.5 mL

This amount is greater than 1 mL so we will round it to the tenth. We will give 1.5 mL to the patient in order to administer 100 mg of phenobarbital.

Method 2: Dimensional Analysis

$$\text{mL} = \frac{1 \text{ mL}}{65 \text{ mg}} \times \frac{100 \text{ mg}}{}$$

$$\text{mL} = \frac{1 \text{ mL}}{65 \text{ mg}} \times \frac{100 \text{ mg}}{}$$

$$\text{mL} = \frac{100}{65} = 1.53 \text{ mL} = 1.5 \text{ mL}$$

Method 3: Formula Method

$$\frac{100 \text{ mg (D)} \times 1 \text{ mL (Q)}}{65 \text{ mg (H)}} = x \text{ mL}$$

$$\frac{100 \cancel{\text{ mg}} \times 1 \text{ mL}}{65 \cancel{\text{ mg}}} = x \text{ mL}$$

$$\frac{100 \times 1}{65} = 1.53 \text{ mL} = 1.5 \text{ mL}$$

This answer, 1.5 mL, is logical based on the information we have. We round this answer to the tenth because it is greater than 1 mL. Therefore, we must calculate to the hundredth in order to round to the tenth. When initially reviewing information at the beginning of the example, we realized we would need more than 1 mL of this medication and the calculations have supported this. We also recognize that this volume (1.5 mL) is an acceptable amount to administer intramuscularly.

Example 2 ■   The physician has given an order for filgrastim 0.25 mg subcutaneous daily. Refer to Figure 12-3 for your available supply, and convert so that the order and supply are in the same unit of measurement.

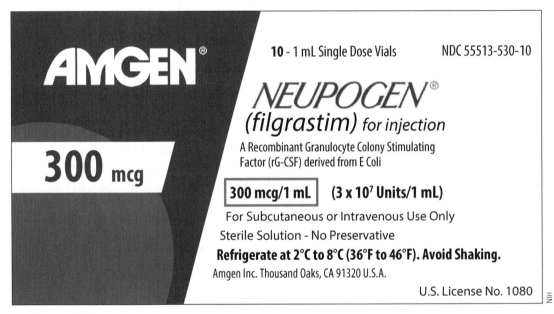

▲ **Figure 12-3**

First, convert mg to mcg, and then calculate the volume of solution to be administered.

Method 1: Ratio and Proportion

In Colon Format

1 mg : 1,000 mcg = 0.25 mg : x mcg

x = 250 mcg

In Fraction Format

$$\frac{1 \text{ mg}}{1,000 \text{ mcg}} = \frac{0.25 \text{ mg}}{x \text{ mcg}}$$

x = 250 mcg

0.25 mg has been converted to 250 mcg and can be replaced in the dosage equations so that the calculation can be completed.

$$300 \text{ mcg} : 1 \text{ mL} = 250 \text{ mcg} : x \text{ mL} \qquad \frac{300 \text{ mcg}}{1 \text{ mL}} = \frac{250 \text{ mcg}}{x \text{ mL}}$$

$$300x = 250 \qquad\qquad 300x = 250$$

$$x = \frac{250}{300} = 0.833 = 0.83 \text{ mL} \qquad x = \frac{250}{300} = 0.833 = 0.83 \text{ mL}$$

Since the calculated amount is less than 1 mL, we calculate to the thousandths and round to the hundredth.

Method 2: Dimensional Analysis

$$\text{mL} = \frac{1 \text{ mL}}{300 \text{ mcg}} \times \frac{1,000 \text{ mcg}}{1 \text{ mg}} \times \frac{0.25 \text{ mg}}{}$$

$$\text{mL} = \frac{1 \text{ mL}}{300 \text{ mcg}} \times \frac{1,000 \text{ mcg}}{1 \text{ mg}} \times \frac{0.25 \text{ mg}}{}$$

$$\text{mL} = \frac{250}{300} = 0.833 = 0.83 \text{ mL}$$

Method 3: Formula Method

First, convert 0.25 mg to mcg. Recall from Chapter 4 that we could move the decimal point three places to the right, converting 0.25 mg to 250 mcg. For purposes of reviewing the methods of calculation, the conversion will also be completed with the formula method.

$$\frac{0.25 \text{ mg} \times 1,000 \text{ mcg}}{1 \text{ mg}} = 250 \text{ mcg}$$

We can now substitute 250 mcg for the doctor's order of 0.25 mg, and this will be our desire. Our have (300 mcg) and quantity (1 mL) will come from the label.

$$\frac{250 \text{ mcg} \times 1 \text{ mL}}{300 \text{ mcg}} = x \text{ mL}$$

$$\frac{250 \times 1}{300} = \frac{250}{300} = 0.833 = 0.83 \text{ mL}$$

As stated previously, the calculated volume is less than 1 mL so we will calculate to the thousandth and round to the hundredth. This result makes logical sense. When we review the order of 250 mcg, we recognize that the volume to administer should be less than the 1 mL volume available in the supply of 300 mcg per 1 mL. We also realize that 0.83 mL is an appropriate volume to administer subcutaneously.

Example 3 ▪   Your patient is to receive furosemide 60 mg IV stat. Refer to Figure 12-4 for your available supply and calculate how many milliliters should be administered.

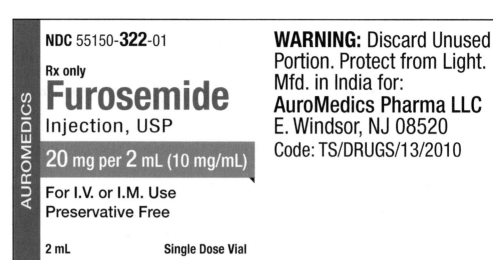

NDC 55150-**322**-01

Rx only

Furosemide

Injection, USP

20 mg per 2 mL (10 mg/mL)

For I.V. or I.M. Use
Preservative Free

2 mL   Single Dose Vial

AUROMEDICS

WARNING: Discard Unused
Portion. Protect from Light.
Mfd. in India for:
AuroMedics Pharma LLC
E. Windsor, NJ 08520
Code: TS/DRUGS/13/2010

▲ **Figure 12-4**

We can either use 20 mg in 2 mL as our available supply or 10 mg in 1 mL. Notice that 10 mg in 1 mL is the same proportion as 20 mg in 2 mL, so the answer will be the same. It is usually easiest to use the information that has reduced the numbers, so we will use 10 mg per mL in our calculations.

Method 1: Ratio and Proportion

In Colon Format

$10 \text{ mg} : 1 \text{ mL} = 60 \text{ mg} : x \text{ mL}$

$10x = 60$

$x = \dfrac{60}{10} = 6 \text{ mL}$

In Fraction Format

$\dfrac{10 \text{ mg}}{1 \text{ mL}} = \dfrac{60 \text{ mg}}{x \text{ mL}}$

$10x = 60$

$x = \dfrac{60}{10} = 6 \text{ mL}$

Method 2: Dimensional Analysis

$$\text{mL} = \dfrac{1 \text{ mL}}{10 \text{ mg}} \times \dfrac{60 \text{ mg}}{}$$

$$\text{mL} = \dfrac{1 \text{ mL}}{10 \text{ mg}} \times \dfrac{60 \text{ mg}}{}$$

$$\text{mL} = \dfrac{60}{10} = 6 \text{ mL}$$

Method 3: Formula Method

$$\dfrac{60 \text{ mg (D)} \times 1 \text{ mL (Q)}}{10 \text{ mg (H)}} = x \text{ mL}$$

$$\dfrac{60 \text{ mg} \times 1 \text{ mL}}{10 \text{ mg}} = x \text{ mL}$$

$$\dfrac{60}{10} = 6 \text{ mL}$$

Our calculations have shown that we need to give 6 mL of the available furosemide to be equivalent to 60 mg. 6 mL may seem like a lot; however, when we look at the route for administration, we realize the volume is appropriate. The intravenous route can accommodate a larger volume than IM or SUBQ.

Parenteral medications can also be measured in alternate measures of international units, units, milliequivalents, and percentages. Ratios may still be present on labels but, recall from Chapter 5, the Food and Drug Administration (FDA) has revised its standards. The FDA now requires that ratios be removed from labels and concentration be expressed as weight per volume. There are really no conversions needed for these alternate measures as the order and supply will be in the same measurement.

Let's look at some examples of these alternate measures as they relate to dosage calculation.

Example 4 ▪   The doctor has ordered 100 units of calcitonin salmon by subcutaneous injection every other day for postmenopausal osteoporosis. Refer to Figure 12-5 for the available supply.

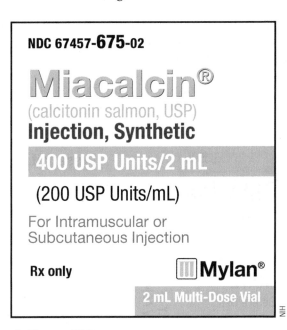

NDC 67457-**675**-02

Miacalcin®
(calcitonin salmon, USP)
Injection, Synthetic

400 USP Units/2 mL

(200 USP Units/mL)

For Intramuscular or
Subcutaneous Injection

Rx only   ‖‖‖**Mylan**®

2 mL Multi-Dose Vial

▲ **Figure 12-5**

Notice the physician's order is in units and the supply is in units. No conversion is necessary as both the order and the supply are in the same unit of measurement.

Method 1: Ratio and Proportion

In Colon Format

200 units : 1 mL = 100 units : x mL

$200x = 100$

$x = \dfrac{100}{200} = 0.5$ mL

In Fraction Format

$$\dfrac{200 \text{ units}}{1 \text{ mL}} = \dfrac{100 \text{ units}}{x \text{ mL}}$$

$200x = 100$

$x = \dfrac{100}{200} = 0.5$ mL

Method 2: Dimensional Analysis

$$mL = \frac{1\ mL}{200\ units} \times \frac{100\ units}{}$$

$$mL = \frac{1\ mL}{200\ \cancel{units}} \times \frac{100\ \cancel{units}}{}$$

$$mL = \frac{100}{200} = 0.5\ mL$$

Method 3: Formula Method

$$\frac{100\ units\ (D) \times 1\ mL\ (Q)}{200\ units\ (H)} = x\ mL$$

$$\frac{100\ \cancel{units} \times 1\ mL}{200\ \cancel{units}} = x\ mL$$

$$\frac{100}{200} = 0.5\ mL$$

We see through our calculations that we would give 0.5 mL of calcitonin salmon sub-cutaneously. This amount is logical and reasonable. We note that the order is half the supply and we realize that 0.5 mL is an appropriate amount to give subcutaneously.

Example 5 ▨   There is an order for potassium chloride 20 mEq to be added to IV fluids for your patient. Refer to Figure 12-6 for your supply.

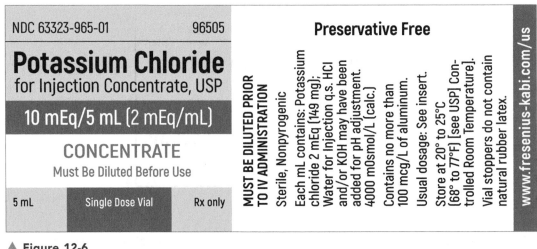

▲ **Figure 12-6**

We need to withdraw a volume of medication that is equivalent to 20 mEq from the vial. Again, notice that the order and the supply are in the same unit of measurement, so no conversions are needed.

Method 1: Ratio and Proportion

In Colon Format	*In Fraction Format*
10 mEq : 5 mL = 20 mEq : x mL	$\dfrac{10\ mEq}{5\ mL} = \dfrac{20\ mEq}{x\ mL}$
$10x = 100$	$10x = 100$
$x = 10$ mL	$x = 10$ mL

Method 2: Dimensional Analysis

$$mL = \frac{5\ mL}{10\ mEq} \times \frac{20\ mEq}{}$$

$$mL = \frac{5\ mL}{10\ \cancel{mEq}} \times \frac{20\ \cancel{mEq}}{}$$

$$mL = \frac{100}{10} = 10\ mL$$

Method 3: Formula Method

$$\frac{20\ mEq\ (D) \times 5\ mL\ (Q)}{10\ mEq\ (H)} = x\ mL$$

$$\frac{20\ \cancel{mEq} \times 5\ mL}{10\ \cancel{mEq}} = x\ mL$$

$$\frac{100}{10} = 10\ mL$$

Through our calculations we determine that we must withdraw 10 mL from the vial of potassium chloride to add to the patient's IV fluids. Potassium chloride will always be diluted and infused, and never given by IV push. If we review our answer, we can see that it is logical based on the information we had—the doctor's order was for 20 mEq and the concentration in the vial was 10 mEq in 5 mL. It is easy to see that the doctor's order is for two times the concentration and thus two times the volume.

We will practice a few more dosage problems in Problems 12.1. Then we will look at the equipment we have available to measure parenteral dosages. There are several different syringes available to us, and we will briefly review some of the most common.

Problems 12.1

Calculate the following orders and answer in mL. Be attentive to the rounding instructions.

1. The physician has ordered atropine 600 mcg IV prior to surgery to decrease secretions. How many mL will be administered? Refer to Figure 12-7 for the available supply and calculate to the tenth place.

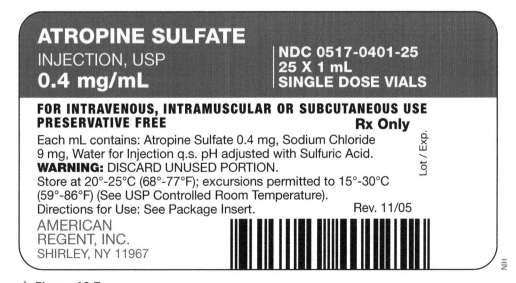

▲ **Figure 12-7**

2. A patient is ordered dexamethasone 15 mg IV prior to chemotherapy. How many mL will be administered? The available supply is 4 mg per 1 mL. Round to the nearest tenth place.

3. Epogen® 1,800 units subcutaneous has been ordered for a patient with anemia. The client will receive how many mL? Refer to Figure 12-8 for the available supply and calculate to the tenth place.

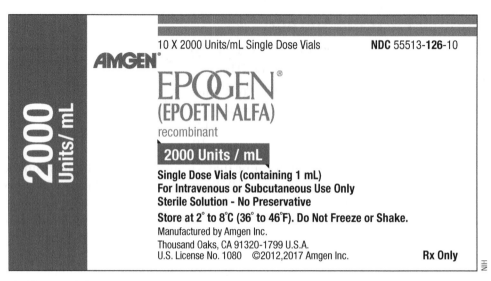

▲ Figure 12-8

4. An order has been written for Ceftriaxone IM 0.75 g for a patient with an infection. How many mL will be administered? The available supply is 350 mg per 1 mL. Calculate to the tenth place.

5. The physician has ordered Ativan® 1.5 mg IV this morning prior to surgery. How many mL will be administered? Refer to Figure 12-9 for available supply and calculate to the hundredths place.

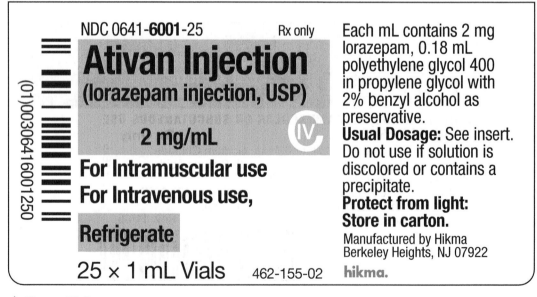

▲ Figure 12-9

6. The physician has ordered levothyroxine 0.075 mg IM for a patient for hypothyroidism. The patient will receive how many mL? The available supply is 200 mcg in 5 mL. Round to the nearest tenth place.

7. A patient has been ordered IV lidocaine 160 mg for arrhythmias. How many mL will be administered? Refer to Figure 12-10 for the available supply.

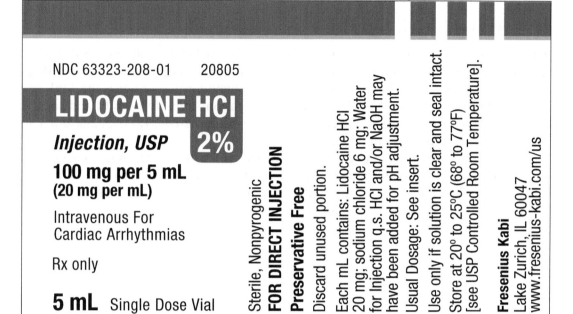

NDC 63323-208-01   20805

LIDOCAINE HCl

Injection, USP   **2%**

100 mg per 5 mL
(20 mg per mL)

Intravenous For
Cardiac Arrhythmias

Rx only

5 mL Single Dose Vial

Sterile, Nonpyrogenic
FOR DIRECT INJECTION
Preservative Free
Discard unused portion.
Each mL contains: Lidocaine HCl 20 mg; sodium chloride 6 mg; Water for Injection q.s. HCl and/or NaOH may have been added for pH adjustment.
Usual Dosage: See insert.
Use only if solution is clear and seal intact.
Store at 20° to 25°C (68° to 77°F) [see USP Controlled Room Temperature].
Fresenius Kabi
Lake Zurich, IL 60047
www.fresenius-kabi.com/us

▲ **Figure 12-10**

8. The physician has ordered cefotaxime 1,500 mg IV for a client with meningitis. How many mL will be administered? The available supply is 2 g in 10 mL. Calculate to the tenth place.

9. Potassium acetate 10 mEq IV has been ordered by the physician to treat a patient with a low potassium level. How many mL will be administered? Refer to Figure 12-11 for available supply.

20 mL Single-dose

POTASSIUM
ACETATE

Injection, USP

K⁺

Rx only

NDC 0409-8183-11

Each mL contains potassium acetate, 196 mg. 4 mOsmol/mL (calc). pH 6.2 (5.5 to 8.0). May contain acetic acid for pH adjustment. Sterile, nonpyrogenic. Usual dose: See insert. Use only if clear and seal is intact and undamaged. Contains no bacteriostat; use promptly, discard unused portion. Contains no more than 200 mcg/L of aluminum.

40 mEq/20 mL (2 mEq/mL)

CAUTION: MUST BE DILUTED.
FOR INTRAVENOUS USE.

Distributed by Hospira, Inc., Lake Forest, IL 60045 USA

RL−7038

▲ **Figure 12-11**

10. A physician has ordered heparin 1,200 units SUBQ daily as an anticoagulant. How many mL will be administered? The available supply is 2,000 units in 1 mL. Calculate to the tenth place.

Standard 3 mL Syringe

The various capacity syringes – 0.5, 1, 3, 5, 10, or 20 mL – will have calibrations that differ from each other. It is important to read a syringe properly and measure your medication dosages accurately. The most commonly used hypodermic syringe is the 3 mL size illustrated in Figure 12-12. Notice the longer calibrations identify zero (0) and each ½ and full mL measure. These longer calibrations are numbered: ½, 1, 1½, 2, 2½, and 3. In most instances, zero (0) is not labeled on syringes.

Next, notice the number of calibrations in each mL, which is 10, indicating that, on this syringe, each mL is calibrated in tenths. When calculating dosages, tenths of a mL are written as decimal fractions – for example, 1.2 mL, 2.5 mL, or 0.4 mL. Also, notice the arrow on this syringe, which identifies a 0.8 mL dosage.

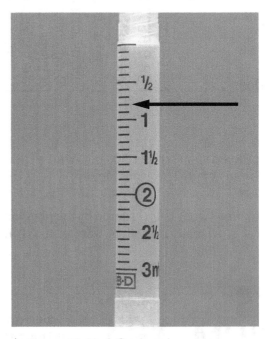

▲ **Figure 12-12** A 3 mL syringe

In addition, most syringes in use today have safety features to prevent needle stick injuries. Several safety syringes have been developed in recent years to reduce the danger of needle sticks. These safety features may include protective needle guards, which are activated after injection by using a single finger to cover the needle with the sheath. Another safety feature may involve pushing on the plunger after the needle has been withdrawn from the patient's skin. When the plunger is pushed, the needle may either retract or a shield may come down over the needle. These are two examples of safety syringes. The practitioner should become aware of the safety features of the syringes that are being used in the clinical setting.

This is important to protect the practitioner from needlestick injury. Protocols are in place to decrease the number of needlestick injuries, but the most important consideration is not to recap a used needle; instead, utilize the safety devices on the syringe and discard immediately in a sharp's container. Examples of safety syringes are shown in Figures 12-13 through 12-15.

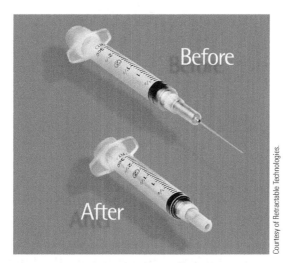

▲ **Figure 12-13** VanishPoint®

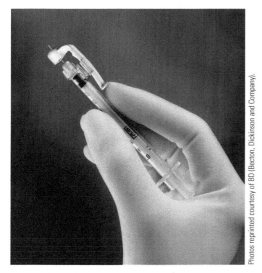

▲ **Figure 12-14** SafetyGlide™ syringe

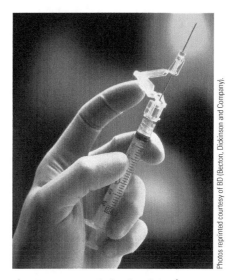

▲ **Figure 12-15** Activating the shield on the Safety syringe.

Remember when looking at 3 mL syringes, the first long calibration on all syringes is zero. It is slightly longer than the 0.1 mL mark and subsequent one-tenth calibrations. Be careful not to mistakenly count it as 0.1 mL. On these syringes, each calibration is 1/10 of a milliliter.

When we look at assembled syringes, the colored suction tip of the plunger has two widened areas in contact with the barrel that look like two distinct rings. Calibrations are read from the top ring or the ring closest to the needle on the syringe and the part of the plunger that is touching the solution. Do not become confused by the second, or bottom, ring or by the raised middle section of the suction tip. Refer to Figure 12-16 for an example of how the solution would be measured in an assembled syringe.

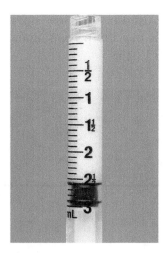

▲ **Figure 12-16**
3 mL syringe measuring 2.6 mL

Problems 12.2

Identify the measurements indicated by arrows on the following standard 3 mL syringes.

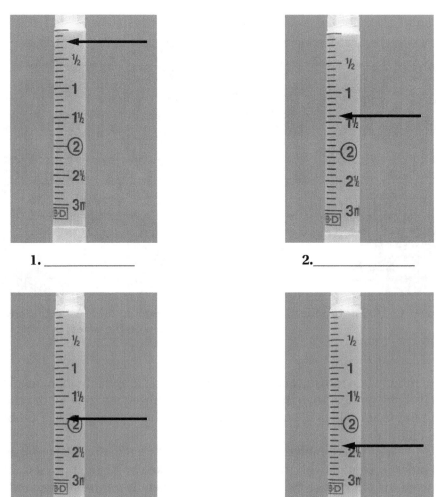

1. _____

2. _____

3. _____

4. _____

Identify the dosage measurements on the following assembled syringes.

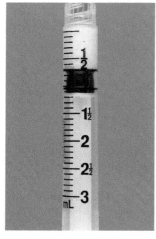

5. _____

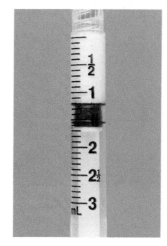

6._____

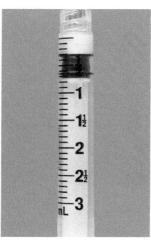

7. _____

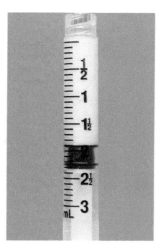

8._____

Draw an arrow on the following syringe barrels to indicate the required dosages.

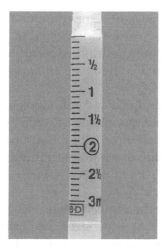

9. 1.3 mL

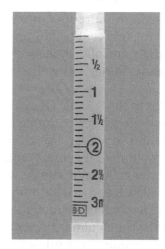

10. 2.4 mL

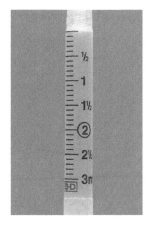

11. 0.9 mL

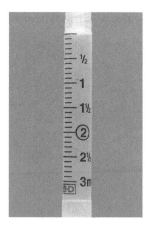

12. 2.1 mL

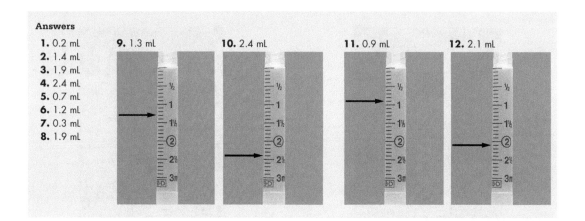

Answers
1. 0.2 mL
2. 1.4 mL
3. 1.9 mL
4. 2.4 mL
5. 0.7 mL
6. 1.2 mL
7. 0.3 mL
8. 1.9 mL
9. 1.3 mL
10. 2.4 mL
11. 0.9 mL
12. 2.1 mL

Tuberculin (TB) Syringe or Small Volume Syringe

When very small dosages are required, they are measured in special tuberculin (TB) 0.5 mL or 1 mL syringes calibrated in hundredths. This is the only syringe that will measure hundredths of a milliliter. Originally designed for the small dosages required for tuberculin skin testing, these syringes are also widely used in a variety of sensitivity and allergy tests. Syringes calibrated in hundredths are commonly used for pediatric dosages, as well as some medications, such as heparin, an anticoagulant drug.

Refer to the 0.5 mL TB syringe in Figure 12-17, and take a careful look at its calibrated hundredth scale. Notice that slightly longer calibrations identify zero, 0.05, 0.1, 0.15, 0.2, and so on, through the 0.5 mL measure. Not all these calibrations are labeled with the volume; therefore, you must be knowledgeable of what the calibrations indicate. Shorter calibrations lie between these to measure the hundredths. Each tenth mL, 0.1, 0.2, 0.3, 0.4, and 0.5, is numbered on this TB syringe.

Take a moment to study the dosage measured by the arrow in Figure 12-18, which is 0.43 mL. Tuberculin syringes are also manufactured in 1 mL sizes. The calibrations remain the same; the 1 mL tuberculin syringe is also calibrated in hundredths and is used to measure very precise doses of medication.

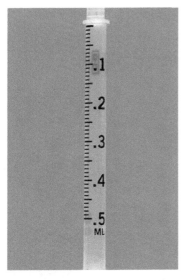

▲ **Figure 12-17** A tuberculin
(TB) syringe

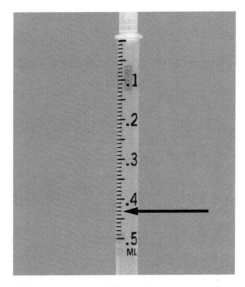

▲ **Figure 12-18** TB syringe measuring
0.43 mL

Since the calibrations are in hundredths, amounts less than 1 mL can be measured very precisely. For example, in Figure 12-19, the dosage identified in this syringe is 0.75 mL. The closeness and small size of TB syringe calibrations mandate particular care and an unhurried approach in TB syringe dosage measurement. In the drawing below, all calibrations before 0.1 mL are obscured by the plunger.

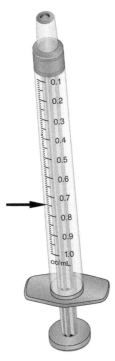

▲ **Figure 12-19** TB syringe measuring
0.75 mL

Problems 12.3

Identify the measurements on the 0.5 mL TB syringes provided.

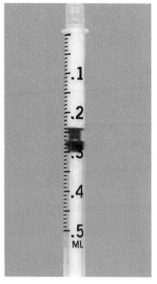

1. _____

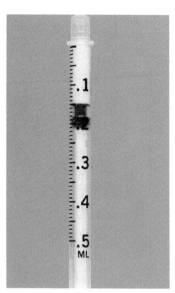

2. _____

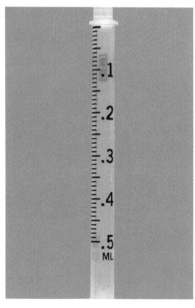

3. _____

Draw an arrow on the syringe barrel to identify the indicated dosages.

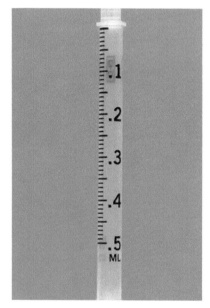

4. 0.06 mL

5. 0.27 mL

Identify the measurements on the 1 mL TB syringes provided.

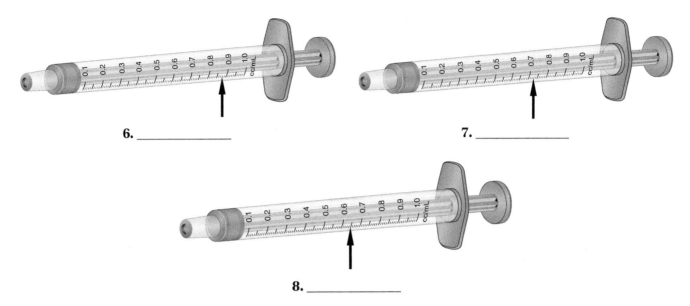

6. _____

7. _____

8. _____

Draw an arrow on the syringe barrel to identify the indicated dosages.

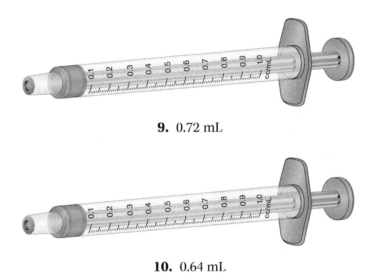

9. 0.72 mL

10. 0.64 mL

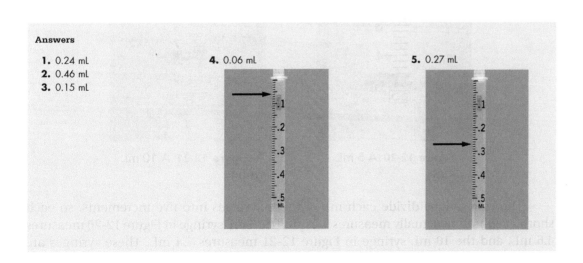

Answers

1. 0.24 mL
2. 0.46 mL
3. 0.15 mL

4. 0.06 mL

5. 0.27 mL

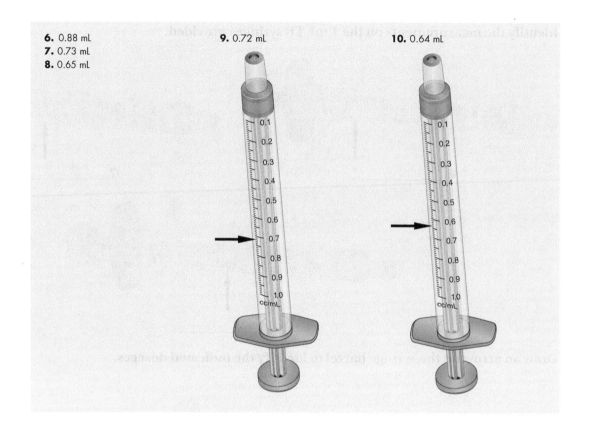

6. 0.88 mL
7. 0.73 mL
8. 0.65 mL

9. 0.72 mL

10. 0.64 mL

Large Volume Syringes (5, 10, and 20 mL Syringes)

When volumes larger than 3 mL are required, a 5 mL, 10 mL, or 20 mL syringe is typically used. Refer to Figures 12-20 and 12-21. Examine the calibrations between the numbered mL to determine how these syringes are calibrated.

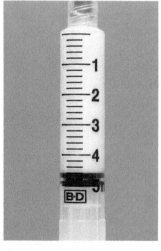

▲ **Figure 12-20** A 5 mL syringe

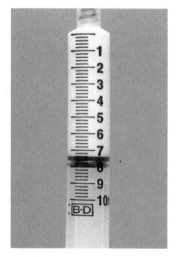

▲ **Figure 12-21** A 10 mL syringe

The calibrations divide each mL of these syringes into five increments, so each shorter calibration actually measures 0.2 mL. The 5 mL syringe in Figure 12-20 measures 4.6 mL, and the 10 mL syringe in Figure 12-21 measures 7.4 mL. These syringes are most often used to measure whole, rather than fractional, dosages. However, we could measure amounts in tenths if they were even numbers. A full range of measurements is included in examples and problems to give you practice with reading the calibrations.

Example ■   Examine the 20 mL syringe in Figure 12-22, and determine how it is calibrated.

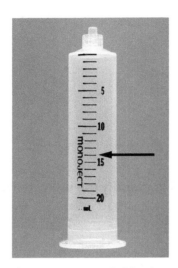

▲ **Figure 12-22** A 20 mL syringe

The syringe in Figure 12-22 shows the arrow measuring **14 mL**.

This syringe is calibrated in 1 mL increments, with longer calibrations identifying the 0, 5, 10, 15, and 20 mL volumes. Syringes with a capacity larger than 20 mL are also calibrated in full mL measures. These syringes are used only for measurement of very large volumes.

Problems 12.4

What dosages are measured on the following syringes?

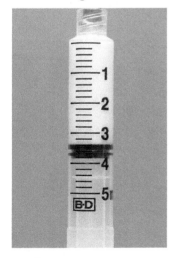 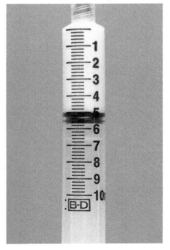 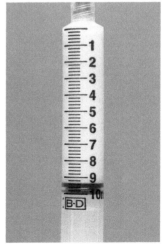

1. _____   2._____   3._____

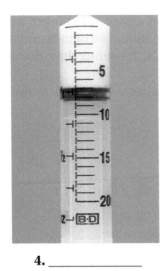

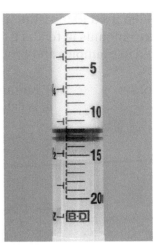

4. _____

5. _____

Draw an arrow on the syringe barrel to identify the indicated dosages.

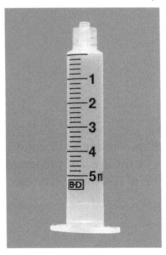

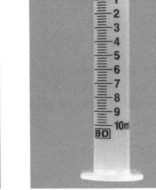

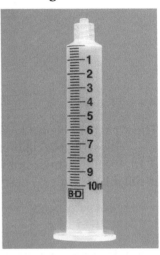

6. 1.4 mL

7. 3.2 mL

8. 6.8 mL

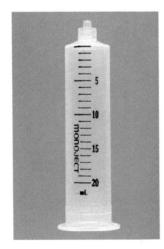

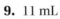

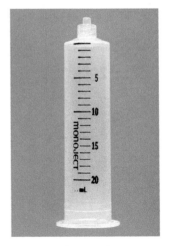

9. 11 mL

10. 9 mL

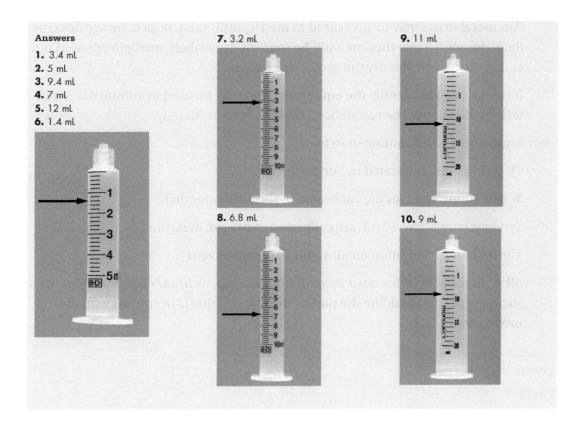

Answers

1. 3.4 mL
2. 5 mL
3. 9.4 mL
4. 7 mL
5. 12 mL
6. 1.4 mL
7. 3.2 mL
8. 6.8 mL
9. 11 mL
10. 9 mL

Summary

This concludes your introduction to parenteral dosage calculations and using medication labels to calculate the volume of medication to be given. Also, included in this chapter is identification of equipment used to measure the volume of parenteral medications. Identification of syringe calibrations is important to measure dosages accurately. The important points to remember from this chapter are:

- The most commonly used parenteral administration routes are IV, IM, and subcutaneous.

- The labels of most parenteral solutions are quite small and must be read with particular care.

- The average IM dosage will be contained in a volume of between 0.5 mL and 3 mL. This can be used as a guideline to accuracy of calculations.

- The average subcutaneous dosage volume is between 0.5 and 1 mL.

- IV medication preparation is usually a two-step procedure: measurement of the dosage, then dilution according to manufacturer's recommendations or a physician's or prescriber's order.

- IV injections are being given into the circulating blood, so the ranges of volume are much broader.

■ Parenteral drugs may be measured in metric, unit, mEq, or percentage dosages. Ratio dosages, while they may still be seen on drug labels, are being phased out and the label will identify the metric equivalents.

■ It is important to identify the equipment that may be used to administer parenteral medications. The calibrations must be read accurately.

■ 3-mL syringes are calibrated in tenths.

■ TB syringes are calibrated in hundredths.

■ 5- and 10-mL syringes are calibrated in fifths (two-tenths).

■ Syringes larger than 10 mL are calibrated in full mL measures.

■ The first long calibration on all syringes indicates zero.

■ All syringe calibrations must be read from the top, or front, ring of the plunger's suction tip. This would be the part of the plunger that is in contact with the medication.

Summary Self-Test

Part I

Calculate the ordered dosages in the following questions using the method of your choice, and draw arrows on the syringe barrel to indicate the calculated dose. Have your instructor check your arrows on the syringes for accuracy. Round mL answers to the nearest tenth (or hundredth where indicated) using the medication labels provided. The route of the order is provided for you.

Dosage Ordered   **mL Needed**

1. terbutaline sulfate 600 mcg subcutaneous   _____

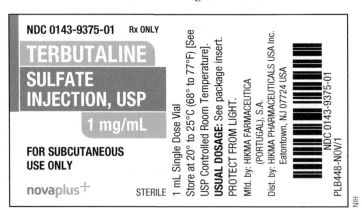

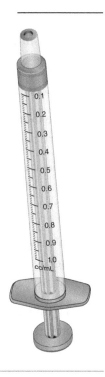

Dosage Ordered   **mL Needed**

2. furosemide 25 mg IV   _____

NDC 70121-**1163**-1

Furosemide
Injection, USP

20 mg/2 mL
(10 mg/mL)
FOR IV OR IM USE

2 mL SINGLE-DOSE VIAL
Rx only

WARNING: USE ONLY IF SOLUTION IS CLEAR AND COLORLESS. PROTECT FROM LIGHT. Store at 20° to 25°C (68° to 77°F); excursions permitted between 15° to 30°C (59° to 86°F) [see USP Controlled Room Temperature]. Directions for Use: See Package Insert. Mfg. Lic. No. G/28/1539
Distributed by:
Amneal Pharmaceuticals LLC
Bridgewater, NJ 08807
Rev. 05-2019-02   Made in INDIA

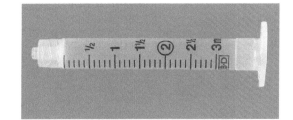

3. dexamethasone 2.5 mg IV (Calculate to the   _____
   hundredth.)

NDC 63323-506-41   PRX500601

Dexamethasone Sodium Phosphate
Injection, USP

10 mg per mL

For IM or IV use only.
Preservative free.
Discard unused portion.
Protect from light.
1 mL Single Dose Vial   Rx only

PREMIERProRx® Mfd. by: Fresenius Kabi

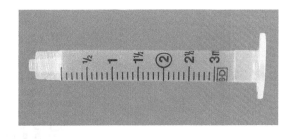

4. fentanyl citrate 0.08 mg IV   _____

NDC 17478-030-02   **2 mL Ampule**

Fentanyl Citrate Injection, USP ©

100 mcg/2 mL (50 mcg/mL)*

FOR INTRAVENOUS OR INTRAMUSCULAR USE   Rx only

***Each mL contains:** 0.0785 mg fentanyl citrate equivalent to 50 mcg fentanyl base.
Mfd. by: **Akorn,** Lake Forest, IL 60045

AFCADL Rev.09/21

Dosage Ordered   **mL Needed**

5. naloxone 150 mcg subcutaneous (Round to the   _____
   hundredth.)

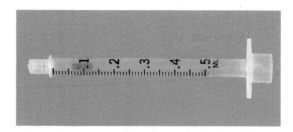

17478-**041**-01
**Naloxone HCl
Injection, USP**
0.4 mg/mL
For I.V., I.M. or S.C. use
1 mL Single-dose Vial

Rx only
Protect from light.

○AKORN
Mfd. by: Akorn Inc.
Lake Forest, IL 60045
NLAAL   Rev. 10/17

6. tobramycin 65 mg IM   _____

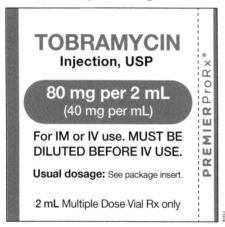

TOBRAMYCIN
Injection, USP

80 mg per 2 mL
(40 mg per mL)

For IM or IV use. MUST BE
DILUTED BEFORE IV USE.

Usual dosage: See package insert.

2 mL Multiple Dose Vial Rx only

PREMIERProRx®

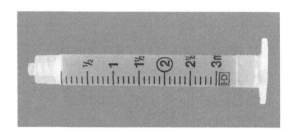

7. Robinul® (glycopyrrolate) 55 mcg IV (Round to the   _____
   hundredth.)

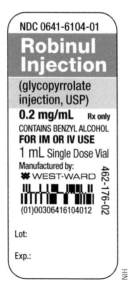

NDC 0641-6104-01
**Robinul
Injection**
(glycopyrrolate
injection, USP)
0.2 mg/mL   Rx only
CONTAINS BENZYL ALCOHOL
FOR IM OR IV USE
1 mL Single Dose Vial
Manufactured by:
❤ WEST-WARD
(01)00306416104012
462-176-02

Lot:

Exp.:

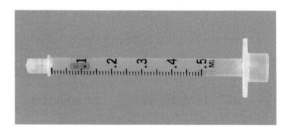

Dosage Ordered   **mL Needed**

8. bumetanide 0.8 mg IV   _____

NDC 65219-**570**-01 **Rx only**

Bumetanide
Injection, USP

1 mg/4 mL (0.25 mg/mL)

For Intravenous or
Intramuscular Use
Contains Benzyl Alcohol
4 mL Single-Dose Vial
Discard unused portion.

Each mL contains bumetanide
0.25 mg, sodium chloride 8.5 mg
and ammonium acetate 4 mg as
buffers, edetate disodium dihydrate
0.1 mg and benzyl alcohol 10 mg
as preservative; pH adjusted to
6.8-7.8 with sodium hydroxide.
This container closure is not made
with natural rubber latex.
Usual Dosage: See package insert.
Store at 20°C to 25°C (68°F to
77°F). Protect from light.

Code No.: TS/DRUGS/2/2015

NIH

9. morphine sulfate 8.5 mg IV   _____

NDC 0641-**6125**-01
Morphine
Sulfate Inj., USP

4 mg/mL Ⓒ

For IV use ONLY
Protect from light
Discard if precipitated

1 mL Single Dose Vial

NIH

10. heparin sodium 10,000 units IV   _____

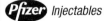

For subcutaneous
or intravenous use.

Derived from
porcine intestinal
tissue

Distributed by
Pfizer Labs
Division of Pfizer Inc
NY, NY 10017

Pfizer *Injectables*

NDC 0069-0137-01

Rx only

HEPARIN
Sodium Injection, USP

NOT FOR LOCK FLUSH

30,000 USP
units per **30 mL**
(1,000 USP units per mL)

Warning: Contains Benzyl Alcohol

Multidose Vial

NIH

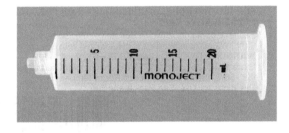

Dosage Ordered

mL Needed

11. phenytoin 0.1 g IM _____

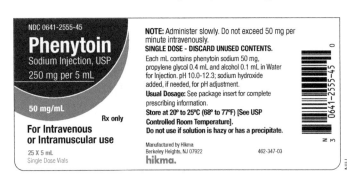

NDC 0641-2555-45
Phenytoin
Sodium Injection, USP
250 mg per 5 mL

50 mg/mL
Rx only

**For Intravenous
or Intramuscular use**

25 X 5 mL
Single Dose Vials

NOTE: Administer slowly. Do not exceed 50 mg per minute intravenously.
SINGLE DOSE - DISCARD UNUSED CONTENTS.
Each mL contains phenytoin sodium 50 mg, propylene glycol 0.4 mL and alcohol 0.1 mL in Water for Injection. pH 10.0-12.3; sodium hydroxide added, if needed, for pH adjustment.
Usual Dosage: See package insert for complete prescribing information.
Store at 20° to 25°C (68° to 77°F) [See USP Controlled Room Temperature].
Do not use if solution is hazy or has a precipitate.

Manufactured by Hikma
Berkeley Heights, NJ 07922   462-347-03
hikma.

12. medroxyprogesterone 0.4 g IM _____

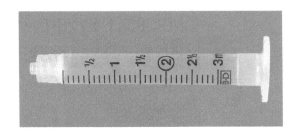

For intramuscular use only
Single-Dose Vial
DOSAGE AND USE:
See accompanying prescribing information.
Shake vigorously immediately before each use. Store upright.
Pharmacia & Upjohn Co
Division of Pfizer Inc, NY, NY 10017

FPO: RSS

NDC 0009-0746-30   Rx only
**Depo-Provera®
Contraceptive
Injection**
medroxyPROGESTERone acetate
injectable suspension, USP
150 mg/mL

13. atropine sulfate 175 mcg subcutaneous _____
     (Round to the hundredth.)

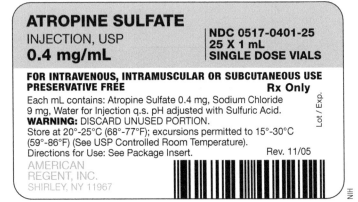

ATROPINE SULFATE
INJECTION, USP
0.4 mg/mL

NDC 0517-0401-25
**25 X 1 mL
SINGLE DOSE VIALS**

**FOR INTRAVENOUS, INTRAMUSCULAR OR SUBCUTANEOUS USE
PRESERVATIVE FREE**   **Rx Only**
Each mL contains: Atropine Sulfate 0.4 mg, Sodium Chloride 9 mg, Water for Injection q.s. pH adjusted with Sulfuric Acid.
WARNING: DISCARD UNUSED PORTION.
Store at 20°-25°C (68°-77°F); excursions permitted to 15°-30°C (59°-86°F) (See USP Controlled Room Temperature).
Directions for Use: See Package Insert.   Rev. 11/05

Lot / Exp.

AMERICAN
REGENT, INC.
SHIRLEY, NY 11967

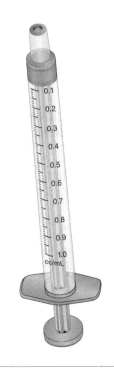

Dosage Ordered   **mL Needed**

14. methotrexate 35 mg IV   _____

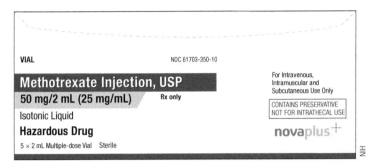

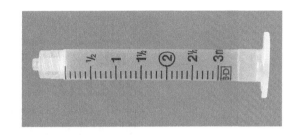

15. ondansetron 12 mg IV   _____

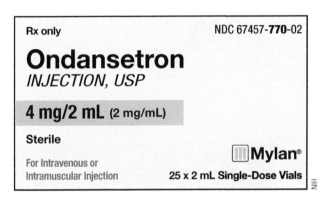

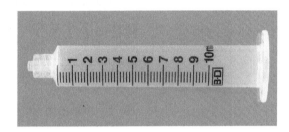

16. methylprednisolone 0.1 g IM   _____

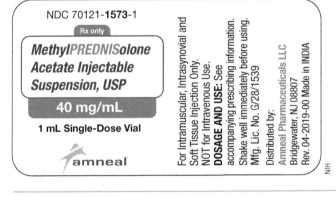

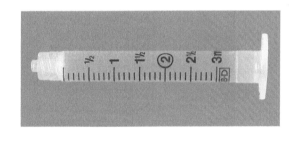

Dosage Ordered   **mL Needed**

17. nalbuphine 15 mg SUBQ (Calculate to the
    hundredth.)   _____

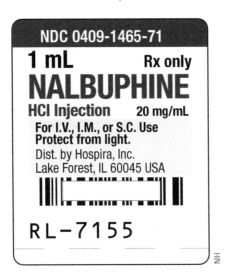
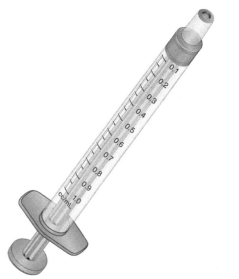

18. hydromorphone 2.5 mg IV   _____

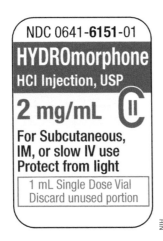
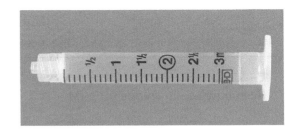

19. digoxin 0.15 mg IV   _____

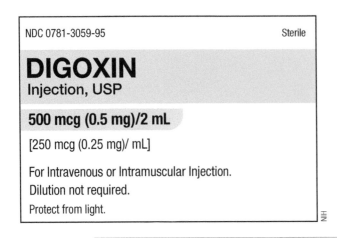
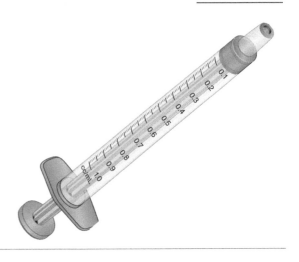

Dosage Ordered   **mL Needed**

20. Aranesp® (darbepoetin alfa) 0.02 mg SUBQ   _____

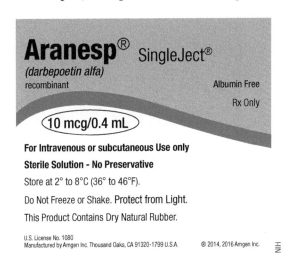

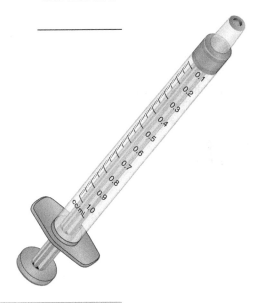

21. sodium chloride 60 mEq IV   _____

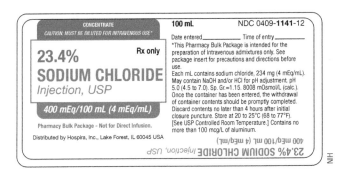

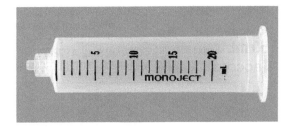

22. octreotide 80 mcg IV   _____

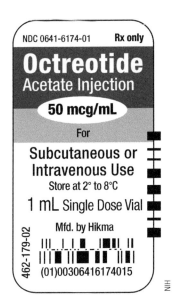

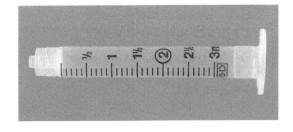

Dosage Ordered   **mL Needed**

23. ranitidine 30 mg IM   _____

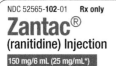

NDC 52565-102-01   **Rx only**

Zantac®
(ranitidine) Injection

150 mg/6 mL (25 mg/mL*)

6 mL Multiple Dose Vial

*For IV or IM injection,
or IV infusion*

Sterile

*Each 1 mL of aqueous solution contains ranitidine 25 mg
(equivalent to 28 mg Ranitidine Hydrochloride, USP);
phenol 5 mg as preservative; monobasic potassium
phosphate and dibasic sodium phosphate as buffers.

See package insert for Dosage and Administration.
Store between 4° and 25°C (39° and 77°F);
excursions permitted to 30°C (86°F).
Protect from light.
Zantac® Injection tends to exhibit a yellow color that may
intensify over time without adversely affecting potency.

Zantac is a registered trademark of
Boehringer Ingelheim Pharmaceuticals, Inc., used under license.

Manufactured by:
Teligent Pharma, Inc., Buena, NJ 08310
C101166   CL-102-00 Rev 04/2019

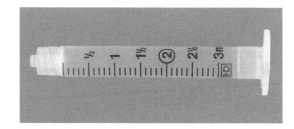

24. CISplatin 10 mg IV   _____

NDC 16729-288-11

CISplatin doses greater than 100 mg/m²
once every 3 to 4 weeks are rarely used.
See Package insert

CISplatin
Injection   **Rx only**

50 mg/50 mL (1 mg/mL)

For Intravenous Use   Sterile

50 mL Multiple Dose Vial

accord

Each mL contains: 1 mg cisplatin and
9 mg sodium chloride in water for injection.
HCl and/or sodium hydroxide added to adjust pH.
The pH range of Cisplatin Injection is 3.5 to 5.0.
Usual dosage: See insert.
Store at 20°C to 25°C (68°F to 77°F); excursions
permitted to 15°C to 30°C (59°F to 86°F) [see
USP Controlled Room Temperature].
DO NOT REFRIGERATE OR FREEZE CISPLATIN
SOLUTION SINCE A PRECIPITATE OR CRYSTAL
WILL FORM. PROTECT FROM LIGHT.

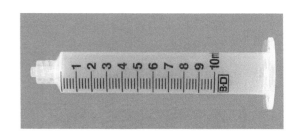

25. diltiazem 20 mg IV   _____

NDC 17478-937-05

DILTIAZEM
Hydrochloride
Injection   **25 mg/5 mL**
                     (5 mg/mL)

5 mL Single-dose Vial   Rx only

For Direct I.V. Bolus Injection and Continuous I.V. Infusion.
Manufactured by: Akorn, Inc.
Lake Forest, IL 60045
DHAEL Rev. 06/16   Sterile

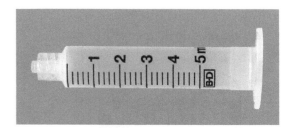

Dosage Ordered	mL Needed
26. acyclovir 120 mg IV	_____

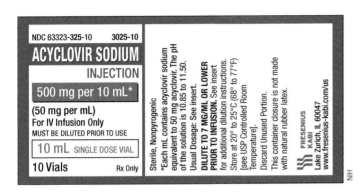

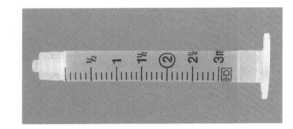

27. phytonadione 10 mg IV _____

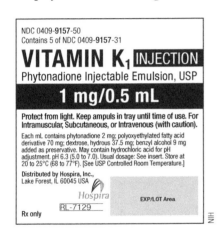

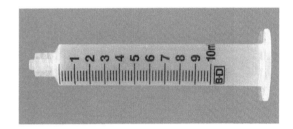

28. penicillin G benzathine 1,000,000 units IM _____

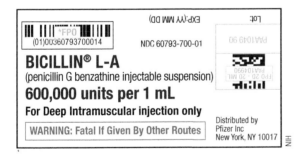

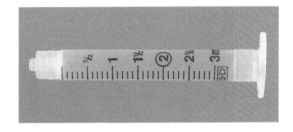

Answers **1.** 0.6 mL **2.** 2.5 mL **3.** 0.25 mL **4.** 1.6 mL **5.** 0.375 = 0.38 mL **6.** 1.62 = 1.6 mL **7.** 0.275 = 0.28 mL **8.** 3.2 mL **9.** 2.12 = 2.1 mL **10.** 10 mL **11.** 2 mL **12.** 2.66 = 2.7 mL **13.** 0.437 = 0.44 mL **14.** 1.4 mL **15.** 6 mL **16.** 2.5 mL **17.** 0.75 mL **18.** 1.25 = 1.3 mL **19.** 0.6 mL **20.** 0.8 mL **21.** 15 mL **22.** 1.6 mL **23.** 1.2 mL **24.** 10 mL **25.** 4 mL **26.** 2.4 mL **27.** 5 mL **28.** 1.66 = 1.7 mL

Part II

Identify the dosages measured on the following syringes.

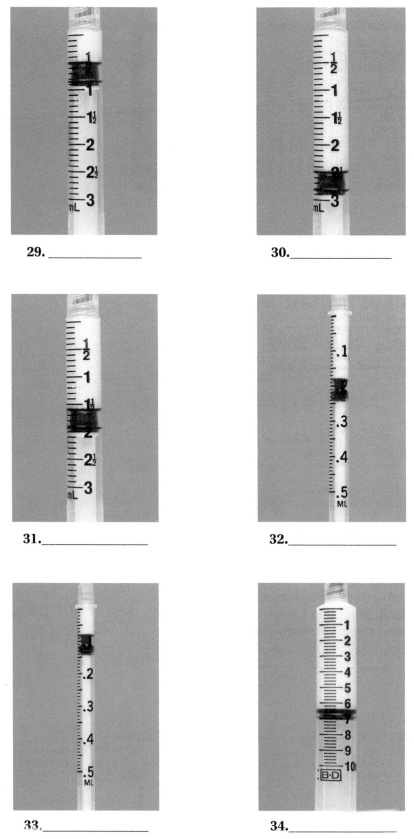

29. _____

30. _____

31. _____

32. _____

33. _____

34. _____

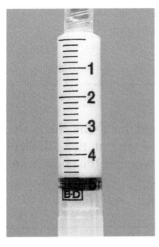

35._____

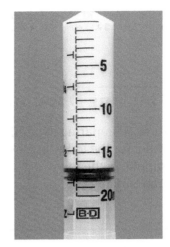

36._____

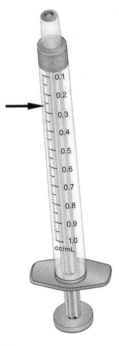

37._____

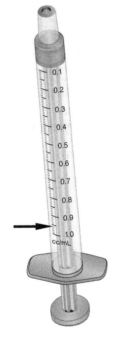

38._____

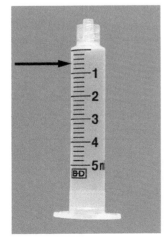

39._____

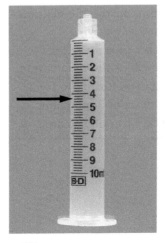

40._____

Critical Thinking Questions

1. The nurse is preparing to administer medications to the client. On the MAR is an order for the following: bumetanide 1.5 mg stat. Refer to Figure 12-23 for your supply. In the following matrix, mark whether the choices are appropriate or inappropriate.

NDC 72572-**040**-01   **Rx only**

Bumetanide
Injection, USP

1 mg/4 mL (0.25 mg/mL)

For IV or IM Use
Contains Benzyl Alcohol

4 mL Single-Dose Vial

Each mL contains bumetanide 0.25 mg, sodium chloride 8.5 mg and ammonium acetate 4 mg as buffers, edetate disodium 0.1 mg and benzyl alcohol 10 mg as preservative; pH adjusted to 6.8-7.8 with sodium hydroxide. Non-Latex.
Usual Dosage: See package insert.
Store at 20° to 25°C (68° to 77°F).
Protect from light.
Mfd for: Civica, Inc., Lehi, UT 84043
Mfd for: Hikma Pharmaceuticals USA Inc.
Cherry Hill, NJ 08003

462-924-00

▲ **Figure 12-23**

Choice	Appropriate Action	Inappropriate Action
Calculate volume to give of 6 mL.		
Administer the medication intravenously.		
Administer the medication intramuscularly.		
Contact pharmacy for a different strength of the medication.		
Divide the dose into two injections of 3 mL each.		
Contact the physician.		

2. The following medication needs to be prepared and administered to your client: heparin 5,000 units subcutaneous every 12 hours. Which of the following would be correct? Select all that apply.

   a. Use the medication in Figure 12-24 and prepare 5 mL.
   b. Use the medication in Figure 12-25 and prepare 0.5 mL.
   c. Use a 1 mL tuberculin syringe to administer the medication.
   d. Use a 5 mL syringe to administer the medication.
   e. Call the physician for clarification.

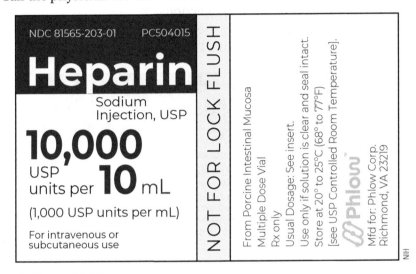

▲ **Figure 12-24**

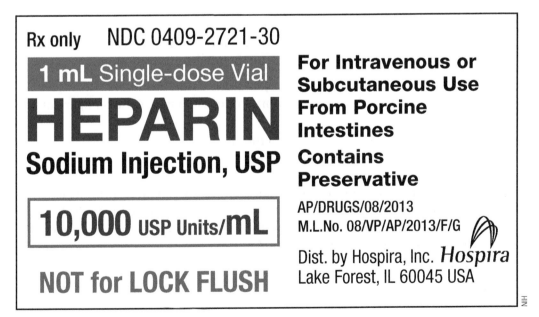

▲ **Figure 12-25**

3. The client has been ordered Neupogen® (filgrastim) 240 mcg subcutaneous once daily for 5 days to treat neutropenia (low white blood count). Refer to Figure 12-26. Without writing out the calculation, the nurse determines the dose is 4 mL. Using critical thinking and clinical judgement for all medication preparation, the nurse determines the following relevant information. Select all that apply.

   a. The calculation is accurate and should be administered as ordered.
   b. The decimal has been misplaced in the calculation.
   c. The subcut route has a limit of 1 mL.
   d. Divide the medication into two injections.
   e. Choose a 5 mL syringe and give the medication.
   f. Recalculate, and choose a 0.5 mL TB syringe.

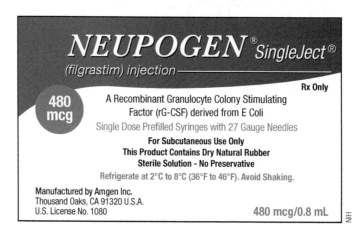

▲ **Figure 12-26**

4. A nurse is preparing the shingles vaccine, Zostavax, to administer to a client. The entire vial of 0.65 mL will be administered. As the medication is withdrawn into the syringe, the nurse will measure the medication solution:

   a. From the top ring of the suction tip closest to the needle.
   b. From the bottom ring of the suction tip closest to where the plunger enters the barrel.
   c. From the raised middle section of the suction tip.
   d. From the second ring of the suction tip.

5. The physician has ordered golimumab 45 mg subcutaneous monthly for a client with rheumatoid arthritis. Refer to Figure 12-27. The nurse reads the order; after calculating the dose and rounding accurately, the nurse will choose which syringe to administer the medication?

   a. either 1 mL syringe or 3 mL syringe
   b. 5 mL syringe
   c. 0.5 mL syringe
   d. 3 mL syringe

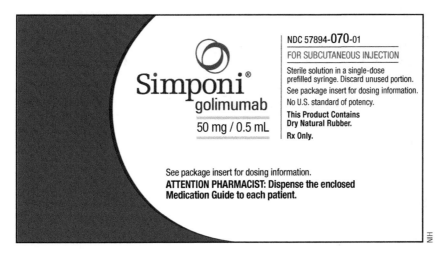

▲ **Figure 12-27**

Answers to Critical Thinking Questions

1.

Choice	Appropriate Action	Inappropriate Action
Calculate volume to give of 6 mL.	X	
Administer the medication intravenously.		X
Administer the medication intramuscularly.		X
Contact pharmacy for a different strength of the medication.		X
Divide the dose into two injections of 3 mL each.		X
Contact the physician.	X	

(Rationale: Calculation of the dose is appropriate and within the nurse's scope of practice. Administer the medication intravenously is not appropriate; there is no route provided in the order and it is not in the nurse's scope of practice to determine the route. Administer the medication intramuscularly is not appropriate; there is no route provided in the order and it is not in the nurse's scope of practice to determine the route. Contacting pharmacy for a different strength is not appropriate as there is no route provided for the order and the different strength would not make a difference. Dividing the dose into two injections is not appropriate; there is no route provided in the order. While 6 mL is too much to give in a single IM injection, it is a realistic amount to administer IV. Contacting the physician is appropriate as the order is incomplete.)

2. b, c. **(Rationale:** A would not be selected because 5 mL is too much to give subcutaneous; d would not be selected because the correct dose is 0.5 mL and this cannot be measured in a 5 mL syringe; e would not be selected because the order is complete and the physician does not need to clarify any aspect of the order.)

3. b, c, f. **(Rationale:** A would not be selected because the calculation is inaccurate; d would not be selected because it will not be necessary to give 2 injections; e would not be selected because this is a subcutaneous injection, and a 5 mL syringe cannot measure 0.5 mL.)

4. a

5. c (0.45 mL – use a 0.5 mL syringe.)

Chapter

13

Reconstitution of Powdered Drugs

Objectives

The learner will:

1. describe the process to prepare solutions from powdered drugs using directions printed on vial labels.

2. describe the process to prepare solutions from powdered drugs using drug literature or inserts.

3. determine the expiration date and time for reconstituted drugs.

4. calculate dosages for reconstituted drugs.

The process of reconstitution involves adding a liquid to a powder or crystals to make a solution of a particular concentration. Reconstitution can be applied to oral or parenteral medications. The drug label, or instructional package insert, will give specific directions for reconstitution of the drug. It is essential to read these with care. This chapter will help you identify the necessary reconstitution information from different types of labels.

Keypoint: Reconstitution directions on vial labels may be small and difficult to read. Reading them with extreme care is essential. When reading the label, it is important to locate the necessary information to prepare the medication, as well as calculate the dosage. It is also important to identify whether the reconstituted solution can be used for multiple doses, or if it is a single-use only vial.

You will need to understand several terms used on the label or insert. Diluent or solvent refers to the liquid used to dilute the powder and put it into solution. The **diluent** may be sterile water, sterile saline, bacteriostatic water with benzyl alcohol, or any other solution specified for reconstitution. Parenteral medications will need reconstituted with sterile solutions, whereas oral medications may specify tap water or distilled water for reconstitution of the powder. Oral medications would not need to be reconstituted with sterile solutions as the GI tract is nonsterile and does not require sterile technique for medication administration. The diluent will vary by type and amount for various medications; therefore, the directions must be read carefully.

The powder in the vial or bottle may be referred to as the solute. The **solute** is the component that will be dissolved. The end product may be referred to as the **constituted solution** or the **reconstituted solution**. These terms are sometimes used interchangeably.

The directions for reconstitution on the label or package insert may also include specific storage instructions after the medication is reconstituted, as well as information about expiration of the reconstituted solution. Follow these instructions completely. Reconstitution instructions will be located on the vial or on the package insert. Instructions may give information to reconstitute to a variety of strengths. Instructions may also differ depending on the route of administration. This chapter will review information found on reconstitution labels and package inserts.

Clinical Relevance: Some medications are unstable in solution form and are supplied by pharmaceutical companies as powders for reconstitution. These medications may be reconstituted by the clinical pharmacy. However, in some clinical settings, it may be the responsibility of the individual who administers the medication to reconstitute it. This responsibility involves careful understanding of directions on the medication label, or the package insert.

The medication label or package insert will give explicit directions for the process of reconstituting. These directions must be followed precisely so that the medication has the potency that is expected. Usually there are several different numbers present within the reconstitution directions, and the individual administering the medication must be clear on the numbers needed to calculate the dosage.

It is also extremely important to carefully read the information on the vial to determine expiration date and time. The powder may come from the pharmaceutical company with an expiration date on the label. However, once reconstituted, the medication in solution may have a different expiration date and time. This process of reconstitution challenges the practitioner to take care in reading the label or insert, as well as carefully following all instructions for reconstituting and storage of the prepared solution.

Single-Strength Solutions with Reconstitution Directions on the Vial Label

Let's review a single-strength solution with the directions on the vial label. Examine the label for the methylprednisolone 500 mg vial in Figure 13-1.

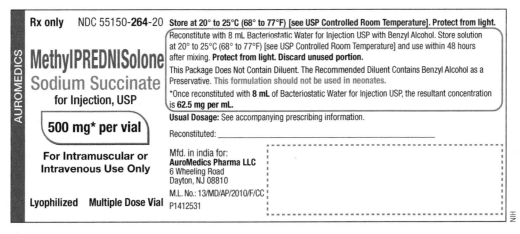

▲ **Figure 13-1**

The first step in reconstitution is to locate the directions. For instructional purposes, these directions are located inside the red circle drawn on this label. On the label in Figure 13-1, for example, the directions indicate to reconstitute with 8 mL Bacteriostatic Water for Injection with Benzyl Alcohol.

Once the type and amount of diluent are identified, the next step in all parenteral reconstitution is to use a sterile syringe and aseptic technique to draw up the volume and type of diluent required. This will then be injected slowly into the vial of powder above the level of medication so there are few air bubbles created during the process. Air bubbles in the final solution can displace medication in the syringe creating a discrepancy in the amount of medication withdrawn for injection. In this case, then 8 mL of Bacteriostatic Water for Injection with Benzyl Alcohol will be drawn up and inserted into this vial of powder. Sometimes, if the diluent volume is large, as in this case, pressure will form in the vial and air may be forced into the syringe from the vial to equalize the pressure. Very large volumes of diluent may have to be injected in divided amounts to keep the internal vial pressure equalized. When all the diluent has been injected, the vial is rotated until all the medication has been dissolved. Do not shake unless directed to do so, because this also can add air bubbles to some medications and distort dosages.

After reconstitution, locate the information that relates to the length of time the reconstituted solution may be stored, and how it must be stored. Refer to the directions circled in red on the label in Figure 13-1 and locate this information. You will find that this solution can be stored at room temperature and that it must be used within 48 hours of reconstitution.

When the reconstitution procedure is completed, the next step is to place a label on the vial to identify the process of reconstitution as complete. This label should include your initials, as the person who reconstituted the drug, and the date and time of preparation. It should also include the new expiration date and time based on the information on the label—48 hours from the time of reconstitution. Assume you reconstituted this vial of methylprednisolone at 2 pm on January 3, 2024. Based on the information on the label, the medication will retain its potency for 48 hours at room temperature. The expiration date and time that would be written on this label would be "Expires January 5, 2024 at 2 pm."

Keypoint: The person who reconstitutes a drug is responsible for labeling it with the date and time of expiration, as well as their initials. This process cannot be overlooked.

After the medication has been reconstituted, identify the information you will use in your dosage equations. There are various numbers on the label in Figure 13-1. It is important to determine which numbers are needed for calculation. On the label, there will be numbers needed for preparation of the medication, as well as for calculation of the dose.

On the vial in Figure 13-1, the total dosage strength is identified as 500 mg. There is no volume associated with this strength, so you need to read further on the label to find a strength associated with a volume. Remember, this information is located on the vial and cannot be made up. Within the information inside the red circle, you will see the statement: the resultant concentration is 62.5 mg per mL. This statement contains the concentration of the solution—62.5 mg in 1 mL.

In this case, the reconstituted volume equals the amount of diluent that was added. Adding 8 mL of diluent, we have 62.5 mg in every mL; 62.5 mg per mL multiplied by 8 mL equals 500 mg, and this is the total amount in the vial as listed on the front of the label.

Reconstituted volumes do not always exactly equal the amount of diluent added; in fact, many do not. This is because the medication itself has a volume, and it usually makes the total volume somewhat larger than the amount of diluent injected. Before we consider another example, let's use the information from the label to calculate based on a physician order.

Example 1 ▣   If the physician orders methylprednisolone 125 mg IM stat, how many mL will we administer? Use the information from the label in Figure 13-1—methylprednisolone 62.5 mg per mL—for the available supply.

Method 1: Ratio and Proportion

| *In Colon Format* | *In Fraction Format* |

$$62.5 \text{ mg} : 1 \text{ mL} = 125 \text{ mg} : x \text{ mL}$$

$$\frac{62.5 \text{ mg}}{1 \text{ mL}} = \frac{125 \text{ mg}}{x \text{ mL}}$$

$$62.5x = 125 \qquad\qquad\qquad 62.5x = 125$$

$$x = \frac{125}{62.5} = 2 \text{ mL} \qquad\qquad x = \frac{125}{62.5} = 2 \text{ mL}$$

Once the medication is reconstituted, we will administer 2 mL of the solution to administer the ordered dose of 125 mg. We will now do this calculation using dimensional analysis and the formula method. Notice that the calculations for medications that require reconstitution follow the same formats as calculations in previous chapters. The challenge will be locating the proper information to place in the equations.

Method 2: Dimensional Analysis

$$mL = \frac{1 \text{ mL}}{62.5 \text{ mg}} \times \frac{125 \text{ mg}}{}$$

$$mL = \frac{1 \text{ mL}}{62.5 \text{ \sout{mg}}} \times \frac{125 \text{ \sout{mg}}}{}$$

$$mL = \frac{125}{62.5} = 2 \text{ mL}$$

Method 3: Formula Method

$$\frac{125 \text{ mg (D)} \times 1 \text{ mL (Q)}}{62.5 \text{ mg (H)}} = x \text{ mL}$$

$$\frac{125 \text{ \sout{mg}} \times 1 \text{ mL}}{62.5 \text{ \sout{mg}}} = x \text{ mL}$$

$$\frac{125 \times 1}{62.5} = 2 \text{ mL}$$

This demonstrates that the calculation process does not change. You have practiced dosage calculation in previous chapters; that process will be the same for reconstitution, provided you locate the correct information on the label or package insert.

    Let's consider a second example and concentrate on identifying the diluent, the volume of diluent, and the final concentration, which may also be called the final yield.

Example 2 ■   Refer to Figure 13-2, an oral suspension medication, where the total volume after reconstitution is greater than the volume of diluent added. We will identify the various pieces of information on this label.

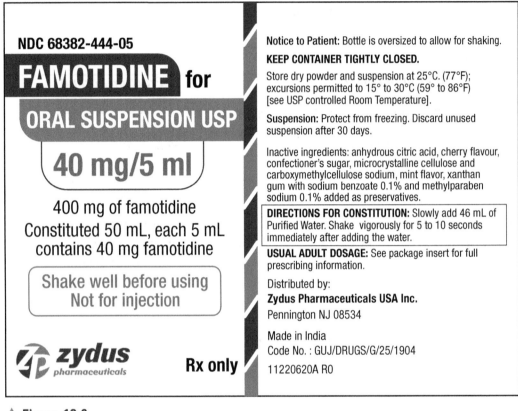

NDC 68382-444-05

FAMOTIDINE for

ORAL SUSPENSION USP

40 mg/5 ml

400 mg of famotidine
Constituted 50 mL, each 5 mL
contains 40 mg famotidine

Shake well before using
Not for injection

zydus
pharmaceuticals   **Rx only**

Notice to Patient: Bottle is oversized to allow for shaking.
KEEP CONTAINER TIGHTLY CLOSED.
Store dry powder and suspension at 25°C. (77°F); excursions permitted to 15° to 30°C (59° to 86°F) [see USP controlled Room Temperature].

Suspension: Protect from freezing. Discard unused suspension after 30 days.

Inactive ingredients: anhydrous citric acid, cherry flavour, confectioner's sugar, microcrystalline cellulose and carboxymethylcellulose sodium, mint flavor, xanthan gum with sodium benzoate 0.1% and methylparaben sodium 0.1% added as preservatives.

DIRECTIONS FOR CONSTITUTION: Slowly add 46 mL of Purified Water. Shake vigorously for 5 to 10 seconds immediately after adding the water.

USUAL ADULT DOSAGE: See package insert for full prescribing information.

Distributed by:
Zydus Pharmaceuticals USA Inc.
Pennington NJ 08534

Made in India
Code No. : GUJ/DRUGS/G/25/1904

11220620A R0

▲ **Figure 13-2**

Notice that there are several numbers on the front of the label, as well as information on the side in the box. The front of the label indicates there are 40 mg/5 mL, and there is a total of 400 mg in this container.

The directions for reconstitution are on the side. The diluent is purified water. Notice, as an oral medication, it is not necessary to add sterile water. The instructions indicate to add 46 mL of purified water and to shake well. This label is a good example of a reconstituted medication, which will have a greater volume after reconstituted than the amount of diluent added. Reviewing the front of the label, we notice that the volume of the constituted (or reconstituted) solution is 50 mL; therefore, the powder has added to the volume by approximately 4 mL. The numbers that you would need for a calculation using this label would be 40 mg per 5 mL. This would be the final concentration, or some labels may refer to this as the final yield.

Keypoint: Reconstituted volumes may exceed the volume of the diluent added since the drug itself has a volume. It is important to remember this and always carefully search your label for the final yield or the final concentration of the solution after dilution.

Problems 13.1

For any dosage calculation questions, please follow the rounding considerations presented earlier in the book—for amounts greater than 1 mL, round to the tenth; for amounts less than 1 mL, round to the hundredth.

Refer to the label in Figure 13-3 to answer the following questions about doxycycline.

1. How should this drug be reconstituted?   _____

2. After reconstitution, what is the final yield?   _____

3. After reconstitution, should it be kept in the refrigerator?   _____

4. What is the route of this drug?   _____

5. How many mL will be administered for a 75 mg dose?   _____

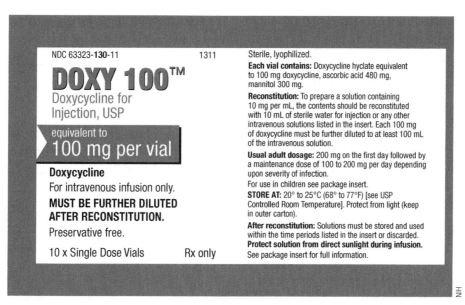

NDC 63323-**130**-11   1311   Sterile, lyophilized.

DOXY 100™
Doxycycline for
Injection, USP

equivalent to
100 mg per vial

Doxycycline
For intravenous infusion only.
**MUST BE FURTHER DILUTED
AFTER RECONSTITUTION.**
Preservative free.

10 x Single Dose Vials   Rx only

Each vial contains: Doxycycline hyclate equivalent to 100 mg doxycycline, ascorbic acid 480 mg, mannitol 300 mg.

Reconstitution: To prepare a solution containing 10 mg per mL, the contents should be reconstituted with 10 mL of sterile water for injection or any other intravenous solutions listed in the insert. Each 100 mg of doxycycline must be further diluted to at least 100 mL of the intravenous solution.

Usual adult dosage: 200 mg on the first day followed by a maintenance dose of 100 to 200 mg per day depending upon severity of infection.

For use in children see package insert.

STORE AT: 20° to 25°C (68° to 77°F) [see USP Controlled Room Temperature]. Protect from light (keep in outer carton).

After reconstitution: Solutions must be stored and used within the time periods listed in the insert or discarded. **Protect solution from direct sunlight during infusion.** See package insert for full information.

▲ **Figure 13-3**

Refer to the label in Figure 13-4 to answer the following questions about cefaclor.

6. How much diluent is needed to mix this medication in the container?   _____

7. How will the diluent be divided to mix the medication?   _____

8. What type of diluent will be used?   _____

9. If the drug is mixed at 4 pm on November 28, 2024, what date and time should the unused portion be discarded?   _____

10. What should always be done with the container prior to use?   _____

11. How many mL will be administered for a 400 mg dose?   _____

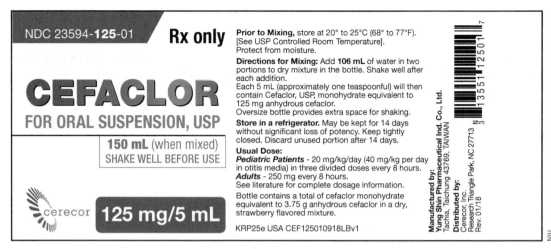

▲ Figure 13-4

Refer to the label in Figures 13-5 and 13-6 to answer the following questions about cefazolin.

12. What are the routes for cefazolin?   _____

13. What is the IM reconstitution instruction for this vial?   _____

14. What is the final concentration after reconstitution
    for the IM injection?   _____

15. Where should the reconstituted drug be stored after 24 hrs?   _____

16. How many mL will be administered for a 300 mg IM dose?   _____

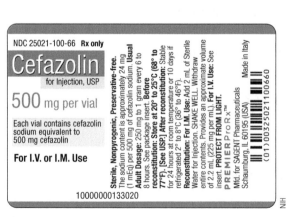

▲ Figure 13-5   ▲ Figure 13-6

Refer to the label in Figure 13-7 to answer the following questions about linezolid.

17. What route will linezolid be given from this container?   _____

18. What type of diluent will be used to mix the powder?   _____

19. What is the total amount of diluent?   _____

20. How will this diluent be distributed to mix the powder?   _____

21. Before using this suspension, what specific action should be taken?   _____

22. How many mL will be administered for a 220 mg dose?   _____

NDC 0054-0319-50

150 mL
(when constituted)

Linezolid for
Oral Suspension

100 mg/5 mL

WARNING: NOT FOR INJECTION.
USUAL DOSAGE: See Package Insert
for Complete Prescribing Information.
Store at 20° to 25°C (68° to 77°F).
[See USP Controlled Room Temperature.]

Mixing Directions: Gently tap bottle to loosen
powder. Add a total of 123 mL distilled water in
two portions. After adding the first half, shake
vigorously to wet all of the powder. Then add the
second half of the water and shake vigorously to
obtain a uniform suspension.

Distributed by: **Hikma**
Pharmaceuticals USA Inc.
Berkeley Heights, NJ 07922

Rx only

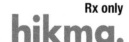

Each 5 mL of suspension contains
linezolid equivalent to 100 mg after
reconstitution.
Gently invert the bottle 3 to 5 times
before using.
DO NOT SHAKE.
Keep container tightly closed.
Protect from light and moisture.
Constituted product may be used for
21 days. Store constituted suspension
at room temperature. Discard unused
portion after 21 days.

3 N
0 0 5 4 - 0 3 1 9 - 5 0
2

c50000713/01

▲ **Figure 13-7**

Reconstitution from Package Insert Directions

Some drug labels will not include the reconstitution directions but will instead reference the package insert for further instruction. This section concentrates on the parts of the package insert that provide the directions for reconstitution. The package insert provides much more information about the medication, including specific use of the drug for diagnosed conditions, such as bacterial meningitis and infections of the gastrointestinal or genitourinary tracts. The insert will also give dosage recommendations, if they are not included on the label. Untoward or adverse reactions may also be included on the package insert. It is important that you understand what information you need from the package insert to reconstitute the medication and what information on the package insert is important for other reasons.

Let's look at an example of a label that refers you to a package insert with reconstitution instructions.

Example ■   The label in Figure 13-8 indicates to look at the package insert for reconstitution directions. The information has been circled in red to draw your attention to it. Refer to Figure 13-9 to review a portion of the package insert. The information on a package insert can be confusing and difficult to find; therefore, it is very important to read the information carefully to identify the reconstitution instructions. Note the bolded information at the bottom of the table—this information indicates that for this 2 g vial, we would dilute with 10 mL of sterile water. This would give an approximate volume of 11.2 mL and result in a concentration of 180 mg per mL.

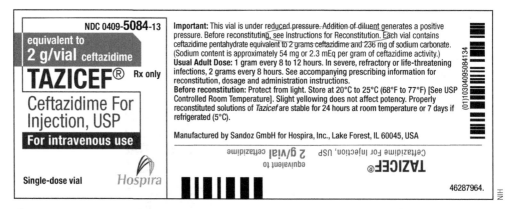

▲ Figure 13-8

Intramuscular Administration
For IM administration, Tazicef should be constituted with one of the following diluents: Sterile Water for Injection, Bacteriostatic Water for Injection, or 0.5% or 1% Lidocaine Hydrochloride Injection. Refer to Table 5.

Intravenous Administration
For direct intermittent IV administration, constitute Tazicef as directed in Table 5 with **Sterile Water for Injection**. Slowly inject directly into the vein over a period of 3 to 5 minutes or give through the tubing of an administration set while the patient is also receiving one of the compatible IV fluids (see COMPATIBILITY AND STABILITY).

For IV infusion, constitute the 1-gram or 2-gram vial and add an appropriate quantity of the resulting solution to an IV container with one of the compatible IV fluids listed under the COMPATIBILITY AND STABILITY section.

Freezing solutions of ceftazidime for injection is not recommended.

Table 5. Preparation of Solutions of Tazicef

Size	Amount of Diluent to be Added (mL)	Approximate Available Volume (mL)	Approximate Ceftazidime Concentration (mg/mL)
Intramuscular			
1 gram vial	3	3.6	280
Intravenous			
1 gram vial	10	10.6	95
2 gram vial	**10**	**11.2**	**180**

▲ Figure 13-9

Problems 13.2

Refer to the nafcillin label in Figure 13-10 and package insert in Figure 13-11 to answer the following questions.

1. Based on the package insert, what are the options for reconstitution solutions? _____

2. What is the instruction for reconstitution for an IM route? _____

3. What is the final yield for an IM or IV injection? _____

4. How many mL will be administered for an 800 mg IV route? _____

5. What are the directions for reconstituting a 2 g vial? _____

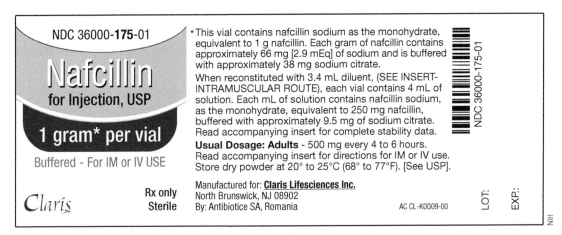

▲ **Figure 13-10**

Reconstitute with Sterile Water for Injection, USP, 0.9% Sodium Chloride Injection, USP or Bacteriostatic Water for Injection, USP (with benzyl alcohol or parabens); add 3.4 mL to the 1 g vial for 4 mL resulting solution; 6.6 mL to the 2 g vial for 8 mL resulting solution. All reconstituted vials have a concentration of 250 mg per mL. The clear solution should be administered by deep intragluteal injection immediately after reconstitution.

▲ **Figure 13-11**

Answers 1. sterile water for injection, USP, 0.9% sodium chloride injection, USP or bacteriostatic water for injection, USP (with benzyl alcohol or parabens) **2.** Add 3.4 mL of diluent **3.** 250 mg/1 mL. **4.** 3.2 mL **5.** Add 6.6 mL of diluent.

In these first two sections, the concentration was specifically on locating vial label and package insert directions for reconstitution. There is no standard way that this information is presented. But the information is all there somewhere, and it is important that you carefully read the information presented on the label and/or the package insert.

Keypoint: Information on labels and package inserts is not presented in a standardized way. It is important to understand that, for dosage equations, you must find the concentration of the solution after reconstitution. This is written as a unit of weight measurement, such as mcg, mg, or g in a certain volume of fluid. There will be numbers present on the label or package insert that will represent directions for preparation, as well as numbers that represent the information needed for calculation. Do not confuse them.

The next section will introduce you to labels that contain directions for reconstitution of multiple-strength solutions. Although multiple-strength solutions are not common, there are still a few medications that may offer a choice of dosage strengths.

Reconstitution of Multiple-Strength Solutions

When powdered drugs offer a choice of dosage strengths, you must choose the strength most appropriate for the dosage ordered. Your decision should be based on considerations, such as route of administration, volume of the reconstituted medication, and the concentration. For example, if the medication order is for intramuscular administration, we know that the limit for administration in one injection would be 3-4 mL, depending on facility protocol and the site of injection. Also, we will consider the concentration of the reconstituted solution. Many times, the more concentrated solutions will be more irritating to the tissues and veins. As an example of a multiple-strength solution, refer to the penicillin label in Figure 13-12. The dosage strengths that can be obtained are shown within the red circle on the label.

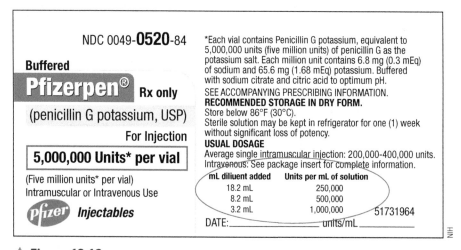

▲ **Figure 13-12**

Notice that there are three options provided for reconstitution of this medication.

1. Add 18.2 mL of diluent to produce a solution of 250,000 units in 1 mL.

2. Add 8.2 mL of diluent to produce a solution of 500,000 units per mL.

3. Add 3.2 mL of diluent to produce a solution of 1,000,000 units per mL.

When you have a multiple-strength vial, it is important to look at the order, and calculate each of the choices to determine the best option for reconstitution.

For example, if the dosage ordered is 500,000 units IM, the most appropriate strength to mix would be 500,000 units/mL. Therefore, according to the label we would add 8.2 mL of diluent to the powder in the vial to obtain a strength of 500,000 units per mL and we would administer 1 mL of the reconstituted solution. The other strengths of 250,000 units per mL and 1,000,000 units per mL could also be mixed, and the amount administered would be different. If we mixed the solution so that there were 250,000 units per mL, then we would administer 2 mL for the order of 500,000 units. If we mixed the solution so that there were 1,000,000 units per mL, then we would administer 0.5 mL for the order of 500,000 units. In this case, any of these options would be appropriate for intramuscular injections, but the 500,000 unit per mL strength would result in a simple calculation of 1 mL to administer.

Sometimes, you will find that not all strengths will be appropriate depending on the order. Using the same label in Figure 13-12, consider what might happen with an order for 1,500,000 units IM. If we were to mix the medication to a strength of 1,000,000 units per mL, we would calculate and determine that the volume to administer would be 1.5 mL. If we reconstituted to a strength of 500,000 units per mL, the volume to administer would be 3 mL. Finally, if we reconstituted to a strength of 250,000 units per mL, the volume to administer would be 6 mL. This last option, 6 mL, would be too large of a volume to administer in one IM injection; therefore, this option would not be the best. One of the other two options would be better choices.

> **Key**point: A multiple-strength solution requires that you add one additional piece of information to the label after reconstitution: the dosage strength that was mixed. This must be added so that any individual using the vial, as mixed, will know the concentration of the solution within the vial.

Vials of multiple-strength solutions have many numbers present on the label. On the label in Figure 13-12, 5,000,000 units per vial is noted on the front. This is the total amount of the medication in this vial. In addition, we see the three choices for reconstitution. These three choices show the volume of diluent to add and the concentration of the solution. This can become very confusing. Carefully, read the label and determine the information provided.

Problems 13.3

Refer to the label in Figure 13-13 to answer the following questions about streptomycin.

1. What is the only route this drug may be given?   _____

2. What is the final concentration if the vial is reconstituted with 4.2 mL?   _____

3. What is the final concentration if the vial is reconstituted with 1.8 mL?   _____

4. How long can prepared streptomycin be kept at controlled room temperature?   _____

5. How many mL will be administered for a 600 mg dose when reconstituting with 3.2 mL?   _____

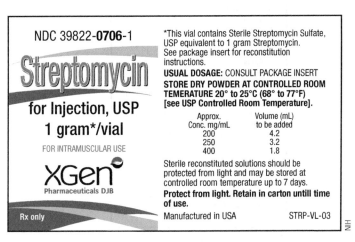

▲ **Figure 13-13**

Refer to the label in Figures 13-14 and 13-15 to answer the following questions about Penicillin G Potassium.

6. What are the routes for this drug?   _____

7. What is the average IM dose range for this drug?   _____

8. What is the final yield when 10 mL of diluent is added to the vial?   _____

9. What is the final yield when 1.8 mL of diluent is added to the vial?   _____

10. Adding 20 mL of diluent, calculate how many mL will be administered for a 400,000 units IV dose.   _____

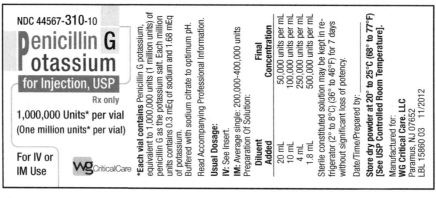

▲ **Figure 13-14**

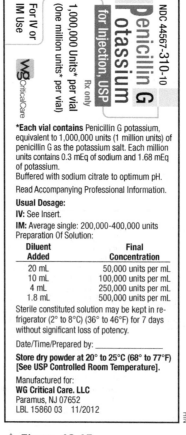

▲ **Figure 13-15**

Other Types of Reconstitution Directions

Reconstitution directions vary based on the route of administration. We identified in Chapter 12 that there are limits on the volume of medication we can administer intramuscularly or subcutaneously. The intravenous route, however, can accommodate larger volumes since the medication is injected into the circulating blood volume. Sometimes directions for reconstitution will consider this difference in acceptable volumes for the IV route. When this occurs, directions for the IM route will produce a more concentrated solution and less volume. Directions for the IV route will produce a less-concentrated solution and more volume.

Example 1 ▪   On the ceftriaxone label in Figure 13-16, there are two sets of directions for reconstitution. The IM directions are in the orange box and the IV directions are in the light green box.

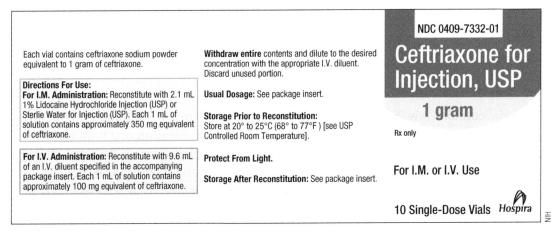

Each vial contains ceftriaxone sodium powder equivalent to 1 gram of ceftriaxone.

Directions For Use:
For I.M. Administration: Reconstitute with 2.1 mL 1% Lidocaine Hydrochloride Injection (USP) or Sterlie Water for Injection (USP). Each 1 mL of solution contains approximately 350 mg equivalent of ceftriaxone.

For I.V. Administration: Reconstitute with 9.6 mL of an I.V. diluent specified in the accompanying package insert. Each 1 mL of solution contains approximately 100 mg equivalent of ceftriaxone.

Withdraw entire contents and dilute to the desired concentration with the appropriate I.V. diluent. Discard unused portion.

Usual Dosage: See package insert.

Storage Prior to Reconstitution:
Store at 20° to 25°C (68° to 77°F) [see USP Controlled Room Temperature].

Protect From Light.

Storage After Reconstitution: See package insert.

NDC 0409-7332-01

Ceftriaxone for Injection, USP

1 gram

Rx only

For I.M. or I.V. Use

10 Single-Dose Vials   *Hospira*

▲ **Figure 13-16**

The IM directions indicate to reconstitute the powder with 2.1 mL of diluent to produce a solution containing 350 mg per mL. The directions for IV administration indicate that the powder should be reconstituted with 9.6 mL of diluent with a resulting solution of 100 mg per mL. The IV solution is less concentrated than the IM solution.

Let's look at what this means for an ordered dose. If ceftriaxone 700 mg IM is ordered, 2 mL would be administered (350 mg per mL; therefore 2 mL would be required to give 700 mg IM). If ceftriaxone 700 mg IV is ordered; 7 mL would be administered (100 mg per mL, therefore 7 mL would be required to give 700 mg IV). Notice the same medication amount results in two different volumes based on the route of administration.

Another type of reconstitution label is one that does not give a final yield or final concentration.

Example 2 ■   On the label in Figure 13-17, the directions for reconstitution are in the green circle.

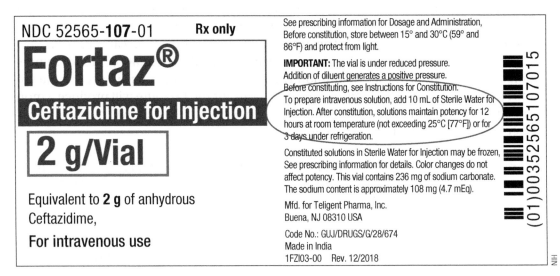

NDC 52565-**107**-01   **Rx only**

Fortaz®

Ceftazidime for Injection

2 g/Vial

Equivalent to **2 g** of anhydrous
Ceftazidime,

For intravenous use

See prescribing information for Dosage and Administration,
Before constitution, store between 15° and 30°C (59° and
86°F) and protect from light.

IMPORTANT: The vial is under reduced pressure.
Addition of diluent generates a positive pressure.
Before constituting, see Instructions for Constitution.
To prepare intravenous solution, add 10 mL of Sterile Water for
Injection. After constitution, solutions maintain potency for 12
hours at room temperature (not exceeding 25°C [77°F]) or for
3 days under refrigeration.

Constituted solutions in Sterile Water for Injection may be frozen,
See prescribing information for details. Color changes do not
affect potency. This vial contains 236 mg of sodium carbonate.
The sodium content is approximately 108 mg (4.7 mEq).

Mfd. for Teligent Pharma, Inc.
Buena, NJ 08310 USA

Code No.: GUJ/DRUGS/G/28/674
Made in India
1FZI03-00   Rev. 12/2018

(01)00352565107015

▲ **Figure 13-17**

This vial contains powder. The instructions are to add 10 mL of the diluent to the powder. Notice that the directions do not provide a final concentration or a final yield. In this case, you must use the only numbers that are available to you on the label. These numbers would be 2 g in the vial as the total weight and 10 mL as the volume—the amount of diluent that was added. Therefore, if the physician ordered 1.5 gram IV, we would administer 7.5 mL of the reconstituted solution.

Problems 13.4

Refer to the label in Figure 13-18 to answer the following questions about vancomycin.

1. How many days can this drug be stored in the refrigerator
   after reconstitution?   _____

2. How much diluent should be used for reconstitution?   _____

3. What type of diluent must be used for reconstitution?   _____

4. What is the final concentration after reconstitution?   _____

5. Calculate the amount of mL for a 900 mg IV dose.   _____

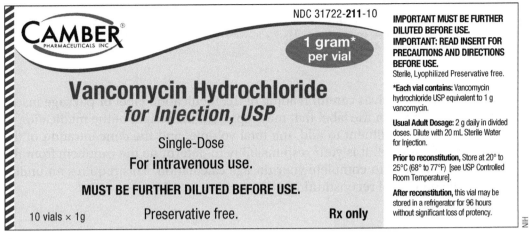

▲ Figure 13-18

Refer to the label in Figure 13-19 to answer the following questions about ceftriaxone.

6. What are the routes for the ceftriaxone? _____

7. How much diluent for reconstitution will be used for IV administration? _____

8. What is the final concentration once reconstituted for IV administration? _____

9. Where will you locate the storage instructions after reconstitution? _____

10. What are the two options of diluent if the medication will be administered IM? _____

11. How much diluent must be used to reconstitute for the IM route? _____

12. What is the final concentration after reconstitution for the IM route? _____

13. Calculate the mL amount for a 650 mg IM order. (Round to the nearest tenth.) _____

14. Calculate the mL amount for a 650 mg IV order. _____

Each vial contains ceftriaxone sodium powder equivalent to 1 gram of ceftriaxone.

Directions For Use:
For I.M. Administration: Reconstitute with 2.1 mL 1% Lidocaine Hydrochloride Injection (USP) or Sterile Water for Injection (USP). Each 1 mL of solution contains approximately 350 mg equivalent of ceftriaxone.

For I.V. Administration: Reconstitute with 9.6 mL of an I.V. diluent specified in the accompanying package insert. Each 1 mL of solution contains approximately 100 mg equivalent of ceftriaxone.

Withdraw entire contents and dilute to the desired concentration with the appropriate I.V. diluent. Discard unused portion.

Usual Dosage: See package insert.

Storage Prior to Reconstitution: Store at 20° to 25°C (68° to 77°F) [see USP Controlled Room Temperature].

Protect From Light.

Storage After Reconstitution: See package insert.

NDC 0409-7332-01
Ceftriaxone for Injection, USP
1 gram
Rx only

For I.M. or I.V. Use

10 Single-Dose Vials *Hospira*

▲ Figure 13-19

Reconstitution involves careful reading of the medication label or package insert. There will be numbers on the label that may represent the weight of the medication in the vial, the volume of diluent to add, the total volume, and the concentration of the solution or the final yield. It is your responsibility to determine the numbers from the label that you will need to complete your dosage calculation. This requires an understanding of the process of reconstitution.

Summary

This concludes the chapter on the reconstitution of powdered drugs. The important points to remember from this chapter are:

- If the medication label does not contain reconstitution directions, these may be located on the medication package insert.

- The type and amount of diluent to be used for reconstitution must be exactly as specified in the reconstitution instructions.

- If directions are given for both IM and IV reconstitution, be careful to read the correct information for the solution you are preparing. The concentration and volume to be administered will be different if there are directions for both routes.

- A vial may be labeled for one time use or multiple uses. If it is a vial that can be used for multiple uses, it is important to read and follow the storage directions carefully.

- The person who reconstitutes a drug must label the vial with their initials and print the expiration time and date on the label, unless all the drug is used immediately.

- If a solution is prepared using multiple-strength medication directions, the strength reconstituted must also be printed on the label.

- Never assume a volume. Always look for specific directions. The powder will occasionally add to the volume of diluent when it is dissolved. Sometimes the volume will be clearly stated in a concentration (i.e., 100 mg/mL). Sometimes you will be directed to use the total volume, or perhaps the volume of diluent with the total weight of the powder in the vial.

Summary Self-Test

For any dosage calculation questions, please follow the rounding considerations presented earlier in the book—for amounts greater than 1 mL, round to the tenth; for amounts less than 1 mL, round to the hundredth.

Refer to the label in Figure 13-20 to answer the following questions about levothyroxine.

1. What is the route of this medication? _____

2. What volume of diluent will be used to reconstitute this medication? _____

3. What is the final concentration after reconstitution? _____

4. How many times may this vial be used to administer medication? _____

5. How many mL will be administered for a dose of 65 mcg? _____

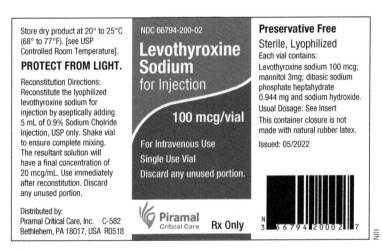

▲ **Figure 13-20**

Refer to the label in Figures 13-21 and 13-22 to answer the following questions about voriconazole.

6. What is the route of this medication? _____

7. What volume of diluent must you add to prepare the solution for use? _____

8. What type of diluent must be used? _____

9. What is the final yield after reconstitution? _____

10. How many mL will be administered for a 150 mg dose? _____

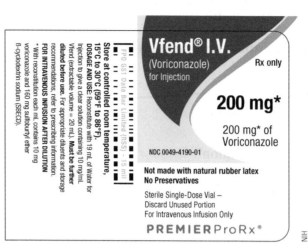

▲ Figure 13-21

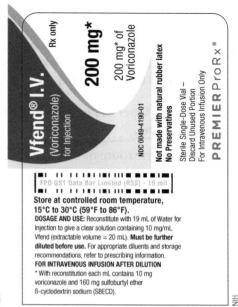

▲ Figure 13-22

Refer to the label in Figure 13-23 to answer the following questions about cefpodoxime.

11. How much diluent is used to reconstitute this medication? _____

12. What type of diluent will be used? _____

13. After reconstitution, how much volume is in the container? _____

14. Where should the reconstituted suspension be stored? _____

15. If the medication is reconstituted for the first dose on October 3, 2024 at 10 a.m., what expiration date must be written on the label? _____

16. How many mL will be administered for a 200 mg oral dose? _____

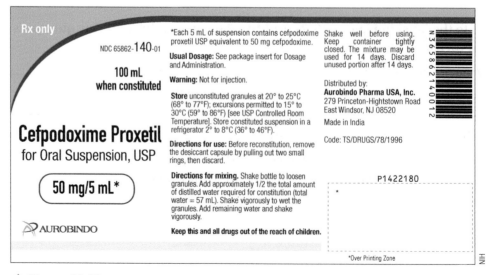

▲ Figure 13-23

Refer to the label in Figures 13-24 and 13-25 to answer the following questions about ampicillin.

17. What are the routes for this medication?   _____

18. How much diluent is required to reconstitute this medication for an IM injection?   _____

19. Where will you find the diluent instructions?   _____

20. What is the strength of each 1 mL of the reconstituted solution?   _____

21. How many mL will be administered for an IM order of 425 mg? _____

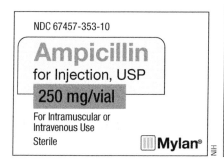

NDC 67457-353-10

Ampicillin
for Injection, USP

250 mg/vial

For Intramuscular or
Intravenous Use
Sterile   ‖‖**Mylan®**

▲ **Figure 13-24**

Each vial contains:
Ampicillin sodium equivalent to Ampicillin 250 mg.
The sodium content is 16.46 mg (0.71 mEq) per 250 mg
of ampicillin.
For IM use, add 1 mL diluent (read accompanying insert).
Resulting solution contains 250 mg ampicillin per mL.
Use solution within 1 hour.
Usual Dosage: Adults - 250 mg to 500 mg IM q. 6h.
READ ACCOMPANYING INSERT for detailed indications,
IM or IV dosage and precautions.
Storage: Store dry powder at 20° to 25°C (68° to 77°F).
[See USP Controlled Room Temperature.]
Protect the constituted solution from freezing.

Manufactured for:
Mylan Institutional LLC
Rockford, IL 61103 U.S.A.
Made in Italy
Code No. : 951030484610

‖‖**Mylan®**
Mylan.com

▲ **Figure 13-25**

Refer to the label in Figure 13-26 to answer the following questions about Penicillin G Potassium.

22. How much diluent will be required to reconstitute this medication for a final yield of 250,000 units per 1 mL?   _____

23. Can this medication be given IM?   _____

24. What must be done after the entire diluent has been added to the vial?   _____

25. What is the final concentration after adding 11.5 mL of diluent?   _____

26. The nurse has added 31.5 mL of diluent to the vial. How many mL of medication will be administered for a 2.5 million units dose IV?   _____

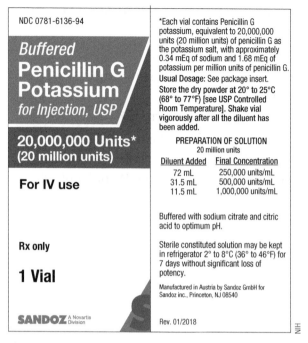

▲ Figure 13-26

Refer to the label in Figure 13-27 to answer the following questions about vancomycin.

27. What is the potency duration after reconstitution?   _____

28. What diluent must be used for reconstitution?   _____

29. How much diluent will be used?   _____

30. What is the final concentration after reconstitution?   _____

31. How many mL will be administered for a 1,000 mg IV dose?   _____

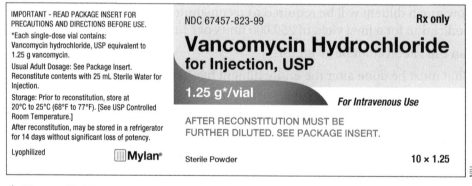

▲ Figure 13-27

Refer to the label in Figure 13-28 and package insert in Figure 13-29 to answer the following questions about cefazolin.

32. What are the routes for cefazolin?   _____

33. What is the IM reconstitution amount for this vial?   _____

34. What is the final yield after reconstitution for the IM injection?   _____

35. For IV administration, what are the complete instructions for dilution, and what total volume will be used?   _____

36. Without refrigeration, how long is the reconstituted solution stable?   _____

37. How many mL will be administered for a 500 mg IM dose?   _____

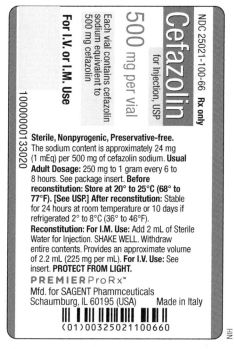

For I.V. or I.M. Use

NDC 25021-100-66 Rx only

Cefazolin
for Injection, USP

500 mg per vial

Each vial contains cefazolin sodium equivalent to 500 mg cefazolin

1000000133020

Sterile, Nonpyrogenic, Preservative-free.
The sodium content is approximately 24 mg (1 mEq) per 500 mg of cefazolin sodium. **Usual Adult Dosage:** 250 mg to 1 gram every 6 to 8 hours. See package insert. **Before reconstitution: Store at 20° to 25°C (68° to 77°F). [See USP.] After reconstitution:** Stable for 24 hours at room temperature or 10 days if refrigerated 2° to 8°C (36° to 46°F). **Reconstitution: For I.M. Use:** Add 2 mL of Sterile Water for Injection. SHAKE WELL. Withdraw entire contents. Provides an approximate volume of 2.2 mL (225 mg per mL). **For I.V. Use:** See insert. **PROTECT FROM LIGHT.**
PREMIERProRx™
Mfd. for SAGENT Phammceuticals
Schaumburg, IL 60195 (USA)   Made in Italy

(01)00325021100660

▲ **Figure 13-28**

Preparation of Parenteral Solution: Parenteral drug products should be SHAKEN WELL when reconstituted, and inspected visually for particulate matter prior to administration. If particulate matter is evident in reconstituted fluids, the drug solutions should be discarded. When reconstituted or diluted according to the instructions below, Cefazolin for Injection is stable for 24 hours at room temperature or for 10 days if stored under refrigeration (5°C or 41°F). Reconstituted solutions may range in color from pale yellow to yellow without a change in potency. Single-Dose Vials: For IM injection, IV direct (bolus) injection or IV infusion, reconstitute with Sterile Water for Injection according to the following table. SHAKE WELL. Discard unused portion.

Vial Size	Amount of diluent	Approximate concentration
500 mg	2 mL	225 mg/1 mL
1 g	2.5 mL	330 mg/1 mL

For Intravenous Administration or Direct (bolus) injection: Follow the reconstitution according to the above table, then further dilute vials with approximately 5 mL Sterile Water for Injection.

▲ **Figure 13-29**

Refer to the label in Figures 13-30 and 13-31 to answer the following questions about ganciclovir.

38. How much diluent is required for this vial?   _____

39. What is the label warning with this drug?   _____

40. How long should the vial be shaken after diluent is added?   _____

41. What should the final concentration be prior to infusion?   _____

42. Once reconstituted, when does the potency expire?   _____

NDC 63323-315-10   315110

GANCICLOVIR
for Injection, USP

500 mg* per vial

For IV Infusion Only

Handle this drug product with great care because it is a potent cytotoxic agent and suspected carcinogen.

25 × 10 mL Vials Rx Only

Sterile, Lyophilized

*Each vial contains: ganciclovir sodium equivalent to 500 mg ganciclovir.

Usual Dosage: See insert for dosage and prescribing information.

Preparation of Solution: Inject 10 mL sterile water for injection, USP, into vial. Shake vial until a clear solution is achieved and use within 12 hours. Dilute a concentration 10 mg or less/mL prior to infusion. See package insert for additional administration instructions.

Store at 20° to 25°C (68° to 77°F) [see USP Controlled Room Temperature].

This container closure is not made with natural rubber latex.

▲ **Figure 13-30**

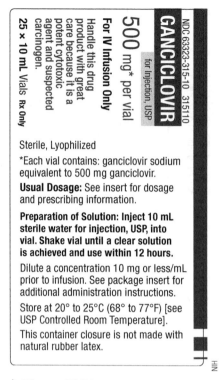

*Each vial contains: ganciclovir sodium equivalent to 500 mg ganciclovir.

Usual Dosage: See insert for dosage and prescribing information.

Preparation of Solution: Inject 10 mL sterile water for injection, USP, into vial. Shake vial until a clear solution is achieved and use within 12 hours.

Dilute a concentration 10 mg or less/mL prior to infusion. See package insert for additional administration instructions.

Store at 20° to 25°C (68° to 77°F) [see USP Controlled Room Temperature].

This container closure is not made with natural rubber latex.

▲ Figure 13-31

Refer to the label in Figure 13-32 to answer the following questions about clarithromycin.

43. What is the total volume of reconstitution solution? _____

44. After reconstitution, how much volume will be in the container? _____

45. What is the final concentration of the solution? _____

46. How is the medication taken in regard to meals? _____

47. How many mL will be administered for a 500 mg dose? _____

Clarithromycin
for Oral Suspension, USP

250 mg* per 5 mL

When reconstituted
*When mixed as directed, each teaspoonful (5 mL) contains 250 mg of clarithromycin in a fruit-punch flavored, aqueous vehicle.

Rx only

50 mL
(when mixed)

SANDOZ

CONSTITUTION INSTRUCTIONS: VOLUME OF WATER 28.5 mL. Measure the required volume of water using a graduated cylinder. Add half the volume of water to the bottle and shake vigorously. Add the remainder of water to the bottle and shake. After mixing store at 20°-25°C (68°-77°F) (see USP Controlled Room Temperature) and use within 14 days. **DO NOT REFRIGERATE.**
Oversize bottle provides shake space.
Usual Dosage: Children - 15 mg/kg/day divided in 2 equal doses. See enclosure for adult dose and full prescribing information. **May be taken before, after or with meals.** Shake well before each use. Store granules at 20°-25°C (68°-77°F) [see USP Controlled Room Temperature]. Keep tightly closed. Contains: Clarithromycin 2.5 g.   Rev. 07-2007
KEEP THIS AND ALL DRUGS OUT OF THE REACH OF CHILDREN.
Manufactured in Romania by Sandoz S.R.L.
Distributed by Sandoz Inc., Princeton,
NJ 08540   328742   0400713

▲ Figure 13-32

Refer to the label in Figure 13-33 and the portion of package insert in Figure 13-34 to answer the following questions about piperacillin/tazobactam.

48. According to the table in the package insert, what is the total diluent for this vial? _____

49. What is the final concentration after reconstitution? _____

50. How many mL will be administered for a 4.5 g dose? _____

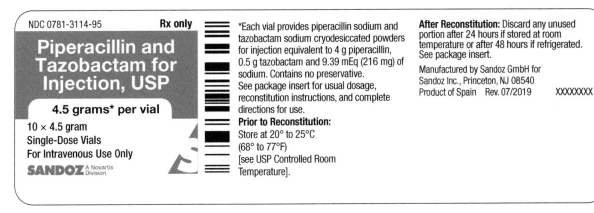

▲ Figure 13-33

Reconstitute vial with a compatible reconstitution diluent, as listed above under the subheading "Compatible Reconstitution Diluents for Single-Dose Vials," using the appropriate volume of diluent, as listed in Table 3 below. Following the addition of the diluent, swirl the single-dose vial until the powder is completely dissolved. Table below: Reconstitution of Single-Dose Vials and Resulting Concentration

Strength of vial	Volume of diluent	Concentration of the Reconstituted Product
2.25 g (2 g piperacillin / 0.25 g tazobactam)	10 mL	202.5 mg/mL (180 mg/mL piperacillin/ 22.5 mg/mL tazobactam)
3.375 g (3 g piperacillin / 0.375 g tazobactam)	15 mL	
4.5 g (4 g piperacillin / 0.5 g tazobactam)	20 mL	

▲ Figure 13-34

Answers to Summary Self-Test
1. IV 2. 5 mL 3. 20 mcg/mL 4. once 5. 3.3 mL 6. IV 7. 19 mL 8. water for injection 9. 10 mg/1 mL
10. 15 mL 11. 57 mL total 12. distilled water 13. 100 mL 14. refrigerator 15. 3/24/2024 at 10am 16. 20 mL
17. IM and IV 18. 1 mL 19. package insert 20. 250 mg 21. 1.7 mL 22. 72 mL 23. No 24. shake vigorously
25. 1,000,000 units/1 mL 26. 5 mL 27. 14 days 28. sterile water 29. 25 mL 30. 1.25 g per 25 mL 31. 20 mL
32. IM and IV 33. 2 mL 34. 225 mg/1 mL 35. 7 mL (2 mL as listed in table, then an additional 5 mL for the IV route)
36. 24 hrs. 37. 2.2 mL 38. 10 mL 39. Handle with care; potent cytotoxic agent. 40. until solution is clear
41. 10 mg or less per 1 mL 42. 12 hrs 43. 28.5 mL 44. 50 mL 45. 250 mg/5 mL 46. before, after, or with meals
47. 10 mL 48. 20 mL 49. 202.5 mg/1 mL 50. 22.2 mL

Insulin

Objectives

The learner will:

1. identify the type of insulin from the label.

2. identify calibrations on 50 units/mL and 100 units/mL insulin syringes.

3. measure single insulin dosages.

4. measure combined insulin dosages.

5. discuss the difference between rapid-, short-, intermediate-, mixed-, and long-acting insulins.

6. discuss insulin injection sites and techniques.

This chapter will introduce you to some of the current insulin preparations available; provide real insulin vial labels to familiarize you with the different insulins; describe the physical appearance of insulins; instruct you in the use of specialized insulin syringes; and provide a step-by-step procedure for the combination of two different insulins in a single syringe, a skill you may use on an ongoing basis throughout your career. We will also describe the process that is used with giving injections using the insulin pen. We will briefly introduce you to insulin action times and injection techniques. This information will be covered in more detail in your nursing courses and pharmacology information. There will also be a brief discussion of noninsulin antidiabetic medications available on the market. Additional information related to insulin can be found in Appendix C.

Clinical Relevance: Insulin is a hormone used to treat diabetes mellitus. This medication has been identified as a high-alert medication by ISMP. As such, it is imperative that special care be used when preparing and administering insulin. Insulin is most commonly supplied as U-100 insulin, meaning there are 100 units per mL. While the order for insulin could be calculated into mL, this practice is not encouraged, and we will not be showing this practice in this book. The accepted practice is to administer U-100 insulin in syringes specially designed for use with this concentration. If a 20-unit dose of U-100 insulin is ordered, we would prepare 20 units in a standard U-100 insulin syringe and no conversion would be needed. Some facilities require two nurses to check the dose of insulin when it is prepared and prior to administration to a client, to prevent medication errors. If an error is made in the administration of insulin, a serious adverse effect can occur. If too much insulin is given, the client may experience low blood sugar; if not enough insulin is given, the client can experience high blood sugar. Both events can be detrimental to the client. It is important to understand the differences between the types of insulin and the practice of administration unique to insulin. This is the only medication that has a specific syringe, which is dedicated for use for insulin preparation and administration.

Types of Insulin and How It Is Supplied

Prior to the 1980s, all insulin was produced from animal sources. Today, most insulins are products of recombinant DNA technology. The two earliest DNA insulins, R (Regular) and N (NPH), are made from recombinant DNA. Both insulins incorporate the suffix -lin in their trade names: Humulin® R and Humulin® N manufactured by the Eli Lilly Co., and Novolin® R and Novolin® N from Novo Nordisk.

Regular insulin is a short-acting clear solution. This is the only insulin that can be given intravenously. NPH insulin is a suspension and is cloudy as the insulin particles are not fully dissolved. This type of insulin will remain cloudy, but there should not be any sedimentation of particles. Mix it thoroughly before use by rotating it in the palm of your hand. It is classified as intermediate-acting, and it has a slower onset but longer action than regular insulin.

Regular and NPH insulin are often combined in a single syringe to reduce the number of injections an individual must have. They may be combined at first to determine an individual's regular (R) and NPH (N) insulin requirements, then ordered in commercially prepared insulin combinations, such as 70/30 and 50/50 mixes, to provide both a fast and more prolonged action. These numbers refer to the percentages of the types of insulin—for example, 70/30 would mean there is 70% NPH and 30% regular insulin combined in each mL of solution. These cannot be separated out; it is how the insulin combination is mixed.

Another type of insulin preparation is the analogs. The analogs are human insulin that have been altered to allow them to be absorbed more quickly. Once again, some of the trade names of these products reflect their origin: the "log" of analog is incorporated in two of the frequently used trade-named insulins: Humalog® and Novolog®. There are also mixtures of these analog insulins. For example, Humalog® 75/25 contains a mix of 75% intermediate insulin and 25% short-acting insulin. Among the analogs whose trade names do not identify their analog structure are Apidra® (insulin glulisine), Lantus® (insulin glargine), and Levemir® (insulin detemir).

Keypoint: The -lin ending of regular and NPH insulin trade names can be used as an additional safeguard in distinguishing them from several of the analogs, which incorporate -log at the end of their trade names. Humulin® insulin is not the same as Humalog® insulin in terms of action and duration.

In addition to injectable insulin, there are also injectable noninsulin medications for people with diabetes. These medications include Byetta® (exenatide), Victoza® (liraglutide), and Trulicity® (dulaglutide). While these medications are not the focus of this chapter, it is important to be aware of these medications and their use in diabetic clients. It is also important to be aware that many of these noninsulin medications are measured in micrograms/mL or milligrams/mL, and not in units.

Insulin is usually an injectable, as it is a hormone. It can be given as a subcutaneous injection, using a syringe. It can also be administered by pen or by pump. Refer to Figure 14-1 for an example of an insulin pump in use.

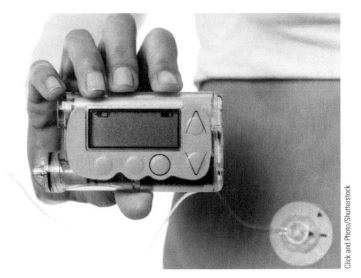

▲ **Figure 14-1** An insulin pump

The insulin pump has a cartridge, which can be filled by the client or can come prefilled for insertion into the pump. The pump is then programmed per physician order and can deliver a constant infusion of insulin, known as a basal rate. It can also be programmed to deliver a bolus dose; an amount delivered right at mealtimes.

Insulin can be given by oral inhalation, as well. This preparation is called Afrezza®. Afrezza® is administered at the beginning of each meal, and it begins to work within 30 minutes. It must be combined with administration of a long-acting subcutaneous insulin. Refer to Figure 14-2 for the components of the inhaler. Refer to Figure 14-3 for its method of use.

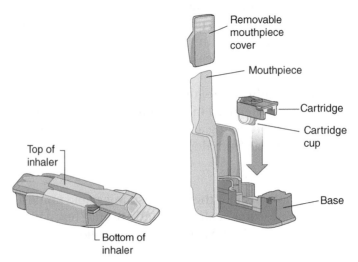

▲ **Figure 14-2** An insulin inhaler closed and one that is open showing the various parts.

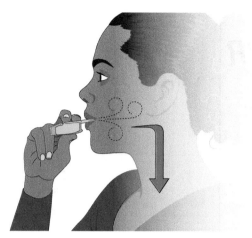

▲ **Figure 14-3** Showing the insulin inhaler in use

Insulin that is given subcutaneously by syringe is usually supplied in a multiple dose vial. Unfortunately, most insulin vials, solutions, and labels appear very similar. It is very easy to confuse the types of insulin. You must always read the label carefully, and identify the characteristics of the medication in the vial or container. Consistently check your medication labels to the order. Do this a minimum of three to four times before you administer the medication and once as you are documenting the medication.

Insulin is a high alert medication. This means that it can cause death or injury to a client. Due to the similarity of vials and the variation of daily doses, especially in hospitalized clients, the risk of error is high. When clients are ill, their insulin requirements will change frequently. Many times, the physician will order insulin based on a sliding scale when the individual is hospitalized. This means that the client's blood sugar will be checked at certain intervals and the client will receive insulin based on the blood sugar. There will be an example of a sliding scale in Appendix C. With a sliding scale, the dose of insulin will vary based on the blood sugar, and the scale must be carefully followed. The classification of insulin as a high alert medication must be taken seriously. Follow all facility protocol with insulin administration and note that any change in dose may need to be confirmed with a colleague.

Like other medications, insulin preparations have both trade and generic names. We will review a few examples of insulin labels. The vials of insulin typically are placed inside a box and the label on the box usually is representative of the label on the vial. Review Figure 14-4 through Figure 14-7.

Notice the labels on these boxes and vials identify the type of insulin with an initial—R for regular insulin and N for NPH insulin. This shows how important it is to read the labels very carefully to ensure you have the proper insulin.

Keypoint: Diligence in the identification of insulin preparations is critical because many vials, solutions, and labels are strikingly similar.

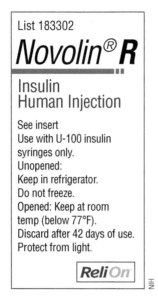

List 183302

Novolin® **R**

Insulin
Human Injection

See insert
Use with U-100 insulin
syringes only.
Unopened:
Keep in refrigerator.
Do not freeze.
Opened: Keep at room
temp (below 77°F).
Discard after 42 days of use.
Protect from light.

ReliOn

NIH

▲ **Figure 14-4**

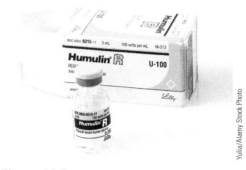

▲ **Figure 14-5**

Yulia/Alamy Stock Photo

List 183411

Novolin® **N**

NPH (isophane
insulin human
suspension)

See insert.
Use with U-100 insulin
syringes only.
To mix, roll gently.
Unopened:
Keep in refrigerator.
Do not freeze.
Opened: Keep at room
temp (below 77°F).
Discard after 42 days of use.
Protect from light.

NSN 6505-01-204-5821

U-100

NIH

▲ **Figure 14-6**

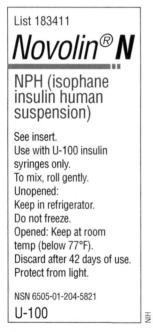

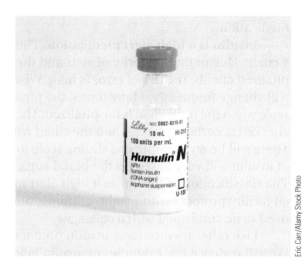

▲ **Figure 14-7**

Eric Carr/Alamy Stock Photo

In addition to vials of insulin, there are insulin pens, which are prefilled self-injection syringes. These pens contain multiple doses of insulin. Refer to Figure 14-8 for an example of an insulin pen.

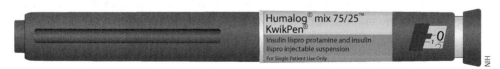

▲ **Figure 14-8**

Figure 14-9 identifies the various parts of the pen. The needle may be separate from the pen cartridge and holder, as shown in this image. The dose knob allows the dose to be adjusted per the individual's needs. The dose that is desired will be set by the individual or the nurse administering it. Then the dose pointer will point to the desired dose in the dose window, allowing the client and/or the nurse to confirm it prior to administration. These pens are labeled as well with the type of insulin contained in the pen. Sometimes it will be only one type, while other times it will be a combination of short- or rapid-acting and intermediate-acting insulins. Pens do not require refrigeration.

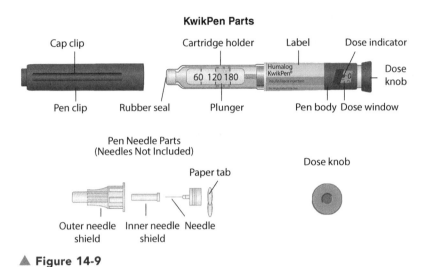

KwikPen Parts

▲ **Figure 14-9**

Pens are used in the clinical setting as well as in the home setting. The nurse must understand how to use the pens in order to teach the clients to use them independently in the home setting. The same label identity checks that are required for other meds are critical prior to administration. Ongoing supervision is essential to determine if a patient, who is being instructed in self-injection, is correctly administering the ordered dosage independently. Pens are prescribed for single client use.

Keypoint: Under no circumstances are insulin pens to be used for anyone other than the patient they are ordered for.

Problems 14.1

Refer to the label in Figure 14-10 to answer the following questions.

1. Where can the Humulin R vial be stored after the first use?   _____

2. How many mL are in this insulin vial?   _____

3. After first opening the vial, when should it be discarded?   _____

4. What routes can this drug be given?   _____

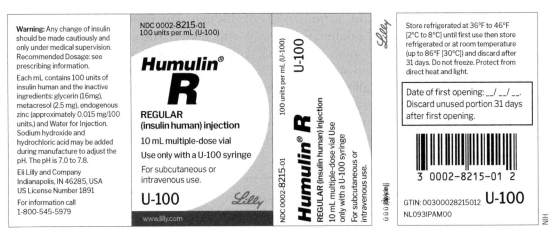

▲ **Figure 14-10**

Refer to the label in Figure 14-11 to answer the following questions.

5. How many insulin pens are in the box?   _____

6. How many mL are in each pen?   _____

7. Where should the pen be stored before the first use?   _____

8. Where should the pen be stored after the first use?   _____

9. When should the pen be discarded?   _____

10. How many units per mL are in this insulin pen?   _____

11. What type of insulin is in this pen?   _____

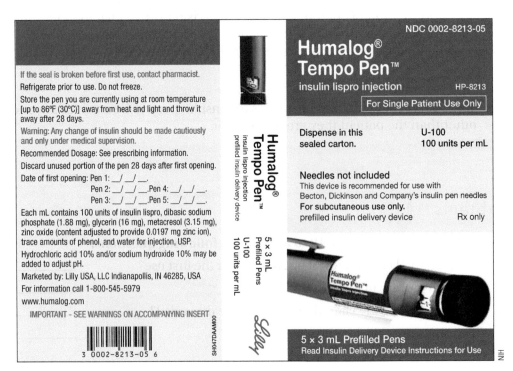

▲ **Figure 14-11**

Refer to the label in Figure 14-12 to answer the following questions.

12. What does the 70 on the label represent? _____

13. What does the 30 identify? _____

14. What company manufactured this insulin? _____

15. How should this vial be mixed? _____

16. Can this medication be administered by IV route? _____

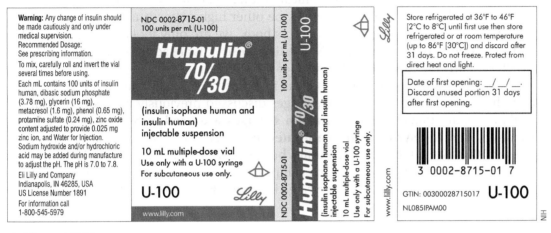

▲ **Figure 14-12**

Refer to the label in Figure 14-13 to answer the following true or false questions.

17. The pen should immediately be put in the freezer. _____

18. The 50/50 stands for a percentage of each type of insulin. _____

19. A needle is already attached to the pen when obtained
from pharmacy. _____

20. This pen can be used without any preparatory action. _____

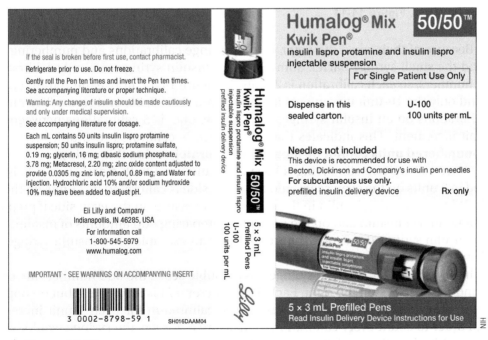

▲ **Figure 14-13**

Insulin Syringes and Sites

Insulin used in medical-surgical clinical settings and for home use have a dosage strength of 100 units per mL. There may be other high-concentration insulins used in critical care areas, but for purposes of this book, we are only looking at insulin with a concentration of 100 units per mL. Notice that these vials are additionally labeled U-100, which similarly identifies the 100 units per mL strength.

Insulin is administered using special insulin syringes calibrated in units. In diameter, these are similar to the 1 mL syringes discussed previously in this book, but the calibrations are totally different. **Insulin syringes are used only for insulin administration, and the syringes are calibrated in units**. These syringes are available in sizes of 100 units, 50 units, and 30 units, but the most common sizes are 100 units and 50 units. Refer to Figure 14-14 for an example of a 100-unit insulin syringe. The calibration associated with the 30 on this syringe indicates 30 units of U-100 insulin.

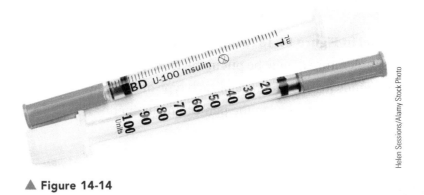

Helen Sessions/Alamy Stock Photo

▲ **Figure 14-14**

Because of their small diameter, insulin syringe calibrations and numbering wrap around the small syringe barrel. Some 100-unit insulin syringes are only calibrated in even numbers, so each calibration is 2 units. In Figure 14-14, notice the 100-unit capacity, and only the 10-unit increments are numbered: 10, 20, 30, and so on. The number of calibrations on an insulin syringe, such as this one, is 5 calibrations between each 10 unit increment. This indicates that the syringe is calibrated in 2-unit increments. **Odd-numbered units cannot be measured accurately using this syringe**.

Other 100-unit insulin syringes have calibrations on both sides—one side is calibrated in 2 units on the even scale, and the other side is calibrated in 2 units on the odd scale. When measuring insulin in these syringes, measure on the even side if preparing even amounts of insulin and on the odd side if preparing odd amounts of insulin. Refer to the insulin syringe drawing in Figure 14-15 for an example of an insulin syringe with odd and even calibrations.

In Figure 14-15, the U-100 syringe has a double scale: the odd numbers are on the left, and the even are on the right. Each 5-unit increment is numbered, but on opposite sides of the syringe. This syringe does have a calibration for each 1-unit increment, but in order to count every calibration to measure a dosage, the syringe would have to be rotated back and forth. This could cause confusion. Therefore, it is best to use the

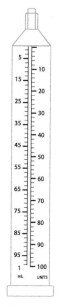

▲ **Figure 14-15**

uneven scale to measure odd-numbered doses, such as 3, 5, 25 units, counting each calibration as 2 units. For even-numbered dosages—such as 6, 10, and 56—use the even scale only, counting each calibration as 2 units. Review the following examples.

Example 1 ▪   To prepare a dosage of 79 units, start at 75 units on the uneven left scale, count the first calibration beyond this as 77 units and the next as 79 units. **Recall that each calibration on the same side measures 2 units**.

Example 2 ▪   To measure a 26-unit dosage, use the even-numbered right-side calibrations. Start at 20 units, move up one calibration to 22 units, another to 24 units, and one more to 26 units. **Recall that each calibration is 2 units**.

The calibrations for the 30- and 50-unit dosage syringes are in 1-unit increments. This makes measurement of small dosages of insulin easier and more accurate. Each 5-unit calibration is numbered 5, 10, 15, etc. The first long calibration on any insulin syringe, as on all other syringes, identifies zero. Figure 14-16 is an example of a 50-unit insulin syringe.

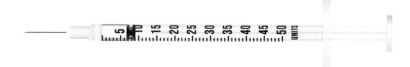

▲ **Figure 14-16** This 50 unit syringe is measuring 7 units.

Insulin is injected subcutaneously. As with other parenteral medications, the injection sites must be rotated, keeping at least an inch away from each previously used site. The most common sites used are the abdomen, posterior upper arm, and the outer side of the upper thigh. There are also subcutaneous sites on the buttocks, but these sites are not readily accessible to most individuals for self-injection. Figure 14-17 illustrates common injection sites.

Insulin injection sites

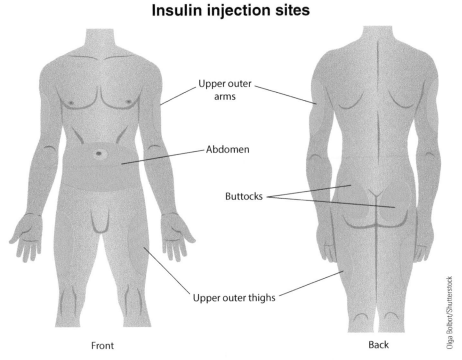

▲ **Figure 14-17** Common subcutaneous injection sites for insulin

The subcutaneous injections will occur either by syringe, or by pen injection. In the hospital setting, regular insulin may be given intravenously if needed for control of blood sugar.

Problems 14.2

Refer to the following 50-unit calibrated syringes and identify the dosages indicated by the arrows.

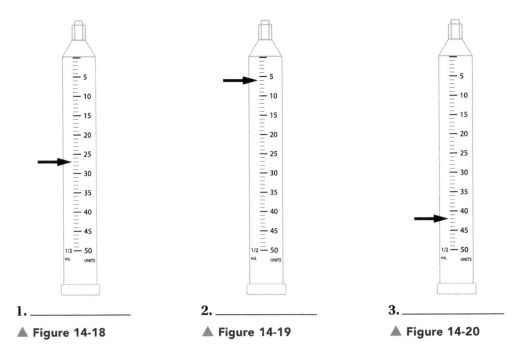

1. _____

▲ **Figure 14-18**

2. _____

▲ **Figure 14-19**

3. _____

▲ **Figure 14-20**

Refer to the following 100-unit calibrated syringes and identify the dosages indicated by the arrows.

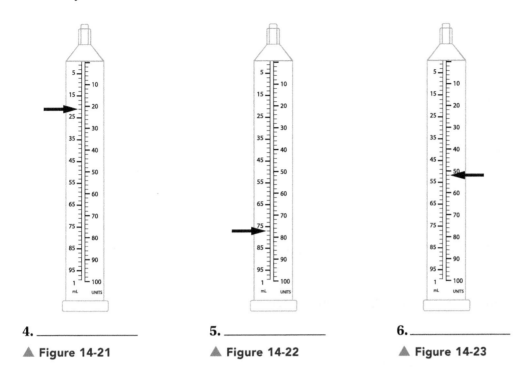

4. _____

▲ **Figure 14-21**

5. _____

▲ **Figure 14-22**

6. _____

▲ **Figure 14-23**

Draw an arrow on the insulin syringe calibrations to indicate the provided dosages.

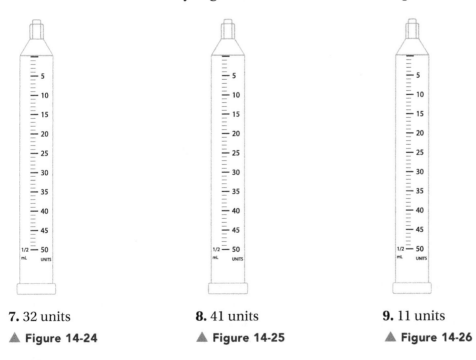

7. 32 units

▲ **Figure 14-24**

8. 41 units

▲ **Figure 14-25**

9. 11 units

▲ **Figure 14-26**

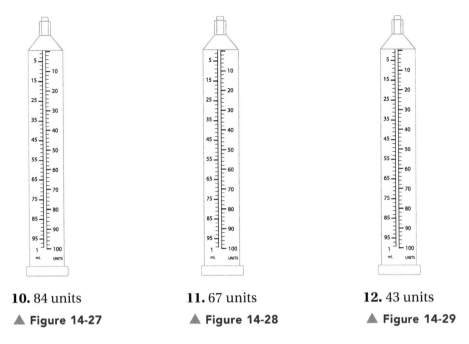

10. 84 units

▲ **Figure 14-27**

11. 67 units

▲ **Figure 14-28**

12. 43 units

▲ **Figure 14-29**

List three common insulin injection sites.

13. _____   **14.** _____   **15.** _____

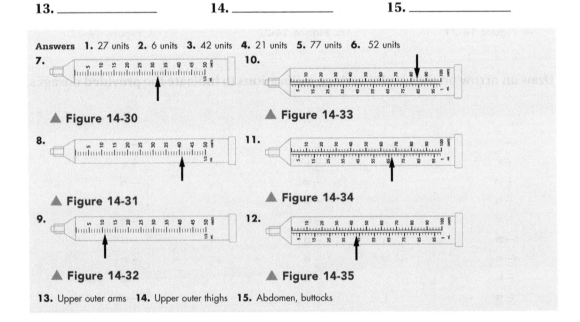

Answers   **1.** 27 units   **2.** 6 units   **3.** 42 units   **4.** 21 units   **5.** 77 units   **6.** 52 units

7.

▲ **Figure 14-30**

8.

▲ **Figure 14-31**

9.

▲ **Figure 14-32**

10.

▲ **Figure 14-33**

11.

▲ **Figure 14-34**

12.

▲ **Figure 14-35**

13. Upper outer arms   **14.** Upper outer thighs   **15.** Abdomen, buttocks

Implications Related to Administration of Insulin

There are some techniques that are specific to insulin therapy. The first technique involves combining two types of insulin in the same syringe. Insulin-dependent individuals may require one or even several subcutaneous injections of insulin per day. To reduce the number of injections an individual needs as much as possible, it is common to combine two insulins in a single syringe: a short-acting R insulin with an intermediate-acting NPH insulin.

Keypoint: When two insulins are combined in the same syringe, the clear R (shortest acting) insulin is drawn up first.

Both insulins will be withdrawn from multiple-dose vials. This requires that an amount of air, equal to the insulin to be withdrawn, be injected into each vial as a preliminary step. This is done to keep the pressure inside the vials equalized after the insulin is withdrawn. An additional step concerns preparation of the insulin itself. Regular insulin, which is clear, does not need to be rotated and mixed. NPH, the most common intermediate-acting insulin used, is cloudy and precipitates out. It must be gently rotated in the palm of your hand to mix.

The smallest volume insulin syringe available is used to measure the dosages ordered, because their larger calibrations provide additional ease and safety in preparing the dose. An example of the actual step-by-step combination procedure follows.

The order is for a dosage of 10 units of R and 28 units of NPH.

Step 1	Locate the correct R and NPH insulin vials. Gently rotate the NPH insulin vial so there are no particles settled out and the solution is consistently cloudy. The clear insulin (R) does not need to be rotated. Use a separate alcohol wipe to cleanse each vial top.
Step 2	Choose the appropriate syringe. The combined dosage, 10 units of R and 28 units of NPH, is 38 units. Use a 50-unit syringe, if available, for ease of preparation.
Step 3	Draw up 28 units of replacement air for the NPH in the syringe and insert the needle tip into the NPH vial. Keep the needle tip above the insulin level so air is not injected into the insulin and no NPH insulin will contaminate the needle. Inject the air and remove the needle.
Step 4	Draw up 10 units of replacement air for the R insulin vial. Insert the needle into the vial, again above the insulin level, and inject the air. Invert the vial, and draw up the 10 units of R insulin. Be very careful to measure the exact amount needed. Remove the needle from the regular insulin vial.

Keypoint: A way to remember which insulin to draw up first is to think **clear before cloudy**. This is in alphabetical order, so clear insulin would be drawn into the syringe before cloudy insulin.

Step 5	Insert the needle into the NPH vial, invert the vial, and draw up exactly 28 units of NPH. Again, be very careful with this process. If you withdraw too much of the NPH, you cannot inject it back into the vial or expel it, as it is now mixed with the regular insulin. If the incorrect amount is withdrawn, you will need to discard everything and begin again.

Keypoint: If, at any time, sterility is compromised, you must again cleanse each vial with an alcohol wipe and obtain all new supplies.

Step 6	Administer the insulin dosage at once so that the NPH has no chance to precipitate out. Chart the administration, including the site where it was administered.

Another procedure for insulin administration that is becoming more common is administration of insulin using the insulin pen. The nurse will administer the insulin pen, but the nurse will also need to understand the step-by-step instructions so the client can be taught to self-administer insulin with the pen. The following are the step-by-step instructions for administration with an insulin pen. When reviewing these steps, please refer back to Figure 14-9 to review the parts of an insulin pen.

Step 1	Obtain the pen and read the label to ensure you have the correct type of insulin as ordered. Remove the cap from the pen.
Step 2	If the insulin in the pen is cloudy, you must prepare the pen according to package directions. Not all instructions for preparation of an insulin pen are the same; you must read the information very carefully. This may require gentle inversion of the pen up and down for 10 to 20 times or for a specified period per the package insert. It may also involve rolling the pen to mix the insulin.
Step 3	Cleanse the rubber seal with an alcohol swab. Attach the needle.
Step 4	Turn the dose knob so that the dose in the dose window shows 2 units. These 2 units will be given as an air shot to prime the needle and ensure the air is removed prior to injecting the ordered dose. The air shot can usually be performed without removing the needle caps. The dose in the dose window should return to 0 and you should see a drop of liquid at the tip of the needle. This shows the needle has been adequately primed. Refer to Figure 14-36.

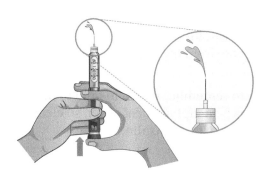

▲ **Figure 14-36**

Step 5	Now, turn the dose knob so that the dose ordered is showing in the dose window. This will be the amount you administer to the client.
Step 6	Remove the needle shields. There may be an outer and an inner needle shield to remove, depending on the manufacturer of the needle.
Step 7	Administer the injection by pushing down on the dose knob. The dose in the dose window should return to 0 (zero). It is important to keep the needle in the skin with the dose knob depressed for at least 6 seconds. This ensures the full dose was administered. Refer to Figure 14-37 for an example of an injection into the abdomen.

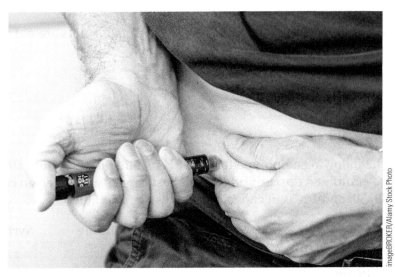

imageBROKER/Alamy Stock Photo

▲ **Figure 14-37**

| Step 8 | Remove the needle and discard it in the sharps container. Replace the cap on the pen. |

Another important consideration with insulin administration is the timing of the insulin dose and consideration of the onset of action, peak, and duration of the insulin being administered. The onset of action is especially important to consider in relation to mealtimes.

Insulin is classified by action as rapid, short, intermediate, or long acting. There is also a combination group where two different types of insulins are premixed by the manufacturer in a vial or insulin pen. Appendix C will include a chart with the various types of insulins and their general onset, peak, and duration. The rapid-acting insulins will have an onset of action within 15 minutes, a peak of 1–2 hours, and a duration of 3–4 hours. Administration of a rapid-acting insulin must be followed immediately by a meal. Failure to immediately ingest food would result in a rapidly lowered blood glucose level and hypoglycemia.

The group of combination insulins have an onset of 15–30 minutes. The peaks vary, but the duration is 24 hours. Due to the onset of 15–30 minutes for the combination group, a meal must be provided immediately.

In comparison, the **short-acting** insulins have an onset of 30–60 minutes, a peak of 2–4 hours, and a duration of 5–7 hours. These also require that the individual **eat immediately after administration** as well.

Keypoint: Rapid-acting insulins, short-acting insulins, and combination insulins must be followed immediately by a meal.

The **intermediate-acting** insulins are moving into the longer action range, with an onset of 2–4 hours, a peak of 4–10 hours, and duration of 10–16 hours. The **long-acting** insulins are in a group that do not share the same onset, peak, and duration. Refer to Appendix C for details. Both intermediate-acting and long-acting insulin administration is unrelated to dietary intake.

Keypoint: Long-acting and intermediate-acting insulins are not administered in relation to immediate food ingestion.

Problems 14.3

For each of the following combined R and NPH insulin dosages, indicate the total volume of the combined dosage and the smallest capacity syringe you can use to prepare it; 30, 50, and 100 unit capacity syringes are available.

	Total Volume	Syringe Size
1. 28 units R, 64 units NPH	_____	_____
2. 6 units R, 16 units NPH	_____	_____
3. 33 units R, 41 units NPH	_____	_____
4. 21 units R, 52 units NPH	_____	_____
5. 13 units R, 27 units NPH	_____	_____

Refer to Figure 14-38 and identify the parts of the insulin pen.

6. _____   8. _____

7. _____   9. _____

60 120 180

Humalog
KwikPen®
Insulin lispro injection
For Single Patient Use Only

9

6

7

8

▲ **Figure 14-38**

Answers 1. 92 units; 100 unit **2.** 22 units; 30 unit **3.** 74 units; 100 unit **4.** 73 units; 100 unit **5.** 40 units; 50 unit **6.** rubber seal **7.** label **8.** dose window/indicator **9.** dose knob

Summary

This concludes the chapter on insulin dosages. The important points to remember from this chapter are:

- Insulin labels must be read with extreme care because they look very similar.

- Insulin is measured using specially calibrated insulin syringes.

- Insulin syringes are available in capacities of 100, 50, and 30 units.

- The smaller 30- or 50-unit capacity syringes provide a greater degree of safety because of their larger calibrations.

- Each calibration on 30- and 50-unit volume syringes measures 1 unit.

▨ Calibrations on 100-unit capacity insulin syringes may measure 1- or 2-unit increments, depending on their design.

▨ Regular (R) and NPH (N) insulin can be mixed in a single syringe. Regular insulin would be drawn up first when combining these in a single syringe.

▨ Insulins that are cloudy must be gently and thoroughly mixed. They contain insoluble particles, so they will never be clear, but should be uniformly cloudy with no sedimentation of particles.

▨ Insulin is administered subcutaneously, and sites are routinely rotated.

▨ Insulin pens are used in both the clinical and home settings. Clients who are prescribed insulin pens must be taught the specific steps for preparation and administration.

▨ The administration of insulin requires knowledge of onset, peak and duration information of the various types of insulin.

Summary Self-Test

Refer to the labels in Figures 14-39 and 14-40 to answer the following questions.

1. What is the generic name of this medication?   _____

2. How many mg does each pen deliver?   _____

3. How often will a client take this medication?   _____

4. How many mL are in each pen?   _____

5. Can trulicity be stored in the freezer?   _____

6. What should be done with each pen after use?   _____

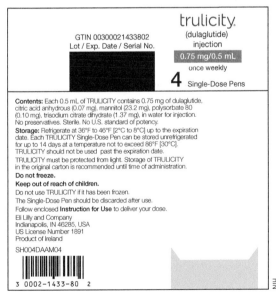

▲ **Figure 14-39**

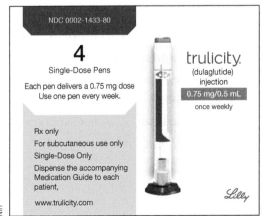

▲ **Figure 14-40**

Refer to the label in Figure 14-41 to answer the following questions.

7. What is the brand name of this medication?   _____

8. How many medications are in this pen?   _____

9. Each mL contains how many mg of liraglutide?   _____

10. Each mL contains how many units of insulin degludec?   _____

11. When should each pen be discarded?   _____

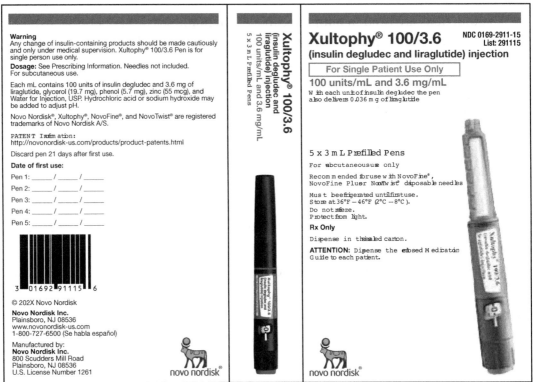

▲ **Figure 14-41**

Refer to the label in Figure 14-42 to answer the following questions.

12. What pharmaceutical company produces this drug?   _____

13. Where should unopened containers be stored?   _____

14. The medication should be used within how many days
    after opening?   _____

15. What is the insulin name of this drug?   _____

16. How many units/mL are in each pen?   _____

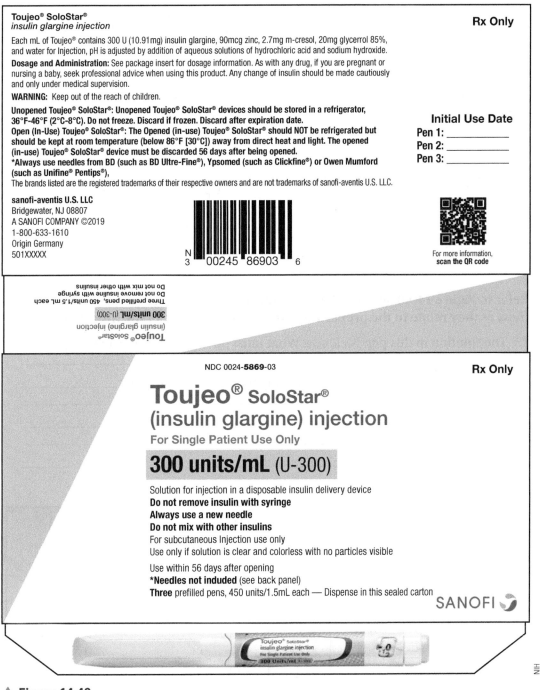

▲ Figure 14-42

Refer to the following 50- and 100-unit calibrated syringes and identify the dosages indicated by the arrows.

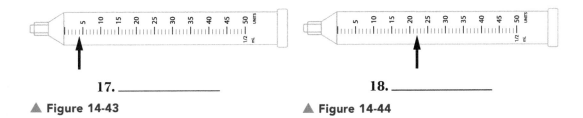

17. _____   18. _____

▲ Figure 14-43   ▲ Figure 14-44

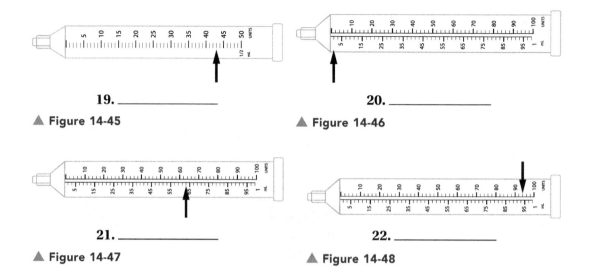

19. _____

▲ Figure 14-45

20. _____

▲ Figure 14-46

21. _____

▲ Figure 14-47

22. _____

▲ Figure 14-48

Refer to Figure 14-49 and the chapter information to answer the following questions as they relate to the preparation and administration of the insulin pen.

23. The solution in this pen is cloudy. What must be done prior to using the pen?

_____

24. What must be done first before attaching the needle to the pen? _____

_____

25. How will this pen be primed? Be specific. _____

_____

26. How long should this pen be refrigerated? _____

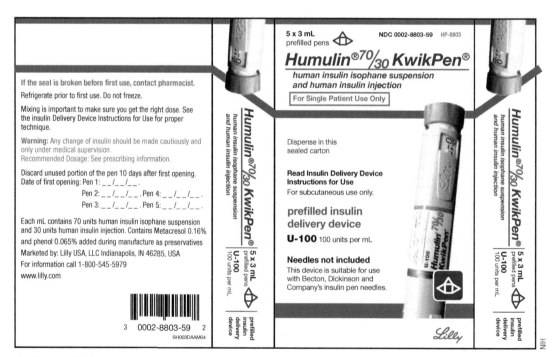

▲ Figure 14-49

Critical Thinking Questions

Refer to the label in Figure 14-50 and chapter information to answer the following questions.

1. A client is ordered Afrezza® to treat diabetes mellitus. Afrezza is an inhaler and the nurse must instruct the patient on the use of this device. Choose the following information from the label and chapter that will be included in the client education. Select all that apply.

    a. Once opened for first use, the inhaler must be discarded after 15 days.
    b. The cartridges may be placed in the refrigerator at any time.
    c. Open the cartridge and place it in the inhaler.
    d. Before use, the cartridge must be at room temp for 10 minutes.
    e. The inhaler will be used at the beginning of each meal.
    f. No other insulin should be used with Afrezza®.

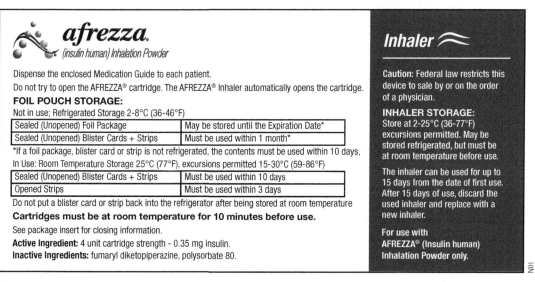

▲ Figure 14-50

2. A physician has ordered 15 units of regular insulin and 38 units of NPH insulin at 8 am. The nurse has obtained the R and NPH vials, and a 100-unit syringe to prepare the insulins. Identify the order of steps, 1 through 8, the nurse must take to accurately prepare the mixture of two insulins.

_____	Inject 15 units of air into the R insulin vial.
_____	Select an approved injection site.
_____	Gently rotate the NPH vial.
_____	Inject 38 units of air into the NPH insulin vial.
_____	Draw up the 38 units of NPH insulin.
_____	Draw up the 15 units of R insulin.
_____	Administer the insulin.
_____	Clean the vial tops with alcohol wipes.

Refer to the label in Figure 14-51 to answer the following questions.

3. The physician has ordered a 34-year-old female client 12 units of Apidra®, a rapid-acting insulin. The nurse is reading the label. Based on the label and chapter information, the nurse should be aware of what relevant information prior to preparing and administering this insulin? Select all that apply.

a. This box contains an insulin pen.
b. If refrigeration is not possible, the container must be discarded.
c. This medication can only be given as a subcutaneous injection.
d. This container is single dosed.
e. Ask the client if she is pregnant.
f. A meal should be available immediately.

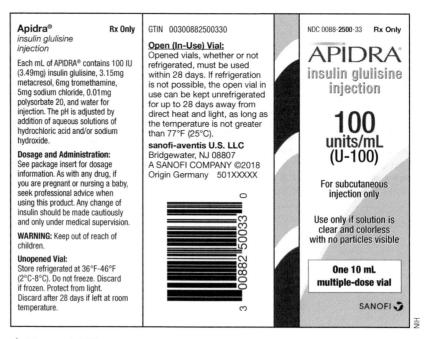

▲ **Figure 14-51**

Answers to Critical Thinking Questions

1. a, d, e. Rationale: a and d are correct per label information, e is correct per chapter information. b is incorrect—once cartridges have been stored at room temperature, they may not be placed in the refrigerator; c is incorrect—the user does not open the cartridge; the inhaler opens the cartridge once it is placed in the inhaler; f is incorrect—Afrezza® must be used with a long-acting insulin (per the chapter information).

2.

4	Inject 15 units of air into the Regular insulin vial.
7	Select an approved injection site.
1	Gently rotate the NPH vial until mixed.
3	Inject 38 units of air into the NPH insulin vial.
6	Draw up the 38 units of NPH insulin.
5	Draw up the 15 units of Regular insulin.
8	Administer the insulin.
2	Clean the vial tops with alcohol wipes.

3. c, e, f. Rationale: c and e are correct per medication label; f is correct per chapter information. a is incorrect—this box contains a vial; b is incorrect—the vial may be kept unrefrigerated for 28 days; d is incorrect—the vial is a multidose vial.

Adult and Pediatric Calculations; Including Body Weight and Body Surface Area

15

Dosages Based on Body Weight

Objectives

The learner will:

1. convert body weight from lb to kg.

2. convert body weight from kg to lb.

3. calculate dosages using mcg or mg per kg, or per lb.

4. determine if dosages ordered are within the dosage range specified by the drug label or drug literature.

Body weight is a major factor in calculating drug dosages for both adults and children. Medications, such as pain medications, antibiotics, and chemotherapy medications may be ordered by body weight. Groups of medications that are used by adults and children use body weight to help individualize the dose and make it safe for the various age groups. Drugs affect children differently from adults due to continued growth, development, and immaturity of various body organs, such as the kidneys and the liver. It is not within the scope of this book to address all the differences in the effects of drugs in children. However, as a general introduction to differences in dosing, it is important to realize that body weight is an important consideration. Body weight is also an important consideration for dosing in some adults, and especially with particular groups of medication. The dosage that will produce optimum therapeutic results for a particular individual, either child or adult, depends not only on dosage, but also on individual variables, including drug sensitivities and tolerance, age, weight, sex, and metabolic, pathologic, or psychologic conditions.

The prescriber will order the drug and dosage. However, it is a nursing responsibility to check each dosage to be sure the order is correct. Each drug label or drug package insert provides specific dosage details, but more information is readily available in drug guides and other medical references on the clinical units. The clinical pharmacist in both inpatient and outpatient settings is also a valuable resource for information.

Individualized dosages may be calculated in terms of mcg per kg or lb; or mg per kg or lb. These calculations may be per dose or per day, so it is extremely important to read the dosing information very carefully. When calculating, make sure you label whether the information is per dose or per day in your end result. If the dose is calculated per day, the total daily dosage may be administered in divided (more than one) dosages. For example, the daily dose may be administered in divided doses every 6 hours or every 8 hours. It is important to be clear how many doses each of these represent. For example, if a daily dose of a medication is divided into doses every 4 hours, then the patient would be receiving 6 doses per day. If the daily dose is divided into doses every 6 hours, then the patient would receive 4 doses a day. If divided into doses every 8 hours, then the patient would receive 3 doses a day.

Because body weight is critical in calculating infant and neonatal dosages, measurement is usually done using a weight scale calibrated in kg. Adult weights may be recorded in either kg or lb; occasionally, conversions between these two measures are necessary.

Clinical Relevance: Dosing of some medications in adults and children is based on body weight. Many times, in the United States, the weight is measured in pounds; however, the dosing may be based on weight in kilograms. It is necessary to be able to convert from pounds to kilograms or from kilograms to pounds. This creates an additional step in which errors can occur. It is important to remember the conversion needed is 2.2 pounds is equivalent to 1 kilogram. Understanding this conversion can help you determine if your calculation is accurate. If we realize that a person's weight in kilograms is approximately half of their weight in pounds, then we can convert and evaluate that number to determine if it makes sense. For example, if a person weighs 120 pounds and we get an answer of 264 kilograms, we should be able to recognize that our calculation is incorrect and should be prompted to recalculate. This critical thinking, while it may seem minor, is very important and can help prevent serious errors. We also must ensure we are reading usual dosing requirements for medications accurately. If the medication label doesn't give adequate information, then we need to remember to look at other drug literature for the information needed to calculate accurate dosages for our patients.

Weight Conversions

It is important to read the order, drug label, or drug literature very carefully to determine if dosing is based on kg or lb for body weight. If body weight is recorded in lb, but the medication information lists dosage per kg, then a conversion from lb to kg will be necessary. Recall that 1 kg can be converted to 2.2 lb. This conversion information means that body weights in kg are a smaller number than body weights in lb.

To convert from lb to kg, divide body weight in pounds by 2.2. You can also use any of the three methods of calculation presented in Chapters 8 through 10. For ease of calculation, fractional pounds may be converted to the nearest quarter and written as decimal fractions instead of oz: ¼ lb (4 oz) as 0.25, ½ lb (8 oz) as 0.5, and ¾ lb (12 oz) as 0.75. If accuracy is more critical and rounding of ounces is not recommended, then the medication information should identify that accuracy is critical and rounding of ounces to the nearest quarter pound should not occur. For purposes of the calculations in this chapter, we will round all weights to the tenth.

 Keypoint: The conversion factor needed for weight conversions is 2.2 pounds is equal to 1 kilogram. When converting, the result will be rounded to the nearest tenth.

The following example includes the three methods of calculation for you to understand a systematic way of converting. However, you can also convert pounds to kilograms by dividing body weight by 2.2.

Example 1 ■   Convert the weight of a 144½ lb adult to kg.

Method 1: Ratio and Proportion

In Colon Format

2.2 lb : 1 kg = 144.5 lb : x kg

2.2x = 144.5

$x = \dfrac{144.5}{2.2} = 65.68 = 65.7$ kg

In Fraction Format

$\dfrac{2.2\ \text{lb}}{1\ \text{kg}} = \dfrac{144.5\ \text{lb}}{x\ \text{kg}}$

2.2x = 144.5

$x = \dfrac{144.5}{2.2} = 65.68 = 65.7$ kg

Method 2: Dimensional Analysis

$$\text{kg} = \dfrac{1\ \text{kg}}{2.2\ \text{lb}} \times \dfrac{144.5\ \text{lb}}{}$$

$$\text{kg} = \dfrac{1\ \text{kg}}{2.2\ \cancel{\text{lb}}} \times \dfrac{144.5\ \cancel{\text{lb}}}{}$$

$$\text{kg} = \dfrac{144.5}{2.2} = 65.68 = 65.7\ \text{kg}$$

Method 3: Formula Method

$$\dfrac{144.5\ \text{lb (D)} \times 1\ \text{kg (Q)}}{2.2\ \text{lb (H)}} = x\ \text{kg}$$

$$\dfrac{144.5\,\cancel{\text{lb}} \times 1\ \text{kg}}{2.2\,\cancel{\text{lb}}} = x\ \text{kg}$$

$$\dfrac{144.5 \times 1}{2.2} = 65.68 = 65.7\ \text{kg}$$

These calculations make logical sense, as we know that the weight in kilograms should be about half of the weight in pounds. Therefore, an answer of 65.7 kg is logical based on the weight of 144.5 lb.

In the following example, to convert to kilograms, divide pounds by 2.2. To ensure that the correct calculation is performed, label numbers with the unit of measure.

Example 2 ■   A child weighs 41 lb 12 oz. Convert to kg.

$$41\ \text{lb}\ 12\ \text{oz} = \dfrac{41.75\,\cancel{\text{lb}}}{2.2\,\cancel{\text{lb}}} = 18.97 = 19\ \text{kg}$$

The kg weight should be a smaller number than 41.75 because you are dividing. We can also estimate that the weight in kilograms will be about half the weight in pounds. 19 kg is smaller, and it is about half of 41.75.

Although it does not occur frequently, there will be times you might have to change kilograms to pounds. The same conversion will be used: 2.2 lb = 1 kg. Pounds will be a larger number and will be approximately twice the number of kilograms. Conversions from kilograms to pounds will be accomplished by multiplying weight in kilograms by 2.2.

The following example uses all three methods of calculation. However, you can also convert kilograms to pounds by multiplying by 2.2.

Example 3 ■   A child weighs 23.3 kg. Convert to lb.

Method 1: Ratio and Proportion

In Colon Format

$1\,\text{kg} : 2.2\,\text{lb} = 23.3\,\text{kg} : x\,\text{lb}$

$x = 51.26 = 51.3\,\text{lb}$

In Fraction Format

$$\frac{1\,\text{kg}}{2.2\,\text{lb}} = \frac{23.3\,\text{kg}}{x\,\text{lb}}$$

$x = 23.3 \times 2.2$

$x = 51.26 = 51.3\,\text{lb}$

Method 2: Dimensional Analysis

$$\text{lb} = \frac{2.2\,\text{lb}}{1\,\text{kg}} \times \frac{23.3\,\text{kg}}{}$$

$$\text{lb} = \frac{2.2\,\text{lb}}{1\,\cancel{\text{kg}}} \times \frac{23.3\,\cancel{\text{kg}}}{}$$

$$\text{lb} = 51.26 = 51.3\,\text{lb}$$

Method 3: Formula Method

$$\frac{23.3\,\text{kg (D)} \times 2.2\,\text{lb (Q)}}{1\,\text{kg (H)}} = x\,\text{lb}$$

$$\frac{23.3\,\cancel{\text{kg}} \times 2.2\,\text{lb}}{1\,\cancel{\text{kg}}} = 51.26 = 51.3\,\text{lb}$$

These calculations make logical sense, as we know that the weight in pounds should be about twice the weight in kilograms. Therefore, 51.3 lb is logical based on the weight of 23.3 kg.

In the following example, convert kilograms to pounds by multiplying the kilograms by 2.2. To ensure that the correct calculation is performed, label numbers with the unit of measure.

Example 4 ■   Convert an adult weight of 73.4 kg to lb.

$$73.4\,\text{kg} = \frac{73.4\,\cancel{\text{kg}}}{1\,\cancel{\text{kg}}} \times 2.2\,\text{lb} = 161.48 = 161.5\,\text{lb}$$

The lb weight should be a larger number than 73.4 because you are multiplying. We can also estimate that the weight in pounds will be about twice the weight in kilograms: 161.5 lb is larger and it is about twice the amount of 73.4 kg.

Problems 15.1

Convert the following body weights from lb to kg. Round to the nearest tenth.

1. $58\frac{3}{4}$ lb = _____ kg
2. $63\frac{1}{2}$ lb = _____ kg
3. $163\frac{1}{4}$ lb = _____ kg
4. $39\frac{3}{4}$ lb = _____ kg
5. $100\frac{1}{4}$ lb = _____ kg
6. $134\frac{1}{2}$ lb = _____ kg
7. $112\frac{3}{4}$ lb = _____ kg
8. $73\frac{1}{4}$ lb = _____ kg
9. $121\frac{1}{2}$ lb = _____ kg
10. $92\frac{3}{4}$ lb = _____ kg

Convert the following body weights from kg to lb. Round to the nearest tenth.

11. 21.3 kg = _____ lb   16. 43.7 kg = _____ lb

12. 99.2 kg = _____ lb   17. 63.8 kg = _____ lb

13. 28.7 kg = _____ lb   18. 57.1 kg = _____ lb

14. 71.4 kg = _____ lb   19. 84.2 kg = _____ lb

15. 30.8 kg = _____ lb   20. 34.9 kg = _____ lb

Answers 1. 26.7 kg **2.** 28.9 kg **3.** 74.2 kg **4.** 18.1 kg **5.** 45.6 kg **6.** 61.1 kg **7.** 51.3 kg **8.** 33.3 kg
9. 55.2 kg **10.** 42.2 kg **11.** 46.9 lb **12.** 218.2 lb **13.** 63.1 lb **14.** 157.1 lb **15.** 67.8 lb **16.** 96.1 lb
17. 140.4 lb **18.** 125.6 lb **19.** 185.2 lb **20.** 76.8 lb

---

Calculation of Dosages Based on Weight

The information you will need to calculate dosages based on body weight will be located on the actual drug label or on the drug package insert. Sometimes, the prescriber will order the medication by body weight as well. Read the information very carefully. Directions to administer 40 mg/kg every 6 hours does not mean the same thing as 40 mg/kg/day in divided doses every 6 hours.

Let's examine these two statements. Administer 40 mg/kg every 6 hours would lead to a calculation of mg per dose. The direction to administer 40 mg/kg/day in divided doses every 6 hours would lead to a calculation of the daily dose, which would then be divided by 4 doses (the number of doses per day) when given every 6 hours. If we are calculating each dose, then the answer we obtain would be the amount of medication to be given for each dose. If we are calculating the daily dose to be divided through-out the day, then it becomes a two-step procedure. First, the total daily dosage is calculated. Then it is divided by the number of doses per day to obtain the actual dose administered at one time.

The following example refers to a label that contains a usual dosage written with mg/kg/day dosage guidelines.

Example 1 ■   Refer to the information written on the left of the Cefaclor label in
                                Figure 15-1 for children's dosages. Notice that the dosage is 20
                                mg/kg/day (or 40 mg/kg/day in otitis media). This daily dosage is
                                to be given in divided doses every 8 hours—or a total of three doses
                                (24 hr ÷ 8 hr = 3 doses).

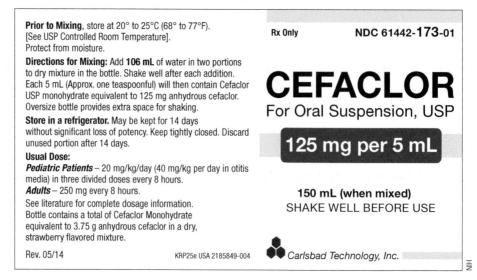

Prior to Mixing, store at 20° to 25°C (68° to 77°F).
[See USP Controlled Room Temperature].
Protect from moisture.

Directions for Mixing: Add **106 mL** of water in two portions to dry mixture in the bottle. Shake well after each addition. Each 5 mL (Approx. one teaspoonful) will then contain Cefaclor USP monohydrate equivalent to 125 mg anhydrous cefaclor. Oversize bottle provides extra space for shaking.

Store in a refrigerator. May be kept for 14 days without significant loss of potency. Keep tightly closed. Discard unused portion after 14 days.

Usual Dose:
Pediatric Patients – 20 mg/kg/day (40 mg/kg per day in otitis media) in three divided doses every 8 hours.
Adults – 250 mg every 8 hours.
See literature for complete dosage information.
Bottle contains a total of Cefaclor Monohydrate equivalent to 3.75 g anhydrous cefaclor in a dry, strawberry flavored mixture.

Rev. 05/14   KRP25e USA 2185849-004

Rx Only   NDC 61442-**173**-01

CEFACLOR
For Oral Suspension, USP

125 mg per 5 mL

150 mL (when mixed)
SHAKE WELL BEFORE USE

♦♦ *Carlsbad Technology, Inc.*

▲ **Figure 15-1**

Once you have located the dosage information, you can calculate the dosage. Let's assume the child you are caring for has otitis media and weighs 40 pounds. The physician indicates the order for the antibiotic should follow the weight-based recommendations on the label.

The first step is to convert the weight to kilograms so the usual dosage can be calculated. The weight in kilograms will be approximately half the weight in pounds; therefore, we divide. Remember, you can also use any method of calculation. Since 2.2 pounds equals 1 kilogram, divide 40 by 2.2.

$$\frac{40 \text{ lb}}{2.2 \text{ lb}} = 18.18 = 18.2 \text{ kg}$$

Once you have the weight of the child, you can calculate the recommended daily dosage from the information on the label. Daily dosage for a child with otitis media equals 40 mg/kg/day.

$$\frac{40 \text{ mg}}{1 \text{ kg}} \times 18.2 \text{ kg} = 728 \text{ mg/day}$$

The recommended dose for this 18.2 kg child with otitis media is 728 mg/day.

Next, calculate how many milligrams the child will receive per dose. For consistency, when calculating, round milligrams to the whole number. The information on the label states the medication is to be given in three divided doses. Therefore, take the calculated dose of 728 mg/day and divide it by 3 doses.

$$728 \text{ mg/day} \div 3 \text{ doses} = 242.66 = 243 \text{ mg per dose}$$

Once you have the recommended dosage for this child, you can follow through with the physician orders. Using the label of the medication, calculate the volume of medication to be administered. Again, you can use any of the three methods of calculation.

Method 1: Ratio and Proportion

In Colon Format	*In Fraction Format*
125 mg : 5 mL = 243 mg : x mL	$\dfrac{125 \text{ mg}}{5 \text{ mL}} = \dfrac{243 \text{ mg}}{x \text{ mL}}$
$125x = 5 \times 243$	$125x = 5 \times 243$
$125x = 1{,}215$	$125x = 1{,}215$
$x = \dfrac{1{,}215}{125} = 9.72 = 9.7 \text{ mL}$	$x = \dfrac{1{,}215}{125} = 9.72 = 9.7 \text{ mL}$

Method 2: Dimensional Analysis

$$\text{mL} = \frac{5 \text{ mL}}{125 \text{ mg}} \times \frac{243 \text{ mg}}{}$$

$$\text{mL} = \frac{5 \text{ mL}}{125 \text{ mg}} \times \frac{243 \text{ mg}}{}$$

$$\text{mL} = \frac{1{,}215}{125} = 9.72 = 9.7 \text{ mL}$$

Method 3: Formula Method

$$\frac{243 \text{ mg (D)} \times 5 \text{ mL (Q)}}{125 \text{ mg (H)}} = x \text{ mL}$$

$$\frac{243 \text{ mg} \times 5 \text{ mL}}{125 \text{ mg}} = x \text{ mL}$$

$$\frac{243 \times 5}{125} = \frac{1{,}215}{125} = 9.72 = 9.7 \text{ mL}$$

Since the physician based the medication order on the label recommendations, you would administer 9.7 mL of cefaclor to the child.

Example 2 ■   Refer to the EryPed label in Figure 15-2.

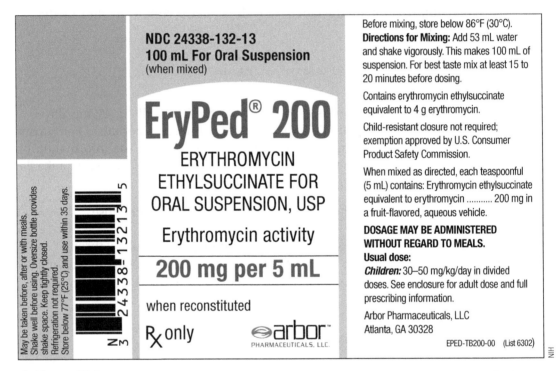

▲ **Figure 15-2**

On this label, notice that the recommended dosage is a range of 30–50 mg/kg/day in divided doses. When there is a range for the recommended dosage, both the lower and the upper number in that range must be calculated. In this example, the patient weighs 55 pounds. The physician has ordered a dose of 300 mg every 6 hours. To determine if this dose is safe, you must compare it to the range that is recommended.

The first step is to convert the weight to kilograms. Since 2.2 pounds equals 1 kg, divide pounds by 2.2 to determine kilograms.

$$\frac{55}{2.2} = 25 \text{ kilograms}$$

Next, calculate the recommended dosage based on the label. You will need to calculate the lower end, or minimum, as well as the upper end, or maximum, number in the range.

$$\frac{30 \text{ mg}}{1 \text{ kg}} \times 25 \text{ kg} = 750 \text{ mg/day}$$

$$\frac{50 \text{ mg}}{1 \text{ kg}} \times 25 \text{ kg} = 1{,}250 \text{ mg/day}$$

You have calculated the minimum dose to be 750 mg/day in divided doses and the maximum dose to be 1,250 mg/day in divided doses. The label does not indicate the intervals for the divided doses, so consult a drug reference to find the recommended frequency. However, based on the information available, you can now determine the safety of the physician's order as it compares to the recommended range.

The doctor has ordered 300 mg every 6 hours. This means the patient will receive 4 doses in a 24-hour period. Therefore, the patient will receive a total of 1,200 mg/day. Compared to the recommended range, this result falls within the range of 750 mg/day to 1,250 mg/day, meaning the ordered dose is safe. You can now determine the volume of medication the patient should receive based on the label. The patient would receive 7.5 mL of the medication per dose.

When comparing a physician's order to a recommended range, it is important to determine if the order falls within the range. If the ordered dose is too high, the individual will receive an overdosage of medication; if the ordered dose is too low, the individual will receive an underdosage, which may be ineffective or nontherapeutic. Sometimes this can also be dangerous, as it doesn't treat the individual effectively. If there is any question regarding a discrepancy in dosage, it is your responsibility to clarify with the provider.

> **Key**point: To determine the safety of an ordered dosage, use body weight to calculate the recommended dosage range, and compare this with the ordered dosage. This emphasizes the importance of labeling calculations as per day or per dose. Assessment should also include the frequency of dosage ordered; for this, you may need to consult drug literature.

It is important to recognize that individuals who are very young, very old, or compromised by illness will be more affected by discrepancies between ordered doses and recommended doses. Some discrepancy may be within accepted practice in your clinical setting. It is important to be familiar with protocols and policies at your clinical site.

There are some medications that use weight in pounds to calculate recommended dosages. Refer to the Tylenol® label in Figure 15-3 on the next page for the following example that uses pounds to calculate recommended dosage.

Example 3 ■   You are administering medications to a 2½-year-old child whose weight was documented as 15 kg. As you are preparing the medications, you notice the physician ordered Tylenol® 160 mg po every 4 hours as needed for fever.

To practice safe medication administration, determine if the ordered dose is safe based on the recommendations on the label. The child's weight is documented as 15 kg. You notice the label identifies recommended dose based on pounds. Your first step will be to convert the weight to pounds. Recall that weight in pounds will be about twice the amount in kilograms, so you must multiply by 2.2.

$$\frac{2.2\ \text{lb}}{1\ \text{kg}} \times 15\ \text{kg} = 33\ \text{lb}$$

Since the weight is now in pounds, you can review the recommended information on the label and determine that for this 2½ year old child, weighing 33 lb, the recommended dose is 5 mL.

To determine safety of the order, calculate the ordered dose and then compare the ordered dose to the recommended dose. There is 160 mg per 5 mL; therefore, you

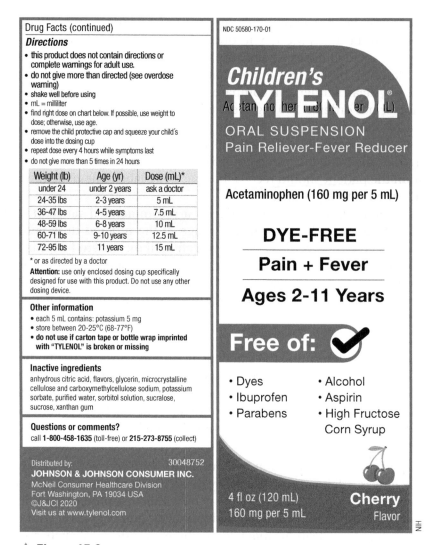

Drug Facts (continued)

Directions

- this product does not contain directions or complete warnings for adult use.
- do not give more than directed (see overdose warning)
- shake well before using
- mL = milliliter
- find right dose on chart below. If possible, use weight to dose; otherwise, use age.
- remove the child protective cap and squeeze your child's dose into the dosing cup
- repeat dose every 4 hours while symptoms last
- do not give more than 5 times in 24 hours

Weight (lb)	Age (yr)	Dose (mL)*
under 24	under 2 years	ask a doctor
24-35 lbs	2-3 years	5 mL
36-47 lbs	4-5 years	7.5 mL
48-59 lbs	6-8 years	10 mL
60-71 lbs	9-10 years	12.5 mL
72-95 lbs	11 years	15 mL

* or as directed by a doctor

Attention: use only enclosed dosing cup specifically designed for use with this product. Do not use any other dosing device.

Other information

- each 5 mL contains: potassium 5 mg
- store between 20-25°C (68-77°F)
- **do not use if carton tape or bottle wrap imprinted with "TYLENOL" is broken or missing**

Inactive ingredients

anhydrous citric acid, flavors, glycerin, microcrystalline cellulose and carboxymethylcellulose sodium, potassium sorbate, purified water, sorbitol solution, sucralose, sucrose, xanthan gum

Questions or comments?

call **1-800-458-1635** (toll-free) or **215-273-8755** (collect)

Distributed by: 30048752
JOHNSON & JOHNSON CONSUMER INC.
McNeil Consumer Healthcare Division
Fort Washington, PA 19034 USA
©J&JCI 2020
Visit us at www.tylenol.com

NDC 50580-170-01

Children's
TYLENOL®
Acetaminophen (160 mg per 5 mL)
ORAL SUSPENSION
Pain Reliever-Fever Reducer

Acetaminophen (160 mg per 5 mL)

DYE-FREE

Pain + Fever

Ages 2-11 Years

Free of: ✓

- Dyes
- Ibuprofen
- Parabens
- Alcohol
- Aspirin
- High Fructose Corn Syrup

4 fl oz (120 mL)   **Cherry**
160 mg per 5 mL   Flavor

▲ **Figure 15-3**

determine that the order is safe based on the recommendation. If you give 5 mL as recommended by the label, you will be giving 160 mg. The recommended frequency on the label is every 4 hours while symptoms last. This is exactly what the physician ordered, and you determine the order is safe.

Sometimes, instead of having recommended dosage information on the medication label, the label will refer you to the package insert or other relevant drug literature to find the relevant information you need. Many parenteral labels will not have the information directly on the label, and they will refer you to package inserts or drug literature.

Adult dosages of medications tend to be standardized dosages based on the weight of an average adult, and you will be comparing the ordered dose to this range. For example, the label or package insert may indicate the adult dosage range is 250–500 mg IM every 6 hours. In this case, you can review the physician's order and compare directly to the range. For example, if the doctor orders 375 mg IM every 6 hours, this order clearly falls in the recommended range and is therefore safe.

However, the safety of some medications, for both children and adults, is determined based on the weight of the individual. It is very important to take the time to do these calculations and determine safety of the ordered dose prior to administering it.

Problems 15.2

Refer to the cefaclor label in Figure 15-4 and answer the following questions regarding a 25-lb child with a urinary tract infection.

1. What is the child's body weight in kg, rounded to the nearest tenth? _____

2. What is the recommended dosage in mg per day for this child? _____

3. How many mg will this be per dose? _____

4. The order is to give 110 mg twice a day. Is this dosage reasonable? _____

5. How many mL will be administered? _____

6. How much water must you add as diluent to prepare this oral suspension? _____

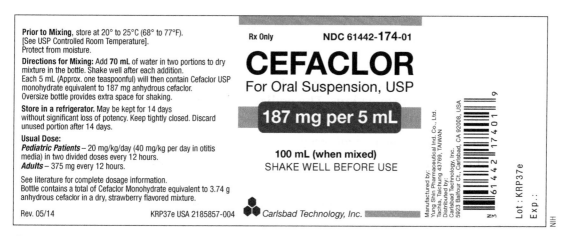

▲ **Figure 15-4**

Refer to the amoxicillin label in Figure 15-5 to answer the following questions.

7. What is the dose range of amoxicillin for a child? _____

8. The pediatric client weighs 34 lb. How many kg does the child weigh? _____

9. Calculate the daily dose range for this client. _____

10. What is the diluent for this powder? _____

11. How will the suspension be prepared? _____

12. The physician has ordered 150 mg q 8 hr. What is the ordered daily dose? _____

13. How should the reconstituted solution be stored? _____

14. Is the ordered daily dose in the calculated dose range? _____

15. If the answer to question 14 is YES, calculate a single dose. If the answer is NO, write NO on the answer line provided. _____

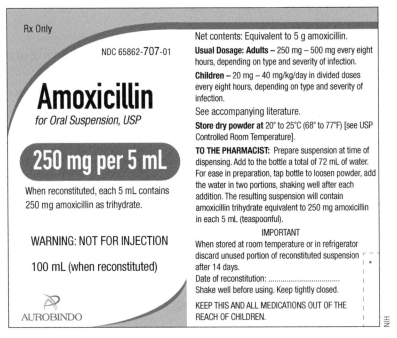

▲ Figure 15-5

Refer to the furosemide label in Figure 15-6 and the package insert in Figure 15-7 to answer the following questions. The pediatric patient weighs 55 lb and is ordered 50 mg PO of furosemide oral suspension.

16. How many kg does the patient weigh?   _____

17. According to the package insert, what is the usual initial dose of furosemide?   _____

18. Calculate how many mg of furosemide this patient can receive as an initial dose.   _____

19. How does this compare to the physician's order?   _____

20. Refer to the label and calculate how many mL the patient will receive.   _____

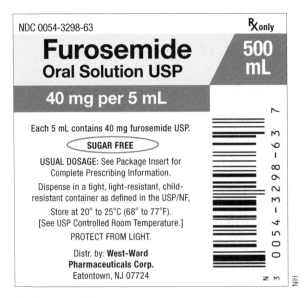

▲ Figure 15-6

Pediatric Patients: The usual initial dose of oral furosemide in pediatric patients is 2 mg/kg body weight, given as a single dose. If the diuretic response is not satisfactory after the initial dose, dosage may be increased by 1 or 2 mg/kg no sooner than 6 to 8 hours after the previous dose. Doses greater than 6 mg/kg body weight are not recommended. For maintenance therapy in pediatric patients, the dose should be adjusted to the minimum effective level.

▲ **Figure 15-7**

Answers   1. 11.4 kg   **2.** 228 mg/day   **3.** 114 mg/dose   **4.** 110 mg per dose would equal 2.9 mL; 114 mg dose would equal 3 mL. It is reasonable. (With any discrepancy, always check the facility policy or clarify with the provider.)   **5.** 2.9 mL   **6.** 70 mL in two portions.   **7.** 20–40 mg/kg/day in divided doses q 8 hr.   **8.** 15.5 kg   **9.** 310–620 mg/day   **10.** Water   **11.** 72 mL in two portions   **12.** 450 mg   **13.** Room temperature or refrigerator   **14.** Yes   **15.** 3 mL   **16.** 25 kg   **17.** 2 mg/kg given as a single dose   **18.** 50 mg   **19.** They are the same.   **20.** 6.3 mL

Summary

This concludes the chapter on dosages based on body weight. The important points to remember from this chapter are:

- Dosages are frequently ordered based on weight, especially for children.

- Medications such as pain medications, antibiotics, and chemotherapy are some of the groups that may have weight-related dosing.

- Individualized dosages may be calculated in terms of mcg per kg or lb; or mg per kg or lb. Dosages may be recommended per dose, or per day, usually administered in divided doses.

- Body weight may need to be converted from kg to lb or lb to kg to correlate with dosage recommendations.

- To convert lb to kg, divide by 2.2; to convert kg to lb, multiply by 2.2; or use one of the methods of calculation covered in Chapters 8 through 10.

- If the recommended dose is a daily amount to be given in divided doses; the calculation will be a two-step procedure. First, calculate the total daily dosage for the weight; then, divide this by the number of doses to be administered.

- Label your calculations to be clear on what the calculation represents—is it per day or per dose?

- To check the accuracy of a prescriber's order, calculate the correct dosage and compare it with the dosage ordered.

- Some discrepancy between the ordered dose and the recommended dose may be permitted in your practice setting. It is your responsibility to know the protocol in your clinical setting. When in doubt, clarify any discrepancy with the provider.

- If the drug label does not contain all the necessary information for safe administration, additional information should be obtained from drug package inserts, other relevant information sources, or the clinical pharmacist.

Summary Self-Test

Convert the following weights and round to the tenth.

1. $100\frac{1}{4}$ lb = _____ kg

2. $54\frac{3}{4}$ lb = _____ kg

3. 135 lb = _____ kg

4. 34.8 kg = _____ lb

5. $22\frac{1}{2}$ kg = _____ lb

6. 75 kg = _____ lb

Refer to the Children's ibuprofen label in Figure 15-8 to answer the following questions. A 4-year-old client is ordered 150 mg of ibuprofen for pain.

7. The physician has ordered a 4-year-old patient 150 mg of ibuprofen every 6 hr. The patient weighs 18.2 kg. Determine how many lb the patient weighs.   _____

8. How many mL is recommended for the weight in lb for this child?   _____

9. How should the medication be given if the patient has experienced stomach upset?   _____

10. What device must be used to measure the mL of the medication?   _____

11. Is the physician's order reasonable? Explain your answer.   _____

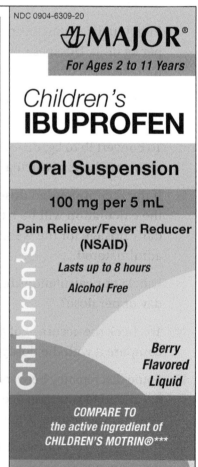

Drug Facts (continued)
• **right before or after heart surgery**
Ask a doctor before use if
• stomach bleeding warning applies to your child
• child has a history of stomach problems, such as heartburn
• child has problems or serious side effects from taking pain relievers or fever reducers
• child has not been drinking fluids
• child has lost a lot of fluid due to vomiting or diarrhea
• child has high blood pressure, heart disease, liver cirrhosis, kidney disease, or had a stroke
• child has asthma
• child is taking a diuretic
Ask a doctor or pharmacist before use if the child is
• under a doctor's care for any serious condition
• taking any other drug
When using this product
• give with food or milk if stomach upset occurs
Stop use and ask a doctor if
• child experiences any of the following signs of stomach bleeding:
   • feels faint
   • vomits blood
   • has bloody or black stools
   • has stomach pain that does not get better
• child has symptoms of heart problems or stroke:
   • chest pain
   • trouble breathing
   • weakness in one part or side of body
   • slurred speech
   • leg swelling
• the child does not get any relief within first day (24 hours) of treatment
• fever or pain gets worse or lasts more than 3 days
• redness or swelling is present in the painful area
• any new symptoms appear

Keep out of reach of children. In case of overdose, get medical help or contact a Poison Control Center right away. (1-800-222-1222)

Directions
• this product does not contain directions or complete warnings for adult use
• do not give more than directed

Drug Facts (continued)
• shake well before using
• mL = milliliter
• find right dose on chart. If possible, use weight to dose; otherwise use age.
• use only enclosed dosing cup. Do not use any other dosing device.
• if needed, repeat dose every 6-8 hours
• do not use more than 4 times a day
• replace original bottle cap to maintain child resistance
• wash dosage cup after each use

Dosing Chart

Weight (lb)	Age (yr)	Dose (mL)**
under 24 lbs	under 2 years	ask a doctor
24-35 lbs	2-3 years	5 mL
36-47 lbs	4-5 years	7.5 mL
48-59 lbs	6-8 years	10 mL
60-71 lbs	9-10 years	12.5 mL
72-95 lbs	11 years	15 mL

**or as directed by a doctor

Other information
• each 5 mL contains: sodium 2 mg
• do not use if printed neckband is broken or missing
• store at 20-25°C (68-77°F)
• do not freeze

Inactive ingredients
anhydrous citric acid, artificial mixed berry flavor, D&C yellow #10, FD&C red #40, glycerin, high fructose corn syrup, hypromellose, polysorbate 80, purified water, sodium benzoate, sorbitol solution, xanthan gum

Questions or comments?
1-800-719-9260

Gluten Free

***Major® Children's Ibuprofen Oral Suspension 100 mg per 5 mL is not manufactured or distributed by Johnson & Johnson Consumer Inc., distributor of Children's Motrin®.

Distributed by: **MAJOR® PHARMACEUTICALS**
17177 N Laurel Park Drive, Suite 233
Livonia, MI 48152 MI 48152
M-05   REV. 07/17   Re-Order No. 700760

NDC 0904-6309-20

⚕MAJOR®

For Ages 2 to 11 Years

Children's
IBUPROFEN

Oral Suspension

100 mg per 5 mL

Pain Reliever/Fever Reducer (NSAID)

Lasts up to 8 hours

Alcohol Free

Berry Flavored Liquid

COMPARE TO
the active ingredient of
*CHILDREN'S MOTRIN®****

120 mL (4 FL OZ)

▲ **Figure 15-8**

Refer to the filgrastim label in Figure 15-9 and the package insert in Figure 15-10 to answer the following questions. A 55-year-old female client is ordered a first dose of filgrastim subcutaneously to treat neutropenia (low neutrophil count). The dose is to be based on the weight recommendations on the label. The client weighs 122 lb.

12. According to the package insert, what is the recommended starting dose per day?   _____

13. What routes are permitted for the starting dose?   _____

14. What is the client's weight in kg?   _____

15. How should this medication be stored?   _____

16. How many mcg will the client receive (round to the whole number)?   _____

17. How many mL will the client receive subcutaneously?   _____

18. What syringe must be used to administer the dose in question 17?   _____

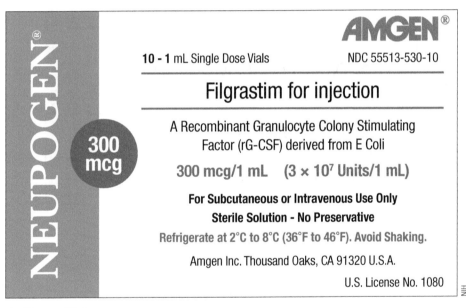

▲ **Figure 15-9**

Dosage in Patients with Cancer Receiving Myelosuppressive Chemotherapy or Induction and/or Consolidation Chemotherapy for AML The recommended starting dosage of NEUPOGEN is 5 mcg/kg/day, administered as a single daily injection by subcutaneous injection, by short intravenous infusion (15 to 30 minutes), or by continuous intravenous infusion.

▲ **Figure 15-10**

Refer to the Tobramycin® label in Figure 15-11 and the package insert in Figure 15-12 to answer the following questions. A 3-year-old male client is ordered 50 mg of Tobramycin IV q 8hrs to treat a staph infection. The client weighs 32.5 lb.

19. What is the kg weight of the client?   _____

20. According to the package insert, and considering the physician's order, what is the recommended dose range?   _____

21. What is this client's dose range?   _____

22. Is there a difference in recommended dosages between the IM and IV routes?   _____

23. What route requires dilution of this medication?   _____

24. Does the order fall within the calculated dose range?   _____

25. If the answer is YES to question 24, calculate the mL to be administered. If the answer is NO, what action should be implemented by the nurse?   _____

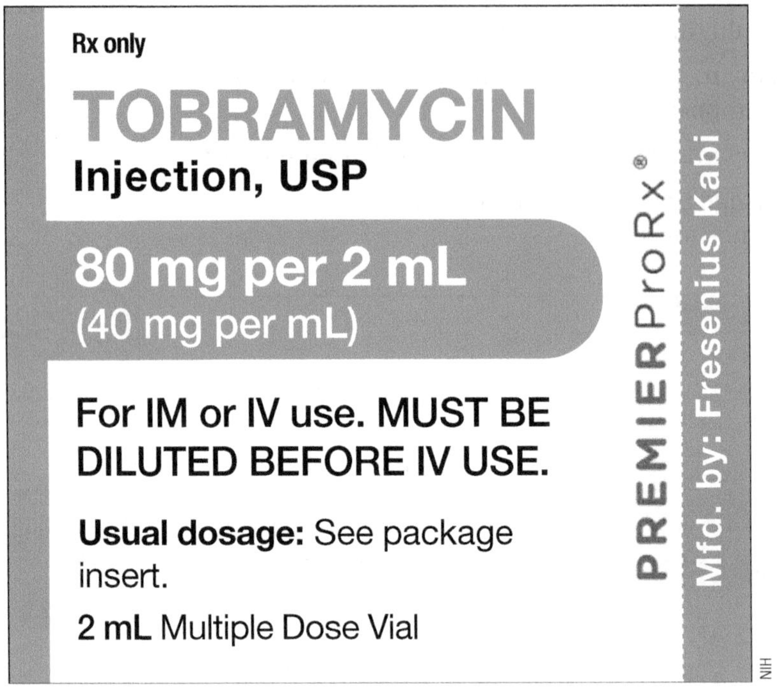

Rx only

TOBRAMYCIN
Injection, USP

80 mg per 2 mL
(40 mg per mL)

For IM or IV use. MUST BE DILUTED BEFORE IV USE.

Usual dosage: See package insert.

2 mL Multiple Dose Vial

PREMIER ProRx®

Mfd. by: Fresenius Kabi

▲ Figure 15-11

DOSAGE AND ADMINISTRATION:

Tobramycin may be given intramuscularly or intravenously. Recommended dosages are the same for both routes. The patient's pretreatment body weight should be obtained for calculation of correct dosage. It is desirable to measure both peak and trough serum concentrations (see WARNINGS box and PRECAUTIONS).

Pediatric Patients (greater than 1 week of age): 6 to 7.5 mg/kg/day in 3 or 4 equally divided doses (2 to 2.5 mg/kg every 8 hours or 1.5 to 1.89 mg/kg every 6 hours).

Premature or Full-Term Neonates 1 Week of Age or Less: Up to 4 mg/kg/day may be administered in 2 equal doses every 12 hours.

▲ Figure 15-12

Critical Thinking Questions

1. The physician has ordered a client high dose Solu-Medrol® one time today. The dose is to be based on the weight recommendations on the label. The client weighs 160 lb. The nurse is preparing the medication. In the following matrix, determine whether the choices are appropriate or inappropriate. Refer to the Solu-Medrol® label in Figure 15-13 and the package insert in Figure 15-14.

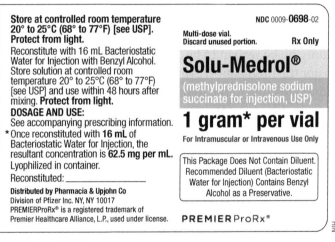

Store at controlled room temperature 20° to 25°C (68° to 77°F) [see USP]. Protect from light.
Reconstitute with 16 mL Bacteriostatic Water for Injection with Benzyl Alcohol. Store solution at controlled room temperature 20° to 25°C (68° to 77°F) [see USP] and use within 48 hours after mixing. **Protect from light.**
DOSAGE AND USE:
See accompanying prescribing information.
* Once reconstituted with **16 mL** of Bacteriostatic Water for Injection, the resultant concentration is **62.5 mg per mL.** Lyophilized in container.
Reconstituted: _____

Distributed by Pharmacia & Upjohn Co
Division of Pfizer Inc. NY, NY 10017
PREMIERProRx® is a registered trademark of
Premier Healthcare Alliance, L.P., used under license.

NDC 0009-**0698**-02

Multi-dose vial.
Discard unused portion.   **Rx Only**

Solu-Medrol®
(methylprednisolone sodium succinate for injection, USP)

1 gram* per vial
For Intramuscular or Intravenous Use Only

This Package Does Not Contain Diluent.
Recommended Diluent (Bacteriostatic Water for Injection) Contains Benzyl Alcohol as a Preservative.

PREMIER ProRx®

▲ **Figure 15-13**

There are reports of cardiac arrhythmias and/or cardiac arrest following the rapid administration of large intravenous doses of SOLU-MEDROL (greater than 0.5 gram administered over a period of less than 10 minutes). Bradycardia has been reported during or after the administration of large doses of methylprednisolone sodium succinate, and may be unrelated to the speed or duration of infusion. When high dose therapy is desired, the recommended dose of SOLU-MEDROL Sterile Powder is 30 mg/kg administered intravenously over at least 30 minutes. This dose may be repeated every 4 to 6 hours for 48 hours.

▲ **Figure 15-14**

Choice	Appropriate action	Inappropriate action
Reconstitute vial with sterile saline.		
Administer the medication intravenously.		
Administer the medication intramuscularly.		
Determine kg weight to be 45 kg.		
Calculate the volume to administer at 34.9 mL.		
Administer the dose over 10 minutes.		

2. A 12-year-old client with a mild skin infection has been ordered 500 mg cephalexin oral suspension daily in four divided doses. The client weighs 80 lb. Utilizing the label in Figure 15-15 and the chapter information, choose the relevant information for preparing and administering this medication. Select all that apply.

   a. Determine the kg weight to be 36.4 kg.
   b. Administer the medication every 4 hr.
   c. Determine the daily range to be 910–1,820 mg.
   d. Reconstitute the container with two portions of 140 mL each and shake well.
   e. Administer 10 mL every 6 hr.
   f. Clarify order with physician prior to administering.

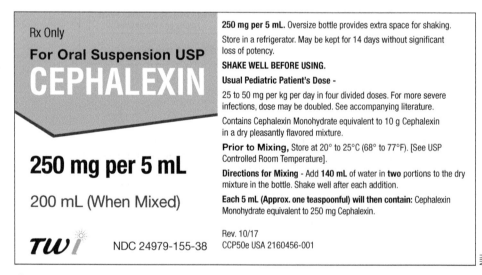

Rx Only

For Oral Suspension USP

CEPHALEXIN

250 mg per 5 mL

200 mL (When Mixed)

TWi   NDC 24979-155-38

250 mg per 5 mL. Oversize bottle provides extra space for shaking.

Store in a refrigerator. May be kept for 14 days without significant loss of potency.

SHAKE WELL BEFORE USING.

Usual Pediatric Patient's Dose -

25 to 50 mg per kg per day in four divided doses. For more severe infections, dose may be doubled. See accompanying literature.

Contains Cephalexin Monohydrate equivalent to 10 g Cephalexin in a dry pleasantly flavored mixture.

Prior to Mixing, Store at 20° to 25°C (68° to 77°F). [See USP Controlled Room Temperature].

Directions for Mixing - Add **140 mL** of water in **two** portions to the dry mixture in the bottle. Shake well after each addition.

Each 5 mL (Approx. one teaspoonful) will then contain: Cephalexin Monohydrate equivalent to 250 mg Cephalexin.

Rev. 10/17
CCP50e USA 2160456-001

▲ **Figure 15-15**

3. An 8-year-old client with an upper respiratory infection has been ordered EryPed® 400. The order is 300 mg EryPed® PO every 8 hr. The client weighs 62 lb. The pharmacy has sent the medication and the nurse is preparing it to

administer to the client. Refer to the EryPed® 400 label in Figure 15-16 and chapter information to choose the appropriate interventions. Select all that apply.

a. Calculate the dose range of this client to be 846–1,410 mg every 8 hr.

b. Administer 3.8 mL per dose.

c. Administer medication without regard to meals.

d. Administer 10 mL every 8 hr.

e. Reconstitute the container with 100 mL of water.

f. Inform the client the medication will taste like fruit.

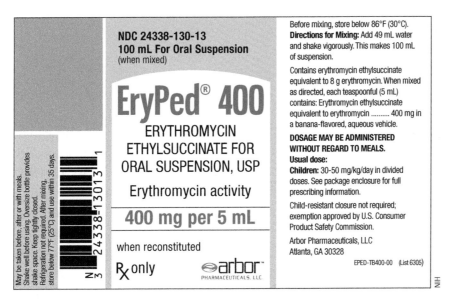

NDC 24338-130-13
100 mL For Oral Suspension
(when mixed)

EryPed® 400
ERYTHROMYCIN
ETHYLSUCCINATE FOR
ORAL SUSPENSION, USP

Erythromycin activity

400 mg per 5 mL

when reconstituted

R︎x only   ⊜arbor
PHARMACEUTICALS, LLC.

May be taken before, after or with meals. Shake well before using. Oversize bottle provides shake space. Keep tightly closed. Refrigeration not required. After mixing, store below 77°F (25°C) and use within 35 days.

Before mixing, store below 86°F (30°C).
Directions for Mixing: Add 49 mL water and shake vigorously. This makes 100 mL of suspension.

Contains erythromycin ethylsuccinate equivalent to 8 g erythromycin. When mixed as directed, each teaspoonful (5 mL) contains: Erythromycin ethylsuccinate equivalent to erythromycin .... 400 mg in a banana-flavored, aqueous vehicle.
DOSAGE MAY BE ADMINISTERED WITHOUT REGARD TO MEALS.
Usual dose:
Children: 30-50 mg/kg/day in divided doses. See package enclosure for full prescribing information.

Child-resistant closure not required; exemption approved by U.S. Consumer Product Safety Commission.

Arbor Pharmaceuticals, LLC
Atlanta, GA 30328

EPED-TB400-00   (List 6305)

▲ **Figure 15-16**

Answers to Critical Thinking Questions

1.

Choice	Appropriate action	Inappropriate action
Reconstitute vial with sterile saline.		X
Administer the medication intravenously.	X	
Administer the medication intramuscularly.		X
Determine kg weight to be 45 kg.		X
Calculate the volume to administer at 34.9 mL.	X	
Administer the dose over 10 minutes.		X

Rationale:

▧ Reconstitute the vial with bacteriostatic water with benzyl alcohol.
▧ Administer the medication intravenously as the package insert instructs for the high dose.
▧ Administer the medication intramuscularly is not appropriate.
▧ This is an inappropriate answer. The kg weight is 72.7.
▧ Calculate the volume to 34.9 mL is appropriate and accurate.
▧ Administer the dose over 10 minutes is not appropriate. Per the package insert, administer over 30 minutes.

2. a, c, f. **Rationale:** b is incorrect—Four divided doses is not every 4 hours; this would be every 6 hours. d is incorrect—Add 140 mL in two portions/70 mL each. e is incorrect because the ordered dose is too low, and it should not be administered. 500 mg a day is too low, and it does not fall within the calculated range of 910–1,820 mg per day. (Call the physician for clarification of the order.)

3. b, c, f. **Rationale:** a is incorrect—This is the daily range. d is incorrect—The dose administered will be 3.8 mL. e is incorrect—Reconstitute the container with 49 mL with a 100 mL resulting solution.

Chapter 16

Dosages Based on Body Surface Area

Objectives

The learner will:

1. calculate BSA using formulas for weight and height.

2. use BSA to calculate dosages.

3. assess the accuracy of dosages prescribed on the basis of BSA.

Body surface area (BSA) is used to calculate dosages of antineoplastic agents for cancer chemotherapy and other medications where increased accuracy of dosing is desired. BSA is also used to describe areas involved in severe burns, as well as for some cardiac and renal functions. The nursing responsibility for checking dosages based on BSA varies widely in clinical facilities; however, nurses are always responsible for ensuring that they are administering medications safely. This chapter covers calculation of BSA, calculation of dosages based on BSA, and assessment of physician orders based on BSA.

BSA is calculated in square meters (m^2) using the patient's weight and height and a calculator that has square root ($\sqrt{\ }$) capabilities. If using a handheld calculator, it is important to identify the square root key and ensure the calculator has one. Refer to Figure 16-1 for an example of a calculator with a square root function.

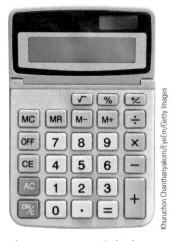

▲ **Figure 16-1** Calculator with square root function.

To correctly use the formulas with a calculator, you must know how to enter the numbers into the calculator to get an accurate answer.

Two formulas are used by physicians and pharmacists: one using kilogram (kg) and centimeter (cm) measurements, and another using pound (lb) and inch (in) measurements. We'll look at these separately.

Clinical Relevance: In Chapter 15, we used body weight to calculate dosages of medication and determine safety of ordered doses. There are some medications that will use BSA to calculate dosages of medications for adults and children. These include most notably chemotherapy medications and some pediatric medications. Body surface area considers height and weight of the individual, and it is calculated using a formula or a nomogram. Using a formula and calculating with a calculator will give the most accurate results and should consistently be used. It is important to know the formulas so that the information can be entered into the calculator; however, there are also online BSA calculators that allow you to enter the height and weight of the individual to calculate the BSA. When the BSA is known, the calculation of a dose of medication based on BSA is completed in the same manner as weight-based calculations since the medication will identify the recommended dose as mg/m^2 or mcg/m^2. The recommended dose may also be identified as any unit of weight of the medication per meter squared. As with any medication that is administered, it is important to check accuracy and safety of the ordered dose. This will require an understanding of body surface area.

Calculation of BSA

The first formula uses kilogram and centimeter measurements. To use this calculation, height and weight must both be in the metric system. You cannot mix up systems. For example, you cannot use height in centimeters and weight in pounds. The calculation will not work.

$$\text{BSA} = \sqrt{\frac{\text{wt (kg)} \times \text{ht (cm)}}{3{,}600}}$$

Example 1 ∎   Calculate the BSA of an adult who weighs **104 kg** and whose height is **191 cm**. For consistency with BSA calculations, multiply the weight times the height and then divide the product by 3,600. We will calculate that number to thousandths but will not round. Finally, we will apply the square root function to determine the answer in m^2. Round BSA to the hundredth.

$$\sqrt{\frac{104 \text{ (kg)} \times 191 \text{ (cm)}}{3{,}600}}$$

$$= \sqrt{5.517}$$

$$= 2.348 = 2.35 \text{ m}^2$$

Calculators may function differently and vary in the way a square root must be obtained. It is important for you to understand how your calculator works.

BSA in m^2 will be rounded to hundredths. Fractional weights and heights are also used in calculations. Refer to Example 2.

Example 2 ■

Calculate the BSA of an adolescent who weighs **59.1 kg** and is **157.5 cm** in height. Round BSA to the hundredth.

$$\sqrt{\dfrac{59.1 \ (kg) \times 157.5 \ (cm)}{3{,}600}}$$

$$= \sqrt{2.585}$$

$$= 1.607 = 1.61 \ m^2$$

The second formula uses pound and inch measurements. Again, you cannot mix systems; you must use both pound and inch measurements, and you cannot use kilogram and inch, or pound and centimeter measurements. The process will be the same; notice, however, that the denominator is different. As with the first formula, multiply the numbers in the numerator and then divide by 3,131. Calculate that number to the thousandths, but do not round. Then, apply the square root function to that number to obtain your answer in m^2. Round BSA to the hundredth.

$$BSA = \sqrt{\dfrac{wt \ (lb) \times ht \ (in)}{3{,}131}}$$

Example 3 ■

Calculate BSA to the hundredth for a child who is 24 inches tall and weighs 34 pounds.

$$\sqrt{\dfrac{34 \ (lb) \times 24 \ (in)}{3{,}131}}$$

$$= \sqrt{0.260}$$

$$= 0.509 = 0.51 \ m^2$$

Example 4 ■

Calculate BSA to the hundredth for an adult who is 61.3 inches tall and weighs 142.7 pounds.

$$\sqrt{\dfrac{142.7 \ (lb) \times 61.3 \ (in)}{3{,}131}}$$

$$= \sqrt{2.793}$$

$$= 1.671 = 1.67 \ m^2$$

In addition to using these formulas, BSA can also be calculated using online BSA calculators. Refer to Figure 16-2 for an example of an online BSA calculator.

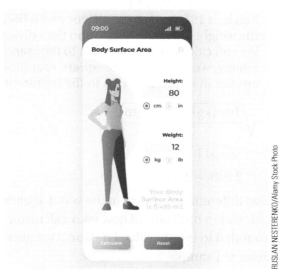

▲ **Figure 16-2** Online BSA Calculator

RUSLAN NESTERENKO/Alamy Stock Photo

This online BSA calculator allows you to put in centimeters and kilograms or inches and pounds to obtain the BSA. Many online calculators allow you to mix systems and use different units of measure for height and weight; you are not restricted to using the same system of measurement for height and weight. For example, you can input pounds for weight and centimeters for height if those are the measurements you have available. If using an online BSA calculator, input the numbers for height and weight, and then the online calculator will determine the BSA in m^2.

Finally, BSA can be approximated by using a nomogram, Figure 16-3. A nomogram is a chart that allows you to plot the height and the weight of the individual. After these measurements are plotted, draw a straight line to connect the two measurements. After the straight line is drawn, identify where the line intersects on the BSA scale, and this will provide the BSA in m^2. A nomogram is not as accurate as the formulas or the online BSA calculator. Therefore, most facilities require the use of the formula and a handheld calculator or an online BSA calculator.

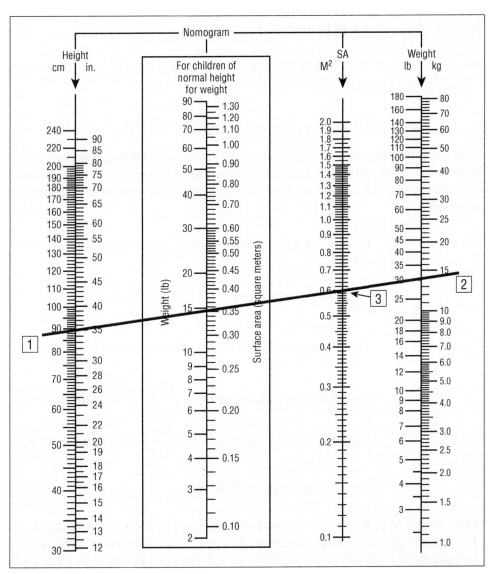

▲ **Figure 16-3** Nomogram depicting (1) height of 35 inches, (2) weight 30 lb, and (3) BSA 0.6 m^2

Problems 16.1

Use the appropriate formula and a handheld calculator to calculate the BSA in m².
Round answers to the hundredth.

1. An adult weighing 59 kg whose height is 160 cm _____
2. A child weighing 35.9 kg whose height is 63.5 cm _____
3. A child weighing 7.7 kg whose height is 40 cm _____
4. An adult weighing 92 kg whose height is 178 cm _____
5. A child weighing 46 kg whose height is 102 cm _____
6. A child weighing 92 lb who measures 35 in _____
7. An adult who weighs 175 lb and measures 67 in _____
8. An adult who weighs 194 lb and whose height is 70 in _____
9. A child who weighs 72.4 lb and measures 40.5 in _____
10. A child who weighs 36 lb and measures 26 in _____

Answers **1.** 1.62 m² **2.** 0.8 m² **3.** 0.29 m² **4.** 2.13 m² **5.** 1.14 m² **6.** 1.01 m² **7.** 1.93 m² **8.** 2.08 m²
9. 0.97 m² **10.** 0.55 m²

Calculation of Dosages Based on BSA

Once you know how to calculate BSA in m², the calculation of dosages based on BSA will be like the calculation of dosages based on body weight. Remember to label all measurements when you are calculating so that you are clear on the unit of measure expressed in your answer.

Example 1 ■   Dosage recommended is 5 mg per m². The child has a BSA of 1.2 m².

$$\frac{5 \text{ mg}}{\text{m}^2} \times 1.2 \text{ m}^2 = 6 \text{ mg}$$

Example 2 ■   The recommended child's dosage is 25–50 mg/m². The child has a BSA of 0.76 m².

Lower dosage (minimum) $\frac{25 \text{ mg}}{\text{m}^2} \times 0.76 \text{ m}^2 = 19 \text{ mg}$

Upper dosage (maximum) $\frac{50 \text{ mg}}{\text{m}^2} \times 0.76 \text{ m}^2 = 38 \text{ mg}$

The dosage range is 19–38 mg.

In the following example, we must use a package insert to calculate a dosage based on BSA. In addition, you may find it necessary to use this information to determine accuracy and safety of a provider's order. Refer to the vinblastine insert in Figure 16-4 for information needed for Example 3.

Adult Patients: It is wise to initiate therapy for adults by administering a single intravenous dose of 3.7 mg/m of body surface area (bsa). Thereafter, white blood cell counts should be made to determine the patient's sensitivity to vinblastine sulfate. A simplified and conservative incremental approach to dosage at weekly intervals for adults may be outlined as follows:

First dose .... 3.7 mg/m^2 bsa
Second dose .... 5.5 mg/m^2 bsa
Third dose .... 7.4 mg/m^2 bsa
Fourth dose .... 9.25 mg/m^2 bsa
Fifth dose .... 11.1 mg/m^2 bsa

The above-mentioned increases may be used until a maximum dose not exceeding 18.5 mg/m bsa for adults is reached. The dose should not be increased after that dose which reduces the white cell count to approximately 3,000 cells/mm. In some adults, 3.7 mg/m bsa may produce this leukopenia; other adults may require more than 11.1 mg/m bsa; and, very rarely, as much as 18.5 mg/m bsa may be necessary. For most adult patients, however, the weekly dosage will prove to be 5.5 to 7.4 mg/m bsa.

When the dose of vinblastine sulfate which will produce the above degree of leukopenia has been established, a dose of one increment smaller than this should be administered at weekly intervals for maintenance. Thus, the patient is receiving the maximum dose that does not cause leukopenia. It should be emphasized that, even though seven days have elapsed, the next dose of vinblastine sulfate should not be given until the white cell count has returned to at least 4,000/ mm. In some cases, oncolytic activity may be encountered before leukopenic effect. When this occurs, there is no need to increase the size of subsequent doses (see PRECAUTIONS).

▲ **Figure 16-4** vinblastine package insert

Example 3 ■

You are caring for an adult patient who is beginning a regimen of vinblastine. Their BSA is 1.66 m^2. The physician has ordered vinblastine 6 mg IV as the first dose. Before you administer the medication, you check the information in the insert and calculate the first dose. Based on that calculation, you will be able to determine accuracy of the physician's order. The information on the package insert indicates the following:

Recommended first dose = 3.7 mg/m^2

You use the patient's BSA to calculate the first dose as follows (rounding the answer to the whole number):

$$\frac{3.7 \text{ mg}}{\text{m}^2} \times 1.66 \text{ m}^2 = 6.14 = 6 \text{ mg}$$

You are now able to compare the physician's order to the amount calculated for this patient. The order and your calculation are the same, so you know the medication is safe to give as ordered. Use the vinblastine label in Figure 16-5 to calculate the volume you will administer to the patient. Complete this using the formula method.

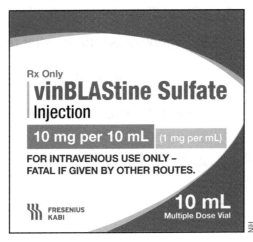

Rx Only

vinBLAStine Sulfate
Injection

10 mg per 10 mL (1 mg per mL)

**FOR INTRAVENOUS USE ONLY –
FATAL IF GIVEN BY OTHER ROUTES.**

FRESENIUS KABI

10 mL
Multiple Dose Vial

▲ **Figure 16-5**

$$\frac{6 \text{ mg (D)} \times 1 \text{ mL (Q)}}{1 \text{ mg (H)}} = 6 \text{ mL}$$

You will administer 6 mL IV to your patient as you have determined the physician order is safe and accurate based on the patient's BSA and the information in the package insert.

Problems 16.2

Refer to the carmustine label in Figure 16-6 and package insert in Figure 16-7 to answer the following questions.

1. What is the dosage per m² if the medication is given as a single dose?   _____

2. If a patient with a BSA of 1.76 m² is receiving carmustine as a single agent, what is the dose range?   _____

3. What is the two-step dilution procedure for carmustine?   _____

4. Should the order of 300 mg as a single agent be clarified by the physician?   _____

5. Once carmustine is reconstituted, where must it be stored?   _____

6. What is the rate for IV infusion for this medication?   _____

7. If crystals are seen in the vial, how can this be resolved?   _____

First, dissolve carmustine for injection, USP with 3 mL of the sterile diluent supplied. Second, aseptically add 27 mL Sterile Water for Injection, USP. Each mL of resulting solution contains 3.3 mg of carmustine for injection, USP in 10% ethanol.

After reconstitution as recommended, carmustine for injection, USP is stable for 24 hours under refrigeration (2°–8°C, 36°–46°F). Reconstituted vials should be examined for crystal formation prior to use. If crystals are observed, they may be redissolved by warming the vial to room temperature with agitation. Protect from light.

USUAL DOSAGE: Read enclosed package insert for indications, dosage, directions for use, and precautions.

Carmustine
for Injection, USP
100 mg per vial

Each carton contains: 1 vial carmustine for injection, USP 100 mg, 1 vial Sterile Diluent for carmustine for injection, USP 3 mL

For intravenous infusion after reconstitution

> **REFRIGERATE IMMEDIATELY**

Single Dose Vial - Discard Unused Portion

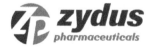 **zydus**
pharmaceuticals

Rx only

NIH

▲ **Figure 16-6**

Recommended Dosage: As a single agent, 150 to 200 mg/m^2 carmustine for injection, USP intravenously every 6 weeks as a single dose or divided into daily injections such as 75 to 100 mg/m^2 on 2 successive days. Adjust dose for combination therapy or in patients with reduced bone marrow reserve.

Administer reconstituted solution only as a slow intravenous infusion over at least 2 hours.

DOSAGE FORMS AND STRENGTHS For injection: 100 mg of carmustine lyophilized powder in a single-dose vial for reconstitution and a vial containing 3mL sterile diluent (Dehydrated Alcohol Injection, USP) (3)

▲ **Figure 16-7**

A 52-year-old female patient has been diagnosed with advanced ovarian cancer. The physician has ordered a chemotherapy treatment. The medication order is Cisplatin 160 mg IV on Day #1 of treatment every 4 weeks. The patient weighs 86.4 kg, with a height of 170.2 cm. Refer to the cisplatin label in Figure 16-8 and the package insert in Figure 16-9 to answer the following questions.

   8. Determine the BSA.   _____

   9. What is the recommended mg/m^2 dose range of Cisplatin?   _____

 10. Where should this vial be stored?   _____

 11. Calculate the dose range for this patient.   _____

 12. How many mL will the patient receive IV?   _____

 13. The answer in question 12 should be diluted in how many liters?   _____

 14. Should the physician be called to clarify the order?   _____

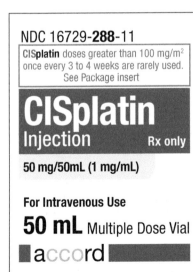

NDC 16729-**288**-11

CISplatin doses greater than 100 mg/m^2 once every 3 to 4 weeks are rarely used. See Package insert

CISplatin
Injection   Rx only

50 mg/50mL (1 mg/mL)

For Intravenous Use

50 mL Multiple Dose Vial

accord

Sterile
Each mL contains: 1 mg cisplatin and 9 mg sodium chloride in water for injection. HCl and/or sodium hydroxide added to adjust pH. The pH range of Cisplatin Injection is 3.5 to 5.0.
Usual dosage: See insert.
Store at 20°C to 25°C (68°F to 77°F); excursions permitted to 15°C to 30°C (59°F to 86°F) [see USP Controlled Room Temperature].
DO NOT REFRIGERATE OR FREEZE CISPLATIN SOLUTION SINCE A PRECIPITATE OR CRYSTAL WILL FORM. PROTECT FROM LIGHT.

Manufactured for: Accord Healthcare Inc., Durham, NC 27703. Manufactured by: Intas Pharmaceuticals Limited, Pharmez, Ahmedabad–382 213, India. Mfg. Lic. No.: G/28/1336 51 25710 713540   INL5026

NIH

▲ **Figure 16-8**

2.3 Advanced Ovarian Cancer Cisplatin injection has been administered at 75 mg/m^2 to 100 mg/m^2 intravenously per cycle once every 3 to 4 weeks on Day 1. Other doses and combination regimens have been used. The drug is then diluted in 2 liters of 5% Dextrose in 1/2 or 1/3 normal saline containing 37.5 g of mannitol, and infused over a 6- to 8-hour period. If diluted solution is not to be used within 6 hours, protect solution from light. Do not dilute cisplatin in just 5% Dextrose Injection. Adequate hydration and urinary output must be maintained during the following 24 hours.

▲ Figure 16-9

Refer to the oxaliplatin label in Figure 16-10 and the package insert in Figure 16-11 to answer the following questions.

15. What is the recommended dose of oxaliplatin on day 1?   _____

16. A patient weighs 63.6 kg and is 161.5 cm. Determine the BSA.   _____

17. Based on the BSA, how many mg will the patient receive?   _____

18. How many mL will be added to the vial for reconstitution?   _____

19. What solution should not be used for reconstitution?   _____

20. How many mL of the medication will be administered?   _____

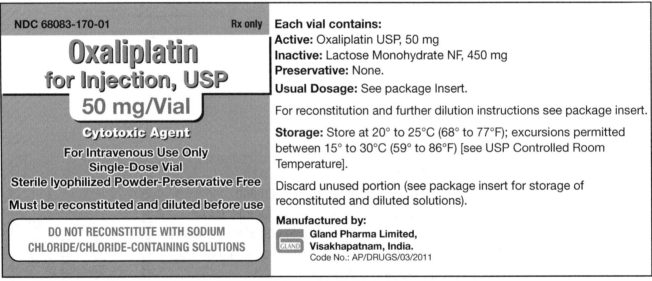

NDC 68083-170-01   **Rx only**

Oxaliplatin
for Injection, USP
50 mg/Vial

Cytotoxic Agent

For Intravenous Use Only
Single-Dose Vial
Sterile lyophilized Powder-Preservative Free

Must be reconstituted and diluted before use

DO NOT RECONSTITUTE WITH SODIUM
CHLORIDE/CHLORIDE-CONTAINING SOLUTIONS

Each vial contains:
Active: Oxaliplatin USP, 50 mg
Inactive: Lactose Monohydrate NF, 450 mg
Preservative: None.
Usual Dosage: See package Insert.

For reconstitution and further dilution instructions see package insert.

Storage: Store at 20° to 25°C (68° to 77°F); excursions permitted between 15° to 30°C (59° to 86°F) [see USP Controlled Room Temperature].

Discard unused portion (see package insert for storage of reconstituted and diluted solutions).

Manufactured by:
GLAND   **Gland Pharma Limited,**
Visakhapatnam, India.
Code No.: AP/DRUGS/03/2011

NIH

▲ Figure 16-10

Administer oxaliplatin for injection in combination with 5-fluorouracil/leucovorin every 2 weeks. For advanced disease, treatment is recommended until disease progression or unacceptable toxicity. For adjuvant use, treatment is recommended for a total of 6 months (12 cycles): **Day 1: Oxaliplatin for injection 85 mg/m^2 intravenous infusion in 250 to 500 mL 5% Dextrose injection, USP and leucovorin 200 mg/m^2 intravenous infusion in 5% Dextrose Injection, USP.**

The lyophilized powder is reconstituted by adding 10 mL (for the 50 mg vial) or 20 mL (for the 100 mg vial) of Water for Injection, USP or 5% Dextrose Injection, USP. Do not administer the reconstituted solution without further dilution. The reconstituted solution must be further diluted in an infusion solution of 250 to 500 mL of 5% Dextrose Injection, USP.

▲ Figure 16-11

Refer to the doxorubicin label in Figure 16-12 and the package insert in Figure 16-13 to answer the following questions. A 68-year-old female patient has been diagnosed with bladder cancer and has been ordered doxorubicin 120 mg as a single agent every 21 days. The patient weighs 140 lb and is 62 in tall.

21. Determine the BSA.   _____

22. What is the recommended dose range of doxorubicin as a
    single agent?   _____

23. Calculate the dose range for this patient.   _____

24. What is the reconstitution instruction?   _____

25. Calculate the dose in mL the patient will receive?   _____

NDC 70121-**1219**-1

|DOXOrubicin
|Hydrochloride for
|Injection, USP

50 mg/vial

FOR INTRAVENOUS USE ONLY

LYOPHILIZED

SINGLE-DOSE VIAL   **Rx Only**

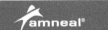

Each vial contains Doxorubicin Hydrochloride, USP 50 mg (equivalent to 46.86 mg of doxorubicin free base) and Lactose Monohydrate 250 mg.
USUAL DOSAGE: See package insert for complete prescribing information.
Reconstitute with 25 mL 0.9% Sodium Chloride Injection, USP.
Store unreconstituted vial at 20° to 25°C (68° to 77°F) [see USP Controlled Room Temperature]. Protect from light. Retain in carton until time of use. Discard unused portion.
WARNING: Severe cellulitis, vesication and tissue necrosis will occur if doxorubicin is extravasated during administration.
Manufactured by: **Amneal Oncology Pvt. Ltd.**
                  Telangana 509301, India
Distributed by: **Amneal Pharmaceuticals LLC**
                  Bridgewater, NJ 08807
Rev. 02-2021-02   Mfg. Lic. No: 7429/A3/2014

▲ **Figure 16-12**

Recommended Dosage for Adjuvant Breast Cancer: The recommended dosage of Doxorubicin Hydrochloride Injection/for Injection is 60 mg/m^2 administered as an intravenous bolus on day 1 of each 21-day treatment cycle, in combination with cyclophosphamide, for a total of four cycles.

Recommended Dosage for Other Cancers: The recommended dosage of Doxorubicin Hydrochloride Injection/for Injection when used as a single agent is 60 mg/m^2 to 75 mg/m^2 intravenously every 21 days. The recommended dosage of Doxorubicin Hydrochloride Injection/for Injection, when administered in combination with other chemotherapy drugs, is 40 mg/m to 75 mg/m intravenously every 21 to 28 days.

▲ **Figure 16-13**

Answers   1. 150–200 mg/m^2 **2.** 264–352 mg   **3.** dissolve with 3 mL and further dilute with 27 mL   **4.** no; falls within the calculated range   **5.** refrigerator   **6.** slowly over 2 hr   **7.** Crystals may be redissolved by warming the vial to room temperature with agitation.   **8.** 2.02 m^2 **9.** 75–100 mg/m^2 **10.** room temperature   **11.** 152–202 mg   **12.** 160 mL   **13.** 2 liters   **14.** no; falls within the calculated range   **15.** 85 mg/m^2 **16.** 1.69 m^2 **17.** 144 mg   **18.** 10 mL   **19.** sodium chloride containing solutions   **20.** 28.8 mL   **21.** 1.66 m^2 **22.** 60–75 mg/m^2 **23.** 100–125 mg   **24.** reconstitute with 25 mL of 0.9% sodium chloride injection USP   **25.** 60 mL

Summary

This concludes the chapter on dosage calculation based on BSA. The important points to remember from this chapter are:

- BSA in m² is calculated from a patient's weight and height.

- BSA is calculated in square meters (m²) using a formula.

- Two formulas for calculation of BSA are available:

  Using kg and cm: $\sqrt{\dfrac{\text{wt (kg)} \times \text{ht (cm)}}{3{,}600}}$ Using lb and in: $\sqrt{\dfrac{\text{wt (lb)} \times \text{ht (in)}}{3{,}131}}$

- After the BSA has been obtained, it can be used to calculate specific drug dosages and assess accuracy of physician orders.

Summary Self-Test

Use the formula method to calculate the following BSAs. Express m² to the nearest hundredth.

1. The weight is 58 lb and the height is 36 in   _____
2. An adult weighing 74 kg and measuring 160 cm   _____
3. A child who is 14.2 kg and measures 64 cm   _____
4. An adult weighing 69 kg whose height is 170 cm   _____
5. An adolescent who is 55 in and 103 lb   _____
6. A child who is 112 cm and weighs 25.3 kg   _____
7. An adult who weighs 55 kg and measures 157.5 cm   _____
8. An adult who weighs 65.4 kg and is 132 cm in height   _____
9. A child whose height is 58 in and whose weight is 26.5 lb   _____
10. A child whose height is 60 cm and weight is 13.6 kg   _____

Calculate the following dosages of vinblastine to the nearest whole number from the information available on the vinblastine label in Figure 16-14 and the package insert in Figure 16-15.

11. Calculate the dosage for an adult's second dose. The patient's BSA is 2.12 m².   _____
12. Calculate the dosage for an adult's third dose. The BSA is 1.91 m².   _____
13. Calculate the adult's fourth dosage. The BSA is 1.44 m².   _____
14. Calculate the adult's fifth dosage for a BSA of 1.53 m².   _____
15. What is the maximum dose of vinblastine for an adult?   _____

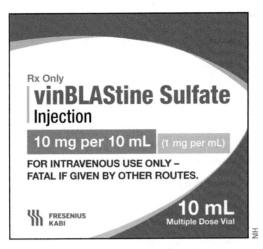

▲ **Figure 16-14**

ADULT PATIENTS: It is wise to initiate therapy for adults by administering a single intravenous dose of 3.7 mg/m² of body surface area (bsa). Thereafter, white blood cell counts should be made to determine the patient's sensitivity to vinblastine sulfate. A simplified and conservative incremental approach to dosage at weekly intervals for adults may be outlined as follows:

First dose .... 3.7 mg/m² bsa
Second dose .... 5.5 mg/m² bsa
Third dose .... 7.4 mg/m² bsa
Fourth dose .... 9.25 mg/m² bsa
Fifth dose .... 11.1 mg/m² bsa

The above-mentioned increases may be used until a maximum dose not exceeding 18.5 mg/m² bsa for adults is reached. The dose should not be increased after that dose which reduces the white cell count to approximately 3,000 cells/mm. In some adults, 3.7 mg/m² bsa may produce this leukopenia; other adults may require more than 11.1 mg/m² bsa; and, very rarely, as much as 18.5 mg/m² bsa may be necessary. For most adult patients, however, the weekly dosage will prove to be 5.5 to 7.4 mg/m² bsa.

When the dose of vinblastine sulfate which will produce the above degree of leukopenia has been established, a dose of one increment smaller than this should be administered at weekly intervals for maintenance. Thus, the patient is receiving the maximum dose that does not cause leukopenia. It should be emphasized that, even though seven days have elapsed, the next dose of vinblastine sulfate should not be given until the white cell count has returned to at least 4,000/ mm. In some cases, oncolytic activity may be encountered before leukopenic effect. When this occurs, there is no need to increase the size of subsequent doses (see PRECAUTIONS).

▲ **Figure 16-15**

Refer to the mitomycin label in Figure 16-16 and the package insert in Figure 16-17 to answer the following questions. A 65-year-old male patient has been diagnosed with stomach cancer and has been ordered mitomycin IV every 6 weeks. The patient weighs 95.5 kg and is 183 cm in height. The dose will be determined according to the BSA.

16. What is the recommended treatment dose?   _____

17. Is the administration of every 6 weeks reasonable?   _____

18. Calculate the BSA of this patient.   _____

19. Calculate the dose for this patient.   _____

20. How many mL will the patient receive?   _____

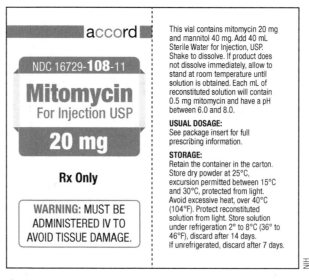

▲ **Figure 16-16**

Mitomycin should be given intravenously only, using care to avoid extravasation of the compound. If extravasation occurs, cellulitis, ulceration, and slough may result. Each vial contains either mitomycin 5 mg and mannitol 10 mg, mitomycin, 20 mg and mannitol 40 mg or mitomycin 40 mg and mannitol 80 mg.

To administer, add Sterile Water for Injection, 10 mL, 40 mL, or 80 mL respectively. Shake to dissolve. If product does not dissolve immediately, allow to stand at room temperature until solution is obtained.

After full hematological recovery (see guide to dosage adjustment) from any previous chemotherapy, the following dosage schedule may be used at 6-to-8-week intervals:

20 mg/m^2 intravenously as a single dose via a functioning intravenous catheter.

Because of cumulative myelosuppression, patients should be fully reevaluated after each course of mitomycin, and the dose reduced if the patient has experienced any toxicities. Doses greater than 20 mg/m^2 have not been shown to be more effective, and are more toxic than lower doses.

▲ **Figure 16-17**

Answers to Summary Self-Test

1. 0.82 m^2 **2.** 1.81 m^2 **3.** 0.50 m^2 **4.** 1.80 m^2 **5.** 1.34 m^2 **6.** 0.89 m^2 **7.** 1.55 m^2 **8.** 1.55 m^2 **9.** 0.70 m^2 **10.** 0.48 m^2 **11.** 12 mg **12.** 14 mg **13.** 13 mg **14.** 17 mg **15.** 18.5 mg/m^2 bsa for adults **16.** 20 mg/m^2 **17.** yes **18.** 2.20 m^2 **19.** 44 mg **20.** 88 mL

Critical Thinking Questions

1. A 16-year-old male client that has been diagnosed with acute myelogenous leukemia (AML) is ordered Oncaspar® intravenously. The dose of Oncaspar® for this client will be based on the BSA. The client weighs 52.3 kg and is 168 cm tall.

Refer to the Oncaspar® label in Figure 16-18 and package insert 16-19 and choose the appropriate interventions in preparing and administering the medication. Select all that apply.

   a. Calculate the BSA to 1.56.

   b. Administer the medication intravenously once daily for 14 days.

   c. Dilute a volume dose of 5.2 mL in 100 mL of an approved solution for IV administration.

   d. Administer the medication IV over 1.5 hr.

   e. Dilute 4.2 mL in 100 mL of an approved solution for IV administration.

DOSAGE: See package insert for complete prescribing information.

Store at 2-8°C (36-46°F). Do not freeze or shake.

Store in carton to protect from light.

ONCASPAR® is a registered trademark of Servier IP UK Ltd, a wholly owned indirect subsidiary of
Les Laboratoires Servier.
Servier and the Servier logo are trademarks of
Les Laboratoires Servier.

Mfd by:
Servier Pharmaceuticals LLC
Boston, MA 02210 USA
U.S. License No. 2125

NDC 72694-954-01

ONCASPAR®
pegaspargase
Injection

3750 International Units Per 5 mL
(750 International Units Per mL)

For intravenous or intramuscular use.

Single-use vial.

Discard unused portion.

Rx Only   SERVIER

NDC 72694-954-01

ONCASPAR®
pegaspargase
Injection

3750 International Units Per 5 mL
(750 International Units Per mL)

ACTIVE INGREDIENTS:
Contains 6.5 mg of L-asparaginase protein (conjugated to multiple 5kDa mPEGs) per mL, *E. coli* is used in the manufacture of the product.

INACTIVE INGREDIENTS:
Dibasic Sodium Phosphate .... 5.58 mg
Monobasic Sodium Phosphate .... 1.2 mg
Sodium Chloride .... 8.5 mg
Water for Injection .... qs to 1.0 mL

No U.S. Standard of Potency
Contains no preservation.

▲ **Figure 16-18**

DOSAGE AND ADMINISTRATION: Recommended Dosage Patients 21 Years of Age or Younger: The recommended dose of ONCASPAR for patients up to and including 21 years of age is 2,500 International Units/m² intramuscularly or intravenously no more frequently than every 14 days. Patients More Than 21 Years of Age: The recommended dose of ONCASPAR for adult patients more than 21 years of age is 2,000 International Units/m² intramuscularly or intravenously no more frequently than every 14 days.

When ONCASPAR is administered intramuscularly: Limit the volume at a single injection site to 2 mL. If the volume to be administered is greater than 2 mL, use multiple injection sites.

When ONCASPAR is administered intravenously: Dilute ONCASPAR with 100 mL of 0.9% Sodium Chloride Injection, USP or 5% Dextrose Injection, USP, using aseptic technique. After dilution, administer immediately into a running infusion of either 0.9% Sodium Chloride, USP or 5% Dextrose Injection, USP, respectively. Administer over a period of 1-2 hours. Do not infuse other drugs through the same intravenous line during administration of ONCASPAR. The diluted solution should be used immediately. If immediate use is not possible, the diluted solution should be stored refrigerated at 2°C to 8°C (36°F to 46°F) for up to 48 hours. Protect infusion bags from direct sunlight.

▲ **Figure 16-19**

2. A physician has ordered a 48-year-old female client with small cell lung cancer, etoposide for 5 days with a dose based on the recommended dosage. The client weighs 128 lb and is 61 in tall. Based on the etoposide label in Figure 16-20 and the package insert in Figure 16-21, what actions are appropriate for the nurse to implement to administer this medication. Select all that apply.

   a. Calculate the BSA to 1.47.
   b. Prepare a dose of 79 mg.
   c. Administer a volume of 4 mL.
   d. Calculate the BSA to 1.58.
   e. Prepare a dose of 55 mg.
   f. Administer a volume of 2.8 mL.

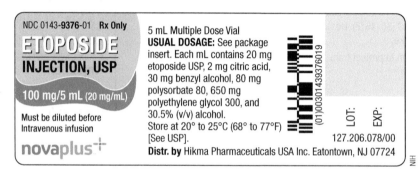

▲ **Figure 16-20**

In small cell lung cancer, the Etoposide Injection dose in combination with other approved chemotherapeutic drugs ranges from 35 mg/m^2 /day for 4 days to 50 mg/m^2 /day for 5 days.

Etoposide Injection must be diluted prior to use with either 5% Dextrose Injection, or 0.9% Sodium Chloride Injection, to give a final concentration of 0.2 to 0.4 mg/mL. If solutions are prepared at concentrations above 0.4 mg/mL, precipitation may occur. Hypotension following rapid intravenous administration has been reported; hence, it is recommended that the etoposide solution be administered over a 30- to 60-minute period. A longer duration of administration may be used if the volume of fluid to be infused is a concern. Etoposide should not be given by rapid intravenous injection.

▲ **Figure 16-21**

Answers to Critical Thinking Questions

1. a, c, d. **Rationale:** b is incorrect—The medication is administered every 14 days; e is incorrect—5.2 is the volume dose to be diluted in 100 mL

2. b, c, d. **Rationale:** a is incorrect—The correct BSA is 1.58; e is incorrect—The dose calculates to 79 mg; f is incorrect—the volume is 4 mL

Pediatric Dosages: Oral, Parenteral, and Intravenous

Two differences between adult and pediatric dosages will be immediately apparent: Most oral drugs are prepared as liquids because infants and small children cannot be expected to swallow tablets easily, if at all; and, for most medications, dosages are dramatically smaller. The oral route is used whenever possible, but when a child cannot swallow or the drug is ineffective given orally, drugs will be administered by a parenteral route. As children approach older adolescence, the dosages are more similar to adult dosages.

Both the subcutaneous and intramuscular routes may be used depending on the type of drug to be administered. However, the smaller size of infants and children limits the use of both routes, as does the nature of the drug being used. Some medications may be given intravenously as their action is more effective by the intravenous route. For example, many antibiotics are administered intravenously rather than intramuscularly.

Clinical Relevance: Pediatrics encompasses a wide range of ages with children in different stages of growth and development. The varying stages of growth and development may mean that certain organ systems, such as the liver and kidneys, are not as mature and developed in children, thus causing differences in the ways medications are metabolized and excreted. Ages for pediatrics range from newborn to 18 or 21, depending on the facility and practice. The wide range of ages and varying stages of growth and development in pediatric care necessitates dosing of medications according to body weight or body surface area in more instances than with adults. Usually, these doses are smaller than doses administered to adults. Therefore, we must consider the form of the medication and the measuring devices used for administration. In addition, as there is not one standard dose or range

Objectives

The learner will:

1. explain how suspensions are measured and administered.

2. calculate pediatric oral dosages.

3. list the precautions of IM and subcutaneous injection in infants and children.

4. calculate pediatric IM and subcutaneous dosages.

5. calculate pediatric IV dosages.

6. compare pediatric dosages to recommended dosages to assess safety.

of doses for a medication used with children, there is also more risk for error. Additional calculations need to be completed, such as mg/kg or mg/m^2, before calculating the volume of medication to administer, or the numbers of tablets or capsules needed. Triple check all calculations for accuracy and, if using a calculator, triple check the entry of all numbers, to prevent errors.

Oral Dosages

Most oral pediatric drugs are prepared as liquids to facilitate ease in swallowing. If the child is old enough to cooperate, these dosages may be measured in a calibrated medication cup. Solutions are also frequently measured using oral syringes, such as the ones shown in Figure 17-1. Notice that oral syringes have the same metric calibrations as hypodermic syringes, but they may also include household measures. For example, oral syringes may have calibrations for teaspoons.

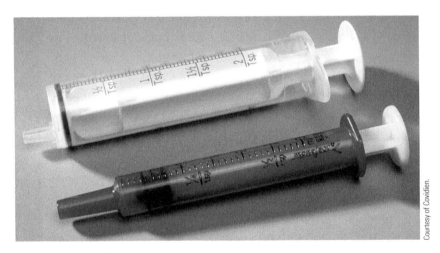

▲ **Figure 17-1** Oral syringes

Oral syringes have different-sized tips to prevent use with hypodermic needles. In addition, the tip of an oral syringe is typically a non-luer lock tip, or a slip tip. This means the needle cannot be screwed on securely, as it can be on a syringe with a luer lock tip. On some oral syringes, the tip is positioned off center, or is an eccentric tip, to further distinguish them from hypodermic syringes. An oral syringe may also be amber-colored to distinguish it from a hypodermic syringe.

While hypodermic syringes have similar calibrations, this book does not advocate the use of a hypodermic syringe to measure oral medications. The use of a hypodermic syringe to measure oral medications could lead to the inadvertent administration of the medication by an incorrect route. This would be detrimental to the client as neither the syringe nor the medication would be sterile.

Measurement of oral liquids in an oral syringe provides accuracy, as well as an excellent method of administering oral liquid drugs to infants and small children. Some oral liquid preparations incorporate a calibrated medication dropper as an integral part of the medication bottle. These may be calibrated in mL, like the dropper shown in Figure 17-2, or in actual dosage—for example, 25 mg or 50 mg. Oral pediatric medication spoons, as shown in Figure 17-3, are also available for measurement and administration of pediatric doses. These spoons are calibrated in mL as well as teaspoons. Household teaspoons or tablespoons should not be used for medication measurement or administration to children.

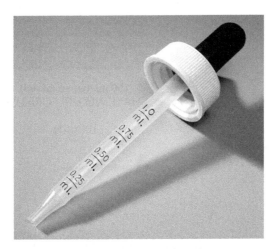

▲ **Figure 17-2** Calibrated dropper

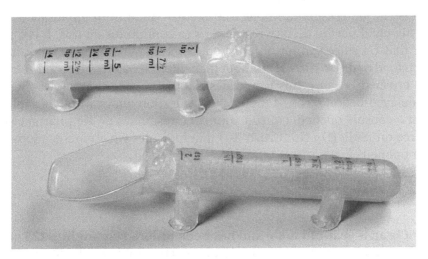

▲ **Figure 17-3** Pediatric medication spoons

Liquid oral medications can be elixirs, syrups, solutions, or suspensions. Care must be taken with liquid oral drugs to identify those prepared as suspensions. A suspension consists of an insoluble drug in a liquid base. The drug in a suspension settles to the bottom of the bottle between uses, and thorough mixing immediately prior to pouring is mandatory. Suspensions must also be administered to the child promptly after measurement to prevent the drug from settling out again and an incomplete dosage being administered. Medication labels of oral suspensions will clearly indicate that the medication is an oral suspension that needs to be mixed thoroughly before use. Refer to the label for cefaclor suspension in Figure 17-4.

Keypoint: Suspensions must be thoroughly mixed before measurement and promptly administered to prevent the settling out of their insoluble particles.

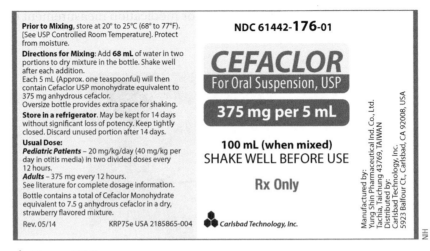

Prior to Mixing, store at 20° to 25°C (68° to 77°F). [See USP Controlled Room Temperature]. Protect from moisture.

Directions for Mixing: Add **68 mL** of water in two portions to dry mixture in the bottle. Shake well after each addition.
Each 5 mL (Approx. one teaspoonful) will then contain Cefaclor USP monohydrate equivalent to 375 mg anhydrous cefaclor.
Oversize bottle provides extra space for shaking.
Store in a refrigerator. May be kept for 14 days without significant loss of potency. Keep tightly closed. Discard unused portion after 14 days.
Usual Dose:
Pediatric Patients – 20 mg/kg/day (40 mg/kg per day in otitis media) in two divided doses every 12 hours.
Adults – 375 mg every 12 hours.
See literature for complete dosage information.
Bottle contains a total of Cefaclor Monohydrate equivalent to 7.5 g anhydrous cefaclor in a dry, strawberry flavored mixture.
Rev. 05/14   KRP75e USA 2185865-004

NDC 61442-**176**-01

CEFACLOR
For Oral Suspension, USP

375 mg per 5 mL

100 mL (when mixed)
SHAKE WELL BEFORE USE

Rx Only

Carlsbad Technology, Inc.

Manufactured by:
Yung Shin Pharmaceutical Ind. Co., Ltd.
Tachia, Taichung 43769, TAIWAN
Distributed by:
Carlsbad Technology, Inc.
5923 Balfour Ct., Carlsbad, CA 92008, USA

NIH

▲ **Figure 17-4**

   Some medications will not be supplied as a liquid and will be administered as a tablet or capsule. When a tablet or capsule is administered, the child's mouth must be checked to be certain the medication has been swallowed. If swallowing is a problem, some tablets can be crushed and given in a small amount of applesauce, ice cream, or juice if the child has no dietary restrictions to contraindicate this. It is important to remember that capsules cannot be crushed; some may be opened, and the contents sprinkled in food or drink. Also, remember that enteric-coated and timed-release tablets cannot be crushed because this would destroy the coating that allows them to function on a delayed-action basis. If there is any question about whether a tablet can be crushed, or a capsule opened, consult your drug resources or the pharmacist. There is also resource on ISMP (Do Not Crush list) that indicates which medications cannot be crushed or opened.

Problems 17.1

The patient is an 8-year-old male and has been ordered cimetidine 225 mg PO with meals and at bedtime to treat a gastric ulcer. The child weighs 58 lb. The recommended dose for a child is 20-40 mg/kg/day in four divided doses.

Refer to the cimetidine label in Figure 17-5 to answer the following questions.

1. What is the recommended daily dose range for this child?   _____

2. Calculate the physician's daily order.   _____

3. The patient is receiving the first dose this morning
   at breakfast. How many mg will the patient receive?   _____

4. Calculate the amount of mL to be administered.   _____

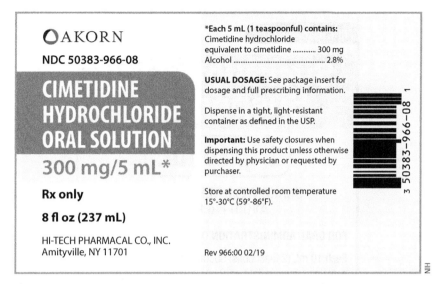

▲ Figure 17-5

5. Draw an arrow to the amount from question 4 on the oral syringe below in Figure 17-6.

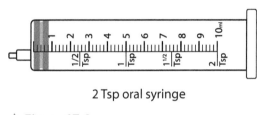

2 Tsp oral syringe

▲ Figure 17-6

The patient is an 11-year-old female and has been ordered sucralfate 2 g daily PO in four divided doses: 1 hr before meals and at bedtime to treat gastroesophageal reflux. The child weighs 81 lb. The recommended dose for a child is 40–80 mg/kg/ day in four divided doses.

Refer to the sucralfate label in Figure 17-7 to answer the following questions.

6. Calculate the kg weight of the child.   _____

7. What is the daily dose range for this patient?   _____

8. Does the physician's daily dose order meet the
   recommended range?   _____

9. Calculate how many tsp will be administered per dose.   _____

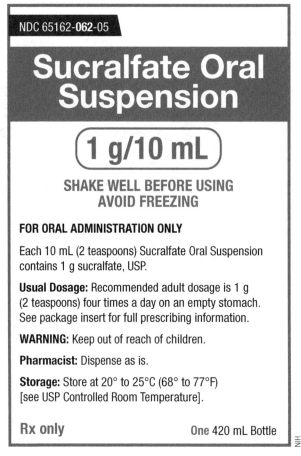

NDC 65162-**062**-05

Sucralfate Oral Suspension

(1 g/10 mL)

SHAKE WELL BEFORE USING
AVOID FREEZING

FOR ORAL ADMINISTRATION ONLY

Each 10 mL (2 teaspoons) Sucralfate Oral Suspension contains 1 g sucralfate, USP.

Usual Dosage: Recommended adult dosage is 1 g (2 teaspoons) four times a day on an empty stomach. See package insert for full prescribing information.

WARNING: Keep out of reach of children.

Pharmacist: Dispense as is.

Storage: Store at 20° to 25°C (68° to 77°F) [see USP Controlled Room Temperature].

Rx only   One 420 mL Bottle

▲ **Figure 17-7**

10. Draw an arrow to the amount in question 7 on the oral syringe in Figure 17-8.

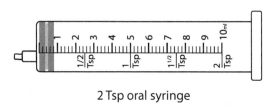

2 Tsp oral syringe

▲ **Figure 17-8**

An 8-year-old male pediatric patient weighs 57.5 lb and has been ordered cefixime oral suspension for pharyngitis in two divided doses. The dose will be weight-based.

Refer to the cefixime label in Figure 17-9 and the package insert in Figure 17-10 to answer the following questions.

11. Determine the kg weight of this patient.   _____

12. How many mg will this patient receive in each dose?   _____

13. How many mL of cefixime will be administered to the patient in each dose?   _____

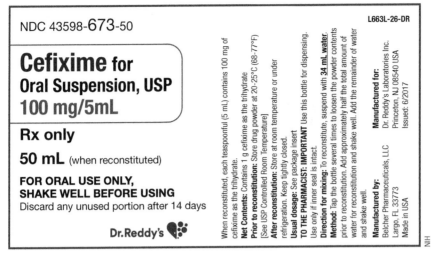

NDC 43598-673-50

L663L-26-DR

Cefixime for
Oral Suspension, USP
100 mg/5mL

Rx only

50 mL (when reconstituted)

FOR ORAL USE ONLY,
SHAKE WELL BEFORE USING
Discard any unused portion after 14 days

Dr.Reddy's

When reconstituted, each teaspoonful (5 mL) contains 100 mg of cefixime as the trihydrate.
Net Contents: Contains 1 g cefixime as the trihydrate
Prior to reconstitution: Store drug powder at 20-25°C (68-77°F)
[See USP Controlled Room Temperature]
After reconstitution: Store at room temperature or under refrigeration. Keep tightly closed.
Usual dosage: See package insert
TO THE PHARMACIST: IMPORTANT Use this bottle for dispensing. Use only if inner seal is intact.
Direction for mixing: To reconstitute, suspend with **34 mL water**.
Method: Tap the bottle several times to loosen the powder contents prior to reconstitution. Add approximately half the total amount of water for reconstitution and shake well. Add the remainder of water and shake well.

Manufactured for:
Dr. Reddy's Laboratories Inc.
Princeton, NJ 08540 USA
Issued: 6/2017

Manufactured by:
Belcher Pharmaceuticals, LLC
Largo, FL 33773
Made in USA

NIH

▲ **Figure 17-9**

The recommended dose of Cefixime is 8 mg/kg/day of the suspension. This may be administered as a single daily dose or may be given in two divided doses, as 4 mg/kg every 12 hours.

▲ **Figure 17-10**

A 7-year-old male child is ordered a 25 mg onetime dose of furosemide oral solution.

Refer to the furosemide label in Figure 17-11 for dosage information.

14. How many mL of furosemide will the client receive?   _____

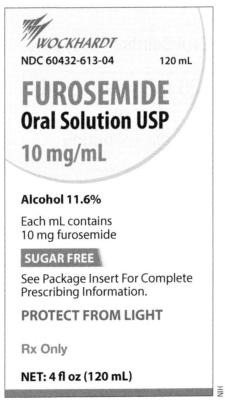

WOCKHARDT
NDC 60432-613-04   120 mL

FUROSEMIDE
Oral Solution USP

10 mg/mL

Alcohol 11.6%

Each mL contains
10 mg furosemide

SUGAR FREE

See Package Insert For Complete
Prescribing Information.

PROTECT FROM LIGHT

Rx Only

NET: 4 fl oz (120 mL)

NIH

▲ **Figure 17-11**

15. Draw an arrow to the teaspoon dose on the dropper in Figure 17-12.

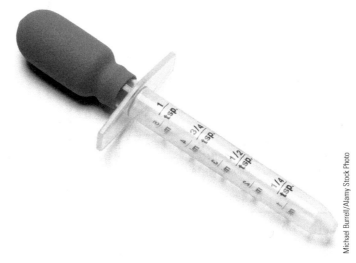

▲ **Figure 17-12**

A 12-year-old female patient is receiving the first dose of potassium chloride oral suspension. The patient is to receive 10 mEq once today and 12 mEq once tomorrow prior to discharge.
Answer the following questions utilizing the label in Figure 17-13.

16. Determine the first dose in mL for this patient.   _____

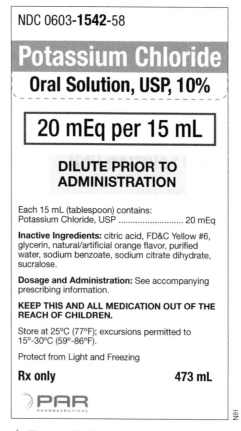

NDC 0603-**1542**-58

Potassium Chloride
Oral Solution, USP, 10%

20 mEq per 15 mL

DILUTE PRIOR TO
ADMINISTRATION

Each 15 mL (tablespoon) contains:
Potassium Chloride, USP .... 20 mEq

Inactive Ingredients: citric acid, FD&C Yellow #6, glycerin, natural/artificial orange flavor, purified water, sodium benzoate, sodium citrate dihydrate, sucralose.

Dosage and Administration: See accompanying prescribing information.

KEEP THIS AND ALL MEDICATION OUT OF THE REACH OF CHILDREN.

Store at 25°C (77°F); excursions permitted to 15°-30°C (59°-86°F).

Protect from Light and Freezing

Rx only   **473 mL**

⟩**PAR**
PHARMACEUTICAL

▲ **Figure 17-13**

17. Draw a line to the correct mL volume on the medicine cup
    below in Figure 17-14.   _____

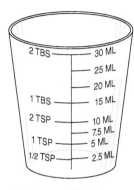

▲ **Figure 17-14**

18. Calculate the dose in mL prior to discharge.   _____

19. Draw a line to the answer in question 18 on the oral syringe in Figure 17-15.

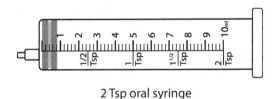

2 Tsp oral syringe

▲ **Figure 17-15**

Answers **1.** 528–1,056 mg/day **2.** 900 mg daily **3.** 225 mg **4.** 3.8 mL **5.** place arrow at 3.8 mL **6.** 36.8 kg
7. 1,472–2,944 mg **8.** yes **9.** 1 tsp **10.** place the arrow at 1 tsp on the oral syringe **11.** 26.1 kg **12.** 104 mg
13. 5.2 mL **14.** 2.5 mL **15.** place arrow at ½ tsp on dropper **16.** 7.5 mL **17.** place arrow at 7.5 mL on medicine cup
18. 9 mL **19.** place arrow at 9 mL on oral syringe

Intramuscular and Subcutaneous Dosages

The medications most often given subcutaneously are insulin and certain immunizations, such as MMR (measles, mumps, rubella) that specifically require the subcutaneous route. Any site with sufficient subcutaneous tissue may be used, with the upper arm being the site of choice for immunizations. The intramuscular route is used most frequently for preoperative and postoperative medications for sedation and pain, and for immunizations such as DPT (diphtheria, pertussis, tetanus), which must be administered deep IM. The intramuscular site of choice for infants and small children is the vastus lateralis, which is located on the anterior lateral aspect of the thigh. The gluteal muscles do not develop until a child has learned to walk. Usually, not more than 1 mL is injected per site, and sites are rotated regularly. This volume may increase as the size of the child increases, but it is usually not more than 3 mL in a large muscle, even in an older child.

Dosage calculation is the same as for adults. The dosages should follow the same rounding recommendations, as well. If the volume is greater than 1 mL, the medication should be rounded to the tenth. If the volume is less than 1 mL, the medication should be rounded to the hundredth. Selection of the syringe will depend on the volume to be administered. If the amount is less than 1 mL, a tuberculin, or 1 mL syringe would be the best choice. If the amount is greater than 1 mL, a 3 mL syringe would be the best choice. (Refer to Chapter 12 if you need to review the calibrations and use of the various syringes). There is less margin for error in pediatric dosages, and calculations and measurements are carefully triple-checked.

Problems 17.2

Answer the following questions utilizing the medication labels.

1. Refer to the amikacin sulfate label in Figure 17-16 and calculate a 200 mg IM dose for a 5-year-old child. _____

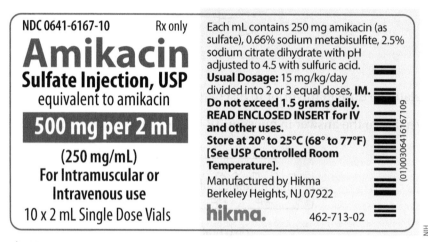

NDC 0641-6167-10   Rx only

Amikacin
Sulfate Injection, USP
equivalent to amikacin

500 mg per 2 mL

(250 mg/mL)
**For Intramuscular or
Intravenous use**
10 x 2 mL Single Dose Vials

Each mL contains 250 mg amikacin (as sulfate), 0.66% sodium metabisulfite, 2.5% sodium citrate dihydrate with pH adjusted to 4.5 with sulfuric acid. **Usual Dosage:** 15 mg/kg/day divided into 2 or 3 equal doses, **IM. Do not exceed 1.5 grams daily. READ ENCLOSED INSERT for IV and other uses. Store at 20° to 25°C (68° to 77°F) [See USP Controlled Room Temperature].** Manufactured by Hikma Berkeley Heights, NJ 07922

hikma.   462-713-02

(01)00306416167109

▲ Figure 17-16

2. Refer to the morphine label in Figure 17-17 and calculate a 2.5 mg subcutaneous dose for a 6-year-old patient. Draw an arrow to the mL on the syringe in Figure 17–18. Round to the nearest hundredth.

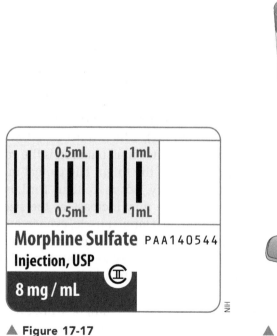

0.5mL   1mL

0.5mL   1mL

Morphine Sulfate PAA140544
Injection, USP
8 mg / mL

▲ Figure 17-17

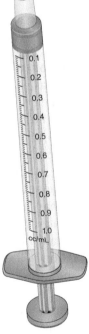

0.1
0.2
0.3
0.4
0.5
0.6
0.7
0.8
0.9
1.0
cc/mL

▲ Figure 17-18

3. Refer to the tobramycin label in Figure 17-19 and calculate a 15 mg IM dose for a pediatric patient. Draw a line on the syringe in Figure 17-20 to the mL volume to be administered.

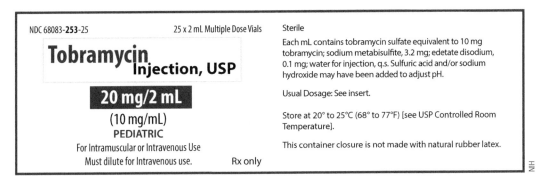

▲ **Figure 17-19**

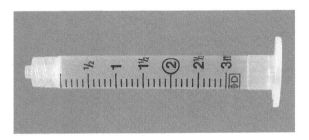

▲ **Figure 17-20**

4. An 8-year-old patient is ordered 1.5 mg of ondansetron IM for nausea. Utilizing the ondansetron label in Figure 17-21, calculate the dose. _____

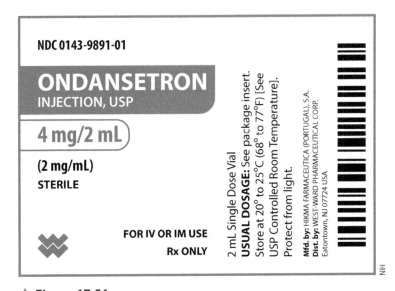

▲ **Figure 17-21**

5. A 12-year-old patient has been ordered 20 mg subcutaneous Lovenox® after surgery. Refer to the Lovenox® label in Figure 17-22 and calculate the amount to be administered. Draw an arrow to the mL dose on the syringe in Figure 17-23.

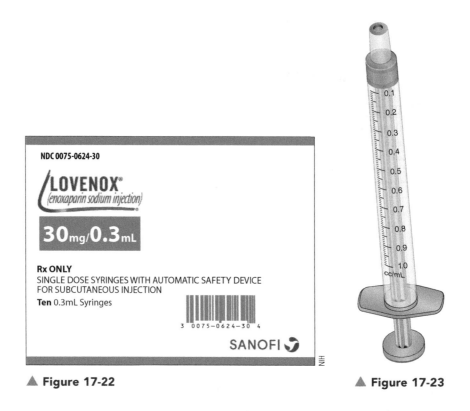

▲ Figure 17-22

▲ Figure 17-23

Answers   **1.** 0.8 mL   **2.** place arrow at 0.31 mL   **3.** place arrow at 1.5 mL   **4.** 0.75 mL   **5.** place the arrow at 0.2 mL

Intravenous Dosages

Pediatric IV medication administration involves a multifaceted challenge and a responsibility. Infants and children, particularly under the age of 4, are not completely developed physiologically, so drug tolerance, absorption, and excretion are ongoing concerns. In addition, infants and acutely ill children can tolerate only a narrow range of hydration, making administration of IV drugs, which are diluted, a critical and exact skill. Drug dilution protocols may specify a range for dilution, and on many occasions the smallest possible volume may have to be used in order to not overhydrate a child. Dosage and dilution decisions may have to be made on a day-to-day or even a dose-to-dose basis and will involve the team effort of nurse, physician, and pharmacist. Additional information regarding pediatric considerations in IV therapy will be presented in the next section of this book.

The veins of infants and children are very fragile. In addition, the irritating nature of many intravenous medications mandates careful site inspection for signs of inflammation and infiltration. This should be done immediately before, during, and after each infusion of IV medication. Signs of inflammation, or phlebitis, include redness, heat, swelling, and tenderness. Signs of infiltration include swelling, coldness, pain, and lack of blood return in the IV tubing. Either complication necessitates discontinuation of the IV and a restart at a new site.

The calculation of pediatric IV doses will be completed using the same methods of calculation as used for adults. Because the IV medications are being administered directly into the circulating blood volume, there are no restrictions on volume due to location, as there are with subcutaneous and intramuscular injections. However, children may be less able to tolerate large volumes of fluid; therefore, the dilution of medications may be limited to prevent overhydration.

It is important to compare dosages ordered with average dosages for a particular medication as discussed in previous chapters. This is a key nursing responsibility to ensure safe medication administration.

 Keypoint: Dosages of pediatric IV medications are usually calculated based on body weight or body surface area (BSA).

In previous chapters we discussed comparing the physician's order to the calculated safe dose for a child based on the weight or body surface area. This concept cannot be stressed enough—as the person administering the medication, you are responsible to ensure the physician's order is safe for the child receiving the medication. The following example will demonstrate how to use the calculated dosage to check safety of dosages ordered by the physician.

Example 1 ▪   A child weighing 22.6 kg has an order for 600 mg of ceftriaxone to be administered IV in 100 mL of D5W every 12 hours. This order means that we will dilute the 600 mg of medication in 100 mL of IV fluids and administer intermittently twice a day. The usual dosage range according to the medication insert is 50–75 mg/kg/day. Determine if the dosage ordered is within the normal range.

Step 1   Calculate the usual daily dosage range for this child, based on the label.

50 mg/day × 22.6 kg = 1,130 mg/day

75 mg/day × 22.6 kg = 1,695 mg/day

The usual range is 1,130 mg/day to 1,695 mg/day. Now we can compare the physician's order to the usual dosage range.

Step 2   Calculate the dosage ordered to infuse in 24 hr. Remember, the dosage will be the amount in milligrams in this example. It will not involve the volume of IV fluids.

600 mg every 12 hr = 1,200 mg in 24 hr

Step 3   Assess the accuracy of the dosage ordered.

1,200 mg in 24 hr is within the 1,130 mg/day to 1,695 mg/day dosage range. Therefore, the medication order is safe, and the remainder of the order can be implemented. Refer to Figure 17-24 to calculate how many mL of medication per dose will be added to the 100 mL of IV fluids.

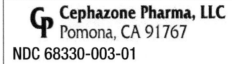

▲ Figure 17-24

Step 4   Using the IV directions on the vial, we would notice that the concentration of the medication is 100 mg per mL after reconstitution. The physician's order is for 600 mg every 12 hours. Therefore, we will withdraw 6 mL from this vial and add it to the 100 mL of IV fluid for administration.

In this example, we have assessed the safety of the IV dose that was ordered by the physician. This same process for assessing the safety of a physician order can be completed for any route of medication administration and is an essential step in safe medication administration.

Another consideration that may apply to children is monitoring fluid intake. A child's fluid intake requirements are typically addressed using the child's weight in kilograms and may include both oral and intravenous fluids. Since volume is associated with IV medications, whether they are given by infusion or by direct injection, this volume must be included in determining if the child's fluid requirements are met. Strict accounting of intake must include the volumes of IV medications being administered. There are various formulas available for determination of required fluid intake for children. Some of these formulas may be used to determine hourly intake, while other formulas will be used to determine daily intake. You must also be clear whether the amount of fluid intake will include both oral and IV fluids. You should follow the protocol in place at your facility.

Problems 17.3

Answer the following questions related to the administration of IV medication to a child.

A child has been ordered furosemide 35 mg IV q 12 hr. The client weighs 22.7 kg. According to the package insert, administer 2–4 mg/kg/day in divided doses every 12 hr IV. Refer to the furosemide label in Figure 17-25 to answer the questions.

1. Calculate the daily dose range for this child.   _____

2. Is the ordered dose safe?   _____

3. Calculate the mL the client will receive
   intravenously per dose.   _____

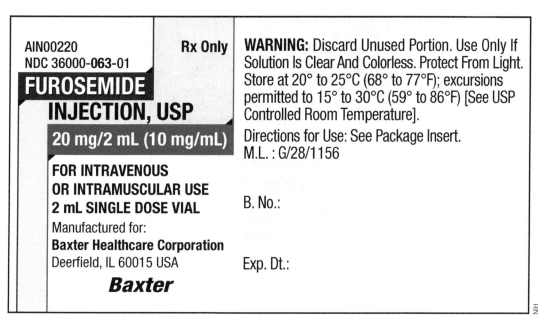

AIN00220   **Rx Only**
NDC 36000-063-01

FUROSEMIDE
INJECTION, USP

20 mg/2 mL (10 mg/mL)

FOR INTRAVENOUS
OR INTRAMUSCULAR USE
2 mL SINGLE DOSE VIAL

Manufactured for:
Baxter Healthcare Corporation
Deerfield, IL 60015 USA

Baxter

WARNING: Discard Unused Portion. Use Only If Solution Is Clear And Colorless. Protect From Light. Store at 20° to 25°C (68° to 77°F); excursions permitted to 15° to 30°C (59° to 86°F) [See USP Controlled Room Temperature].

Directions for Use: See Package Insert.
M.L. : G/28/1156

B. No.:

Exp. Dt.:

▲ **Figure 17-25**

A pediatric patient has been ordered ampicillin 135 mg to be given IV BID. The recommended dosage on the package insert is 5–10 mg/kg/dose. The patient weighs 14.2 kg. The availability of ampicillin is 200 mg per 2 mL.

4. Calculate the safe range per dose for the patient.   _____

5. Is the ordered dose safe?   _____

6. Calculate the mL to be administered IV if the order
   is safe. If it is not safe, answer NO to the question.   _____

A 10-year-old patient has been admitted to the pediatric unit with hypothyroidism. The physician has ordered levothyroxine 0.12 mg IV once daily. The recommended daily dose according to the package insert is 2–4 mcg/kg/day. The patient weighs 70 lb. Refer to the levothyroxine label in Figure 17-26 to answer the following questions.

7. What is the daily dose range recommended for this patient?   _____

8. If the order is safe, calculate the mL to administer IV daily. If it is not safe, what will you do?   _____

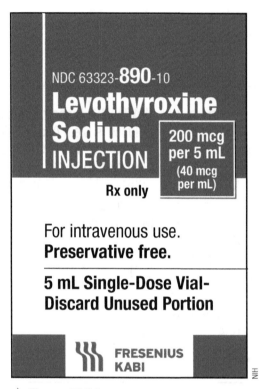

▲ **Figure 17-26**

A 16-year-old male client is being treated for anemia. The physician has ordered epoetin alfa IV 4,200 units three times weekly. The client weighs 140 lb. According to the package insert, the recommended dose is 50–400 units/kg two to three times weekly. Refer to the epoetin alfa label in Figure 17-27 to answer the following questions.

9. Calculate the recommended dose range for this client.   _____

10. Assess the physician's order for safety.   _____

11. Calculate the mL to administer IV per dose if the answer to question 10 is safe. Otherwise, answer NO to this question.   _____

12. If the order is safe, how many vials would be needed per IV dose?   _____

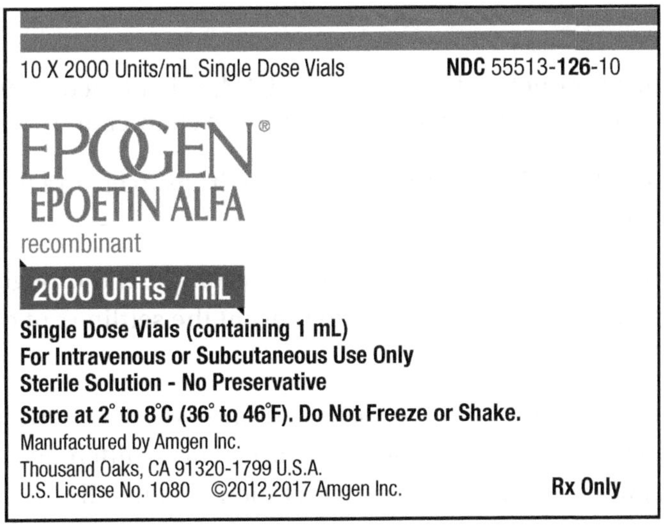

10 X 2000 Units/mL Single Dose Vials   NDC 55513-**126**-10

EPOGEN®
EPOETIN ALFA
recombinant

2000 Units / mL

Single Dose Vials (containing 1 mL)
For Intravenous or Subcutaneous Use Only
Sterile Solution - No Preservative
Store at 2° to 8°C (36° to 46°F). Do Not Freeze or Shake.
Manufactured by Amgen Inc.
Thousand Oaks, CA 91320-1799 U.S.A.
U.S. License No. 1080   ©2012,2017 Amgen Inc.   **Rx Only**

▲ **Figure 17-27**

A newborn baby weighs 8 lb and is diagnosed with an irregular heartbeat. The cardiologist has ordered digoxin 100 mcg IV as an initial dose. According to the package insert, the recommended initial dose in this age group is 20–30 mcg/kg IM or IV. Refer to the label in 17-28 to answer the following questions.

13. What is the safe dose range for this patient?   _____

14. Does the ordered dose fall within the safe range?   _____

15. If the answer to question 14 is yes, calculate the IV mL dose
     the patient will receive as an initial dose. If not, answer
     NO to this question.   _____

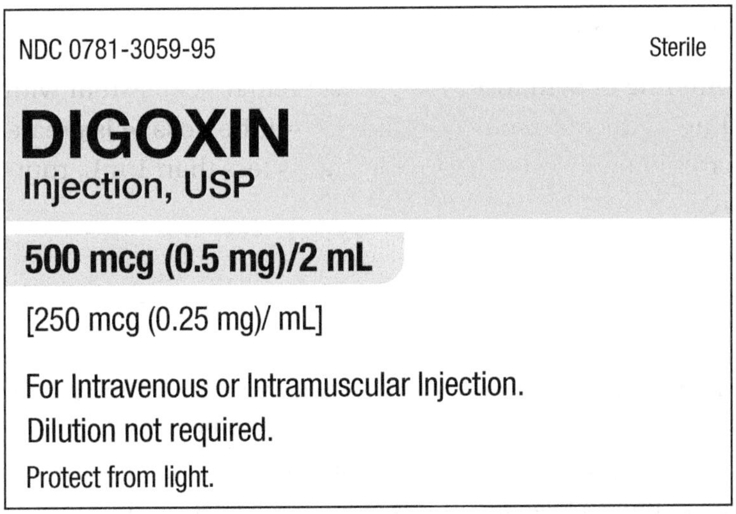

NDC 0781-3059-95   Sterile

DIGOXIN
Injection, USP

500 mcg (0.5 mg)/2 mL

[250 mcg (0.25 mg)/ mL]

For Intravenous or Intramuscular Injection.
Dilution not required.
Protect from light.

▲ **Figure 17-28**

Answers 1. 45–91 mg/day **2.** yes **3.** 3.5 mL **4.** 71–142 mg/dose **5.** yes **6.** 1.4 mL **7.** 64–127 mcg/day **8.** safe, 3 mL **9.** 3,180–25,440 units 2-3 times weekly **10.** safe **11.** 2.1 mL **12.** 3 vials **13.** 72–108 mcg for initial dose **14.** yes **15.** 0.4 mL

Summary

This concludes the introduction to pediatric oral, IM, subcutaneous, and intravenous dosages. The important points to remember from this chapter are:

- Care must be taken when administering oral drugs to ensure that the child has swallowed the medication.

- If liquid medications are prepared as suspensions, mix thoroughly prior to measurement, and administer promptly to prevent the settling out of any insoluble particles.

- Care must be taken not to confuse oral syringes, which are unsterile, with hypodermic syringes, which are sterile. There is usually a difference in the tip of the oral syringe, which prevents secure attachment of a needle.

- The IM site of choice for infants and small children is the vastus lateralis.

- Usually not more than 1 mL is injected per IM or subcutaneous site, and sites are rotated regularly. The volume may increase as the child grows; however, it is usually less than 3 mL in a larger muscle.

- Many IV medications are diluted for administration, and it is important to include this volume of fluids in the child's intake.

- Recommended dosage ranges are used to verify safety of the physician's order for any medication administered by any route. Many times, these dosage ranges are calculated per kg, per lb, or per m^2.

- Children's veins are very fragile, and intravenous sites must be checked for inflammation and infiltration immediately before, during, and after each medication administration.

- The rounding of pediatric dosages will remain consistent with the rounding we recommended for adults—if the dosage is greater than 1 mL, round to the tenth; if the dosage is less than 1 mL, round to the hundredth.

Summary Self-Test

Utilize the medication labels provided to calculate the following pediatric dosages. Calculate in mL and place your answer on the line provided.

1. Prepare a 20 mg dose of Protonix® IV. Directions for reconstitution according to the package insert is to add 10 mL 0.9% sodium chloride solution to the powder in the vial. _____

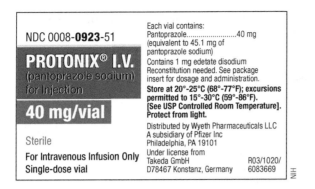

2. Prepare a 150 mg PO dosage of penicillin V potassium.   _____

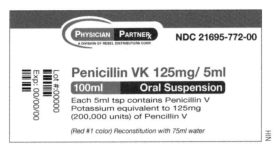

3. Prepare 100 mg of amoxicillin PO.   _____

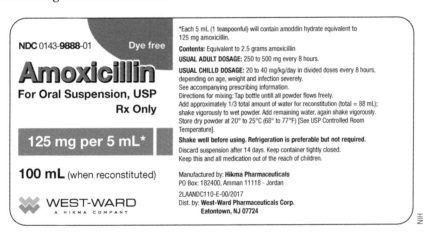

4. Prepare 85 mg cefpodoxime PO.   _____

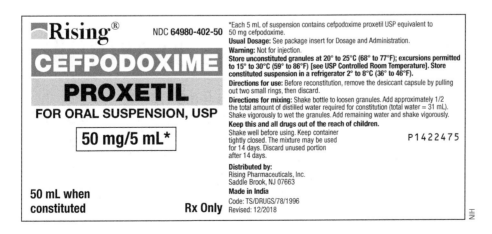

5. Prepare etanercept 32 mg subcutaneous (for label purposes, the child weighs 65 kg). _____

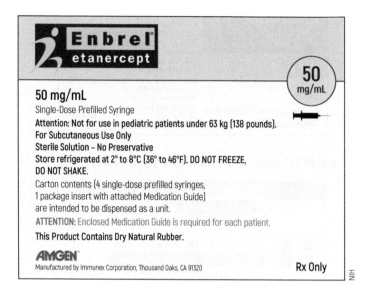

6. Prepare carbamazepine 160 mg PO. _____

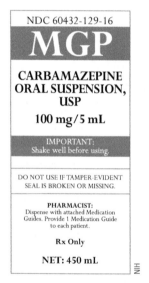

7. Prepare clindamycin 125 mg IM. _____

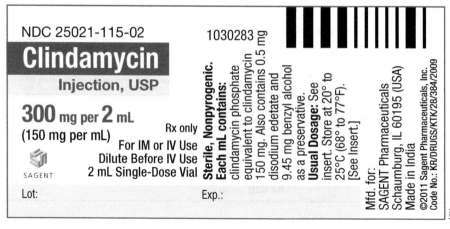

8. Prepare heparin 410 units IV.   _____

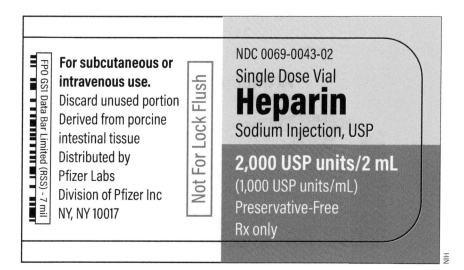

9. Prepare gentamicin 50 mg IM.   _____

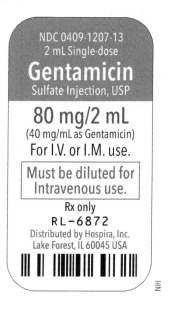

10. Prepare dexamethasone 3 mg IM.   _____

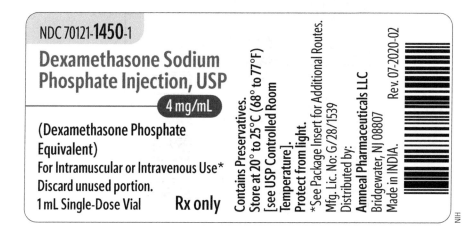

11. Prepare darbepoetin 9 mcg subcutaneous. _____

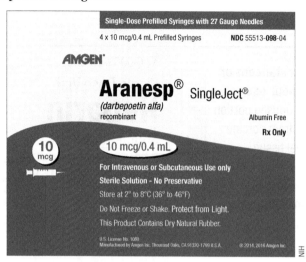

12. Prepare a PO dose of 45 mg of phenobarbital. _____

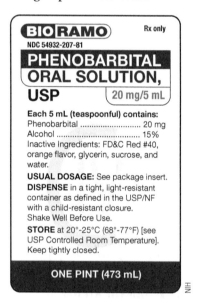

13. Prepare a 6 mg dosage of propranolol PO. _____

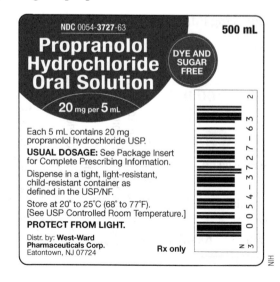

14. Prepare a 15 mg IM dose of ranitidine.   _____

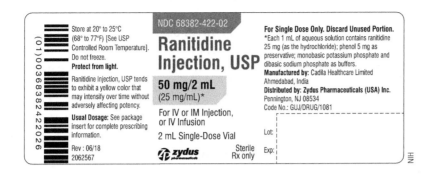

15. Prepare ondansetron 3 mg IV.   _____

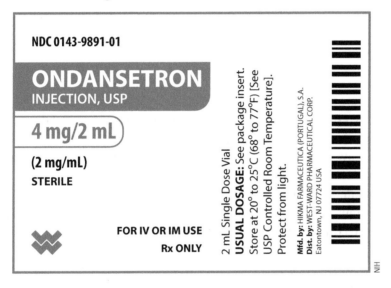

Answers to Summary Self-Test

1. 5 mL	**4.** 8.5 mL	**7.** 0.83 mL	**10.** 0.75 mL	**13.** 1.5 mL
2. 6 mL	**5.** 0.64 mL	**8.** 0.41 mL	**11.** 0.36 mL	**14.** 0.6 mL
3. 4 mL	**6.** 8 mL	**9.** 1.3 mL	**12.** 11.3 mL	**15.** 1.5 mL

Critical Thinking Questions

1. Nurses caring for pediatric clients must be aware of multiple factors related to the safety of administering parenteral medications. What knowledge is essential when administering parenteral medications to this age group? Select all that apply.

   a. Follow the same calculation rounding rules as with adults.

   b. Administer a maximum of 2 mL until the gluteal muscle is developed.

   c. Safe dose calculations are for antibiotics and chemotherapy only.

   d. The risk of overhydration is more significant in a child than in an adult.

   e. Immature liver and kidneys affect pharmacokinetics.

   f. Dilution of IV medications may be made on a dose-to-dose consideration.

2. A 9-year-old female client is ordered a onetime preprocedure IV dose of vanco-mycin based on weight. The client weighs 63 lb. According to the package insert, a single dose of 20 mg/kg must be administered IV one hour prior to a proce-dure. Dilute the dose in at least 100 mL of 0.9% NaCl or D5W and infuse over 60 min. Refer to the vancomycin label in Figure 17-29 for information to answer the question. Choose the appropriate interventions to prepare and administer vancomycin IV. Select all that apply.

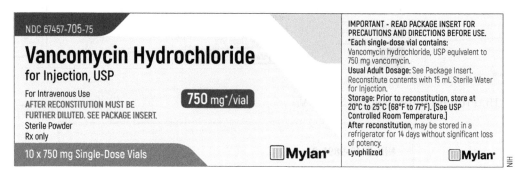

▲ **Figure 17-29**

   a. Calculate the weight at 28.6 kg.
   b. Use the concentration of 750 mg/100 mL to calculate the dose.
   c. Calculate the mg dose at 572 mg.
   d. Withdraw 11.4 mL from the vial and add it to the 100 mL IV bag for administration.
   e. Calculate the weight at 138.6 kg.
   f. Withdraw 0.76 mL from the vial and add it to the 100 mL IV bag for administration.
   g. Use the concentration of 750 mg/15 mL to calculate the dose.

Answers to Critical Thinking Questions

   1. a, d, e, f **(Rationale:** b is incorrect—The maximum dose is 1 mL; c is incorrect—There are no limitations for checking the safety of all pediatric medication orders.)

   2. a, c, d, g **(Rationale:** b is incorrect—refer to the label for the 750mg/15 mL concentration; e is incorrect—the kg weight is 28.6; f is incorrect—11.4 mL will be withdrawn from the vial.)

Intravenous Calculations

Introduction to IV Therapy

Objectives

The learner will:

1. differentiate between primary, secondary, peripheral, and central IV lines.

2. explain the function of IV drip chambers, roller and slide clamps, and needleless injection ports.

3. identify considerations with intermittent infusion ports.

4. differentiate between strengths used for heparin flush solutions and strengths used for therapeutic heparin injections.

5. differentiate between IV infusion pumps, syringe pumps, and patient-controlled analgesia (PCAs).

6. identify the abbreviations used for IV fluid orders.

Calculations associated with IV therapy will be easier to understand with some general understanding of IV therapy. Intravenous fluid and medication administration is one of the most challenging of all nursing responsibilities. There are many different types of IV fluids, as well as many additives that are used with IV fluids, such as medications, electrolytes, and vitamins. It is important to accurately follow the prescriber's order for IV therapy and medication administration. There are also many different types of IV administration sets and components, as well as different models of electronic infusion devices used to infuse and monitor IV fluids. Understanding some basic concepts will make IV therapy less daunting. It is beyond the scope of this book to provide in-depth information about IV therapy, but this chapter will cover some general concepts and terms related to IV therapy to provide a foundation to build on.

Keypoint: The choice of IV fluids and additives is a physician's responsibility. Preparation of IVs containing additives may be the pharmacist's responsibility or may be the responsibility of the nurse, depending on the policy of the clinical setting. The nursing responsibility in all clinical settings will be to double-check for the correct solution and set and regulate IV flow rates of the solutions ordered. Inpatient settings may use pumps to regulate IV flow rates, but there are some settings, such as home care and emergency settings, where gravity flow is still the method in use.

Clinical Relevance: Initiating and monitoring IV therapy is an important nursing function. To initiate IV therapy, a break in skin integrity is involved. Therefore, initiation of IV therapy will not only involve ensuring the correct fluids and medications are administered based on physician order, but it will also involve monitoring the IV site for signs and symptoms of complications, such as infiltration, phlebitis, or infection.

These complications can occur when an IV is infusing by gravity or by IV infusion pump. The IV infusion pump does not prevent these complications. The nurse will also need to monitor the patient for their response to the IV therapy, similar to monitoring a patient for their response to various medications they are receiving. As with medication labels, it is essential to verify that the correct IV fluid is obtained and administered based on physician order. The names of fluids can be very similar; it involves careful comparison of the label to the order. For example, normal saline (NS) and $\frac{1}{2}$ NS could easily be confused, but both fluids have different effects on the body. Treat IV therapy as a medication order and consistently follow all the "rights" for safe medication administration: right patient, right medication (fluid), right dose (rate), right route (IV), right frequency (continuous or intermittent), and right documentation. The onset of action of medications and fluids administered intravenously occurs immediately; therefore, there is no room for error.

IV Administration Sets and Sites

A typical primary IV line connecting an IV fluid bag or bottle to the needle or cannula in a vein is shown in Figure 18-1. The IV tubing is connected to the IV solution bag (using sterile technique), and the bag is hung on an IV stand.

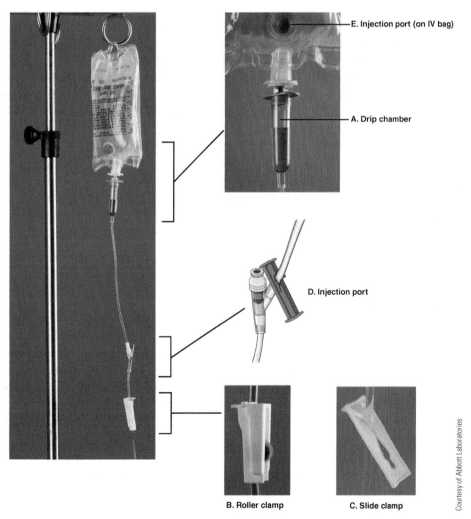

E. Injection port (on IV bag)

A. Drip chamber

D. Injection port

B. Roller clamp

C. Slide clamp

Courtesy of Abbott Laboratories

▲ **Figure 18-1**

Keypoint: Close all roller clamps on the IV tubing before connecting it to the solution bag. This step prevents air bubbles from entering the tubing and prevents the loss of large amounts of fluid when priming the tubing and removing the air from the tubing.

The drip chamber, Figure 18-1A, is then squeezed to half-fill it with fluid. This level is very important with gravity-infused IVs because IV flow rates are set and monitored by counting the drops falling in this chamber. If the chamber is too full, the drops cannot be counted. If the outlet at the bottom of the chamber is not completely covered, air can enter the tubing during infusions and subsequently enter the vein and circulatory system.

Keypoint: The correct fluid level for IV drip chambers is half-full to allow drops to be counted and prevent air from entering the tubing.

Next, the roller clamp, Figure 18-1B, is adjusted to set the flow rate while the drops falling in the drip chamber are counted. A second type of clamp, called a slide clamp, Figure 18-1C, is present on all IV tubings. The slide clamp can be used to temporarily stop an IV without disturbing the rate set on the roller clamp. The roller clamp provides an extremely accurate control of rate, whereas the slide clamp will only stop and start the flow.

Next, identify the needleless injection port, Figure 18-1D. Needleless ports are in several locations on the tubing, typically near the cannula end, drip chamber, and middle of the line. When injecting into these ports, the needle must be removed and the luer lock tip of the syringe will be secured onto the needleless port. These ports allow injection of medication directly into the line. They also allow for attachment to the primary line of secondary IV lines containing compatible IV fluids or medications. There is an injection port on the IV bag as well, Figure 18-1E. This allows for additives to be placed into the IV bag. The injection port on the IV bag will not be needleless.

Intravenous fluids may be on an infusion pump, or they may run by gravity flow. If they are infusing by gravity flow, the IV solution bag will be hung above the patient's heart level to exert sufficient pressure to infuse. Three feet above heart level is considered an average height.

Keypoint: When a pump is not used, the height of an IV bag will affect the flow rate. The higher the bag is hung, the greater the pressure and the faster the IV will infuse.

This pressure differential also means that if the flow rate is adjusted while the patient is lying in bed, it will slow down if they sit or stand, and it changes slightly with each turn from side to side. For this reason, monitoring IV flow rate is ongoing. If the IV is infusing by pump, you will be able to retrieve volumes infused from the pump. If it is infusing by gravity, you will need to check the infusion flow rate frequently, especially after position changes. The goal is to check the rate and site every hour; however, facility policies may vary.

It is your responsibility to use critical thinking to determine the frequency of checking the IV infusion. Several variables will affect frequency of your checks: the condition of the patient, including mental state and physiological concerns; the type of fluid or medication infusing; and the location of the site. In addition to checking flow rate, it is important to check the IV site for signs of complications. These complications may include phlebitis (inflammation of the vein), infiltration (caused by fluid leaking out of the vein into the surrounding tissues), and infection.

There are two additional terms relating to primary lines that you must know: peripheral and central lines. If an arm or hand (or, less commonly, leg) vein is used for an infusion, it is referred to as a **peripheral line**. Figure 18-2 shows a peripheral IV site with a needleless port.

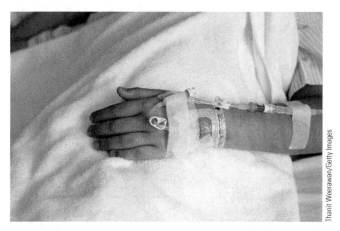

▲ **Figure 18-2** Peripheral IV site with needleless ports.

A **central line** uses a special catheter where the tip is located centrally in a deep chest vein. Central lines may access the subclavian vein directly through the chest wall. Refer to Figure 18-3 for a diagram of a central line entering the chest wall to access the subclavian vein.

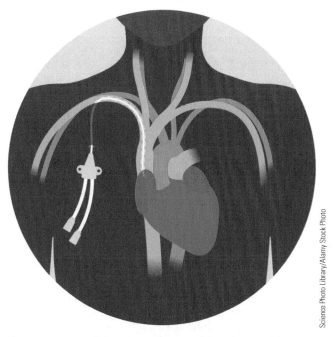

▲ **Figure 18-3** Diagram of central line inserted through chest wall into subclavian vein.

A central line may also be placed via the jugular vein in the neck or through a peripheral vein in the arm. The IV catheter in all these sites would be positioned in the superior vena cava. If the chest vein is accessed through a peripheral vein, the term *PICC* may be used. This means peripherally inserted central catheter. The PICC line is the only central line that starts in a peripheral vein. Refer to Figure 18-4 for a diagram of a PICC line.

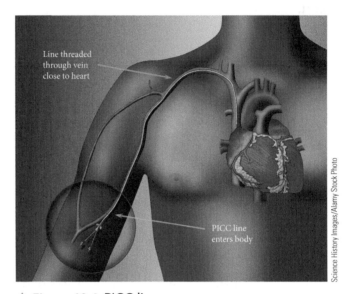

▲ **Figure 18-4** PICC line.

Central lines that go directly into the subclavian vein through the chest wall may include single, double, or triple lumen catheters. Refer to Figure 18-5 for an example of a double lumen catheter. The double or triple lumen catheters have two or three distinct lumens with separate injection ports and exit sites. This is beneficial as multiple fluids and medications can be given at the same time without mixing with each other, thus preventing medication or fluid interactions.

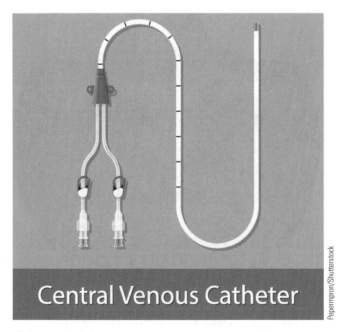

Central Venous Catheter

▲ **Figure 18-5**

Secondary lines attach to the primary line at an injection port. They are used primarily to infuse medications, frequently on an intermittent basis. For example, an antibiotic may be ordered intravenously every 6 to 8 hours. The medication would be prepared in a secondary bag and administered through the injection port on the primary IV. Secondary lines may also be used to infuse other compatible IV fluids through the primary line to prevent the need for another IV site. Secondary lines are commonly referred to as IV piggybacks, abbreviated IVPB. Refer to Figure 18-6 for an illustration of a primary and secondary line setup.

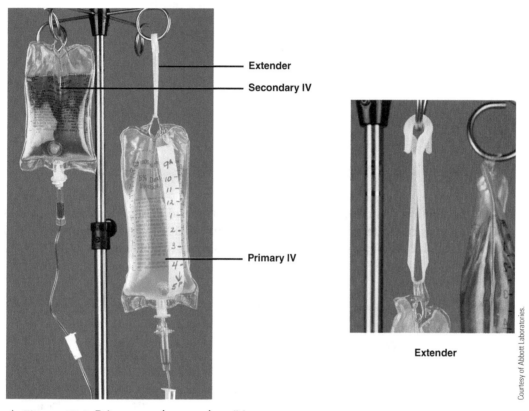

Extender

Secondary IV

Primary IV

Extender

Courtesy of Abbott Laboratories.

▲ **Figure 18-6** Primary and secondary IV setup.

The IVPB is connected to a port located below the drip chamber on the primary line. The IV in Figure 18-6 is infusing by gravity. Notice that the IVPB bag is hanging higher than the primary. This gives it greater pressure and causes it to infuse first. Each IVPB set includes a plastic or metal extender, which is used to lower the primary solution bag to obtain this pressure differential. The flow rate for the IVPB is set by a separate roller clamp located on the secondary line. When the IVPB bag has emptied, the primary line will automatically resume its flow. Secondary medication bags are usually much smaller than primary bags. Volumes of 50–250 mL bags are used for IV piggybacks. If administering a secondary line through an IV infusion pump, check the information manual to determine if you must hang the secondary higher than the primary or if they need to be at the same level. This will vary depending on the IV infusion pump being used.

Another type of secondary medication setup is the ADD-Vantage System® (Figure 18-7). This system is a specially designed IV fluid bag that contains a medication vial port.

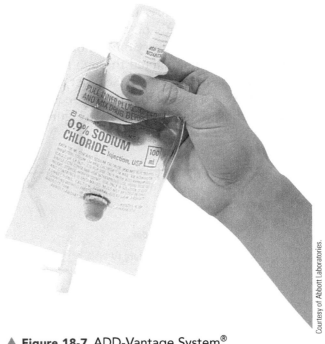

Courtesy of Abbott Laboratories.

▲ **Figure 18-7** ADD-Vantage System®.

The medication vial containing the ordered drug and dosage is inserted into the port. The process of using an ADD-Vantage System® is illustrated in Figure 18-8A–D. The drug (frequently in powdered form) is mixed using IV fluid as the diluent. Once the

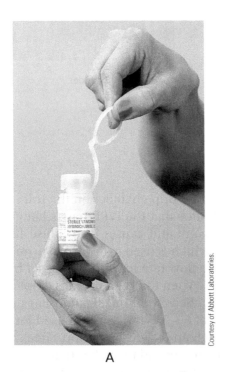

A

Courtesy of Abbott Laboratories.

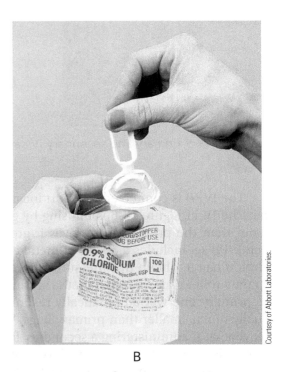

B

Courtesy of Abbott Laboratories.

▲ **Figure 18-8** ADD-Vantage® System **A**, The ADD-Vantage® medication vial is opened first. **B**, The medication vial port on the IV bag is opened. **C**, The vial top is inserted into the IV bag port and twisted to lock tightly in place. **D**, The vial stopper is removed "inside" the IV bag, and the medication and solution are thoroughly mixed before infusion.

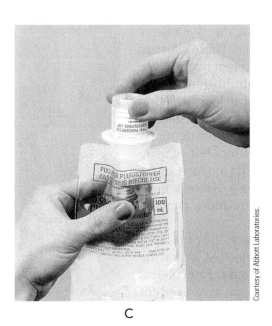

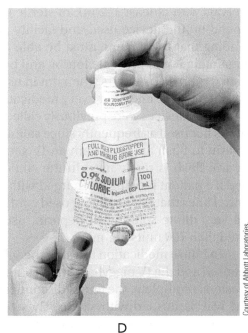

C   D

▲ **Figure 18-8** (Continued)

powder has fully dissolved, the contents of the vial are returned into the infusion bag and thoroughly mixed in the total solution before infusion. The vial remains in the solution bag port throughout the infusion, making it possible to cross-check the vial label for drug and dosage at any time.

If a drug is not available in either a prepackaged or ADD-Vantage® format, it is often prepared and labeled by the hospital pharmacy. An IV medication may also be prepared and added to the appropriate IV fluid by the nurse who initiates the infusion. When this is done, the medication must be thoroughly mixed, labeled, and initialed by that nurse.

When administering small-volume IV medications and fluids by gravity, a calibrated burette chamber, Figure 18-9 (on the next page), may be used for greater accuracy. The total capacity of burettes varies from 100–150 mL, calibrated in 1 mL increments. Many burettes are calibrated to deliver very small drops (microdrops), which contributes to their accuracy. Burette chambers are most often connected to a secondary solution bag and used as a secondary line, but they can also be primary lines.

Burettes are most commonly used in pediatric and intensive care units. When medication is ordered, it is injected into the burette through its injection port. The exact amount of IV fluid is then added as a diluent. After thorough mixing, the flow rate is set using a separate clamp on the burette line. Although most facilities use infusion pumps to deliver IV fluids and medications, burette chambers allow for precise measurement and control of fluid and medication infusions, which are delivered by gravity.

Additionally, it is important to differentiate between an IV site used for a continuously infusing IV and a site used for intermittently infusing IVs or IV medications. When a continuous IV is not necessary, but intermittent IV medication administration is, an infusion port adapter (Figure 18-10, on the next page) can be attached to an indwelling cannula in a vein. Infusion ports are frequently referred to as saline locks, or IPIDs (intermittent peripheral infusion devices). The ports must be flushed at specified intervals with at least 1–2 mL of sterile saline. The volume will depend on the device used and facility policy, with the understanding that the volume must be able to clear the IV catheter to maintain it and prevent clotting and blockage. These sites are flushed every 6 to 8 hours when not in use. When in use, the site is flushed before and after every medication administered.

These devices were previously called heparin locks, but that term is not used as frequently since saline is now used instead of heparin to flush and maintain an IV site used intermittently. A heparin flush is rarely used in the clinical setting, but may be used if a patient is being discharged with an IPID in place, or for central lines that are not being used continuously. Heparin flush is a very dilute solution of heparin, usually no more concentrated than 100 units per mL.

To infuse medication through the saline lock, the port top is cleansed and the IV piggyback medication is attached. When the infusion is complete, the line is disconnected and the needleless port will be flushed with saline. These ports are also used for direct injection of medication using a syringe, which is called an IV push. Flushing protocols before and after this IV push medication will remain in place. The flush after the medication is administered is given at a slower rate to ensure all medication is cleared from the port. It is important to follow facility policy.

If heparin is used to flush the IPID or a central line that is being used for intermittent IV fluids or medications, it is imperative that the heparin label be checked very carefully. There are many different strengths of heparin, but the only strengths for flushes are 10 units/mL or 100 units/mL. Heparin is an anticoagulant, and an incorrect strength may result in a hemorrhage. Due to similarity of vial sizes and colors on the vial, there have been several instances of preventable heparin overdosage. The overdoses could have been avoided if the labels on the medication vials had been verified and compared to the physician's order. Careful reading of any label and comparison to the physician's order is a critical step in preventing errors, which can be life threatening. Heparin anticoagulant therapy will be discussed in a later chapter.

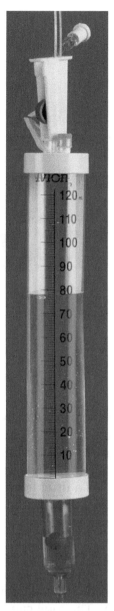

▲ **Figure 18-9** A calibrated burette chamber.

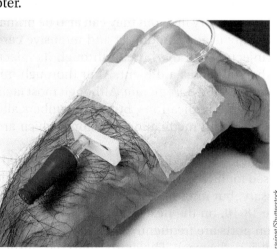

▲ **Figure 18-10** Intermittent peripheral infusion device.

Keypoint: Remember, if heparin is used to flush an IV line, the average heparin flush dosage strength is 10 units/mL and never exceeds 100 units/mL.

Problems 18.1

Answer the questions about IV administration sets and IV sites as briefly as possible.

1. What is the correct fluid level for an IV drip chamber?   _____

2. Which clamp is used to regulate IV flow rate?   _____

3. When might a slide clamp be used?   _____

4. What is a peripheral line?   _____

5. What is a central line?   _____

6. What is the common abbreviation for an intravenous piggyback?   _____

7. Is the intravenous piggyback a primary or secondary line?   _____

8. What must the height of a primary solution bag be when a secondary bag is infusing by gravity?   _____

9. When is a saline lock or IPID used?   _____

10. What are the two strengths of heparin flush solutions available?   _____

11. What is the benefit of a double or triple lumen IV catheter?   _____

12. What does PICC mean?   _____

Answers   1. chamber half-full **2.** roller clamp **3.** stop the IV temporarily without disturbing the rate set on the roller clamp **4.** a site in an arm, hand, or leg vein **5.** IV catheter inserted into a deep chest vein **6.** IVPB **7.** secondary **8.** primary bag must be lower than secondary bag **9.** for intermittent infusions when a continuous IV is not necessary **10.** 10 units/mL and 100 units/mL **11.** Multiple fluids and medications can be given at the same time without mixing with each other **12.** Peripherally inserted central catheter

Intravenous Pumps Used to Administer Fluids and Medications

There are several different types of infusion pumps. Infusion pumps offer an advantage over gravity control IVs as they allow for precise delivery of IV fluids and medications, even at very slow rates. But you must always remember that technology is only as good as the person who programs it, and it is important to be familiar with any equipment you are using and program it very carefully. Smart pumps have decreased some errors that occur when programming pumps, as commonly used medications and dosages can be programmed into the pump with alerts to prevent medication errors. Some pumps are only able to infuse a single IV line, whereas other pumps can have multiple channels attached to infuse more than one IV line. An Alaris® dual-channel infusion pump is shown in Figure 18-11.

    Different types of infusion pumps look similar, but the functions of different models vary widely. Most models will have alarms built in for common problems with IV therapy. For example, the infusion pump may alarm when air is detected in the

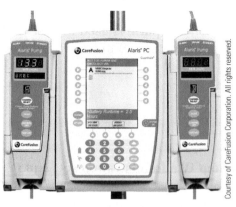

▲ **Figure 18-11** Alaris® dual pump.

tubing, when an infiltration is sensed due to increasing resistance and pressure, or when the infusion has reached its volume limit. These alarms are not perfect, as some infusion pump models may continue to pump fluids even if an IV infiltrates.

Because of the wide variation in pump models and their functions, caution is mandatory when they are used. It is estimated that a significant number of IV medication errors result from errors in pump programming. Ongoing in-services and continuing education are important to maintain competence with infusion pumps.

 Keypoint: Hospital or clinical in-service education is required for the use of all infusion devices. Infusion pumps also have instruction manuals, which should be consulted if there is any doubt surrounding use of the pump.

Infusion devices are also widely used for IV medication administration, and their precautions in use apply less to the difficulty of the skill than in becoming familiar with the specific infusion model being used. There may be more than one model in use at a clinical facility and it is an ongoing nursing responsibility to learn how to use each model. It is also important never to assume the pump is programmed correctly.

 Keypoint: Double checking of programming is mandatory in the use of infusion devices. Do not assume the person caring for the patient prior to you programmed the pump correctly according to physician orders. Always check the physician orders and compare them to the pump settings.

Errors in infusion device programming are factors in IV medication errors, and it is good practice to double check all programming. Smart infusion pumps have built-in libraries of usual drug dosages, offer customizable drug libraries for facility specific needs, and are capable of alerting users to programming errors outside hospital defined parameters. These features help to considerably decrease the risk of error, and these alerts should not be ignored.

Another type of pump used for intravenous administration is the syringe pump. Syringe pumps, as their name implies, are devices that use a syringe to administer medications or fluids (Figure 18-12). Syringe pumps are particularly valuable when drugs that cannot be mixed with other solutions or medications must be administered at a controlled rate over a short period of time; for example, 5, 10, or 20 minutes. The drug is measured in the syringe, which is inserted into the device, and the medication is infused at the rate set.

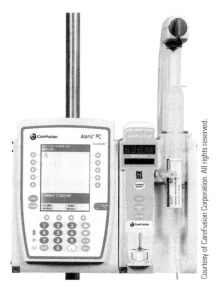

▲ **Figure 18-12** Alaris® System with syringe module.

PCA pumps, Figure 18-13, are syringe pumps that allow a patient to self-administer medication to control pain. A prefilled syringe or medication bag containing pain medication is inserted into the device, and the dosage and frequency of administration ordered are set, based on the physician's orders. The patient is then able to press the control button as medication is needed, and the medication is administered and recorded by the PCA pump. The physician will order a maximum amount of medication that can be self-administered; therefore, the patient may not receive a dose each time they push the button.

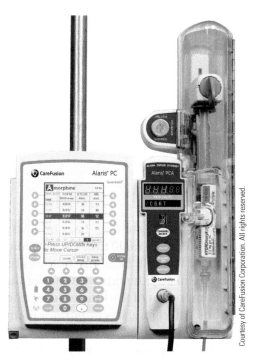

▲ **Figure 18-13** Alaris® Systems with CareFusion PCA pump.

The PCA device keeps a record of the number of times a patient attempts to use it, as well as the number of injections actually given. This provides a record of the effectiveness of the dosage prescribed. If a patient's pain is not being relieved, new orders must be obtained and the PCA pump must be reset to administer the new dosage. Facilities may require that two licensed practitioners be present to make any changes to a PCA pump, therefore decreasing the chance of programming errors.

> **Key**point: All electronic devices must be monitored frequently to be sure they are functioning properly. It is not only gravity IVs that must be monitored. Never assume that an electronic pump is perfect.

At set intervals, we must monitor the IV infusions. This may be every hour, or another interval of time set by clinical site policy. We need to check whether the IV is infusing at the rate that was set. We also need to check the patient's response to the IV therapy. Are there any complications related to the medication that is infusing or to the fluids that are infusing? Is the site free of complications, such as phlebitis or infiltration? Is the patient who activates a PCA pump getting relief of pain? If not, is it possible the PCA pump itself is malfunctioning? Electronic devices have been in use for many years and are relatively reliable, but if the desired goal is not being obtained, in the absence of other obvious reasons, the possibility of malfunction must always be considered. Accurate programming and monitoring of the infusion and site are important nursing responsibilities with infusion pumps.

Problems 18.2

Answer the questions about infusion devices as briefly as possible.

1. What is the function of an infusion pump? _____

2. List two major nursing responsibilities in the use of infusion pumps. _____

3. When might a syringe pump be used? _____

4. What is a PCA? _____

Answers **1.** delivery of IV fluids and medications at precise rates **2.** accurate programming; rate and site monitoring **3.** to infuse small volumes of drugs that are not compatible with other drugs and/or fluids **4.** patient-controlled analgesia device

Introduction to Types of IV Fluids

Intravenous fluids are prepared in plastic solution bags or glass bottles in volumes that typically range from 50 mL (bags only) to 1,000 mL. The 500 and 1,000 mL sizes are the most commonly used for primary IVs. The bags and bottles are labeled with the complete name of the fluid they contain, and the fine print under the solution name identifies the exact amount of each component of the fluid. Orders and charting, however, are usually done using abbreviations. Therefore, it is important to understand the abbreviations used with IV fluids.

Solutions may be abbreviated in different ways – for example, D_5W, 5%D/W, D5%W, or other combinations. But the initials and percentage have identical meanings regardless of the way they are abbreviated. Normal saline, identified by NS, is 0.9%

sodium chloride (NaCl). Normal saline can have varying concentrations such as ½ normal saline, which would be 0.45% NaCl. Normal saline solutions combined with dextrose, identified as D, are written with the following abbreviations: D_5NS (5% dextrose with 0.9% NaCl), $D_5½NS$ (5% dextrose with 0.45% NaCl), or $D_5¼NS$ (5% dextrose with 0.225% NaCl).

 Keypoint: In IV fluid abbreviations, D identifies dextrose; W identifies water; NS identifies normal saline; and numbers identify percentage (%) strengths.

Another commonly used solution is Lactated Ringer's, a balanced electrolyte solution, also called Ringer's lactate solution. This solution is abbreviated LR or RL. It can also be used in combination with dextrose, such as D_5LR. Electrolytes may also be added to IV fluids. One electrolyte so commonly added that it must be mentioned is potassium chloride, abbreviated as KCl, measured in milliequivalents (mEq). An example is 1,000 mL D_5W with 20 mEq KCl.

The numbers associated with dextrose and saline solutions indicate the percentages present in the fluid. Recall from Chapter 5 that percentages used with solutions indicate the number of grams of solute per 100 mL of fluid. This means that a 5% dextrose solution will have 5 g of dextrose in each 100 mL. A 500 mL bag of a 5% solution will contain 5 g × 5, or 25 g of dextrose, whereas 500 mL of a 10% solution contains 10 g × 5, or 50 g of dextrose. Normal saline is 0.9% NaCl. Therefore, there are 0.9 grams of NaCl in 100 mL of fluid. 1,000 mL of NS will contain 9 grams of NaCl (0.9 × 10). The fine print on IV labels always lists the name and amount of all components (Figure 18-14). Review the components of this intravenous solution, which includes 30 mEq potassium in 1,000 mL of 5% dextrose and 0.45% sodium chloride.

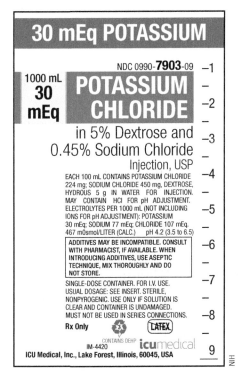

▲ **Figure 18-14** IV solution label: $D_5½$ NS with 30 mEq KCl.

Percentages and the components present in IV fluids make them significantly different from each other. As with drugs, it is critically important to read labels and make sure that the IVs are administered as ordered.

Problems 18.3

List the components and percentage strengths of the IV solutions.

1. $D_{10}NS$ _____
2. D_5NS _____
3. ½NS   _____
4. D_5 ¼NS   _____
5. $D_{20}W$ _____
6. D_5NS with 20 mEq KCl   _____
7. ¼ NS   _____
8. D_5LR _____
9. Identify what D_5W means. Include the number of grams of dextrose in 1 liter of fluid.   _____
10. Identify what 0.9% NaCl means and include the number of grams of NaCl in 500 mL of NS solution.   _____

Answers 1. 10% dextrose in 0.9% saline (NaCl) **2.** 5% dextrose in normal (0.9%) saline (NaCl) **3.** 0.45% saline (NaCl) **4.** 5% dextrose in 0.225% saline (NaCl) **5.** 20% dextrose in water **6.** 5% dextrose in 0.9% saline (NaCl) with 20 mEq potassium chloride **7.** 0.225% saline (NaCl) **8.** 5% dextrose in Lactated Ringer's solution **9.** This means 5% dextrose in water. There are 5 grams of dextrose per 100 mL; therefore, there are 50 grams of dextrose in 1000 mL (5 g × 10) **10.** 0.9% NaCl is the same as NS. There are 0.9 g of NaCl per 100 mL, therefore there are 4.5 grams of NaCl in 500 mL of NS solution.

Summary

This concludes your introduction to IV therapy. The important points to remember from this chapter are:

- Sterile technique is used to set up all IV solutions, tubings, and devices.
- The correct fluid level for an IV drip chamber is half full.
- Injection ports on an IV line are used to connect secondary lines and to administer medications.
- A peripheral line refers to an IV infusing in a hand, arm, or leg vein.
- A central line refers to an IV infusing into a deep chest vein.
- IVs may infuse by gravity; the higher the solution bag, the faster the IV will infuse.
- The average height for an IV solution bag above the patient's heart level is 3 feet.

■ Secondary solution bags must hang higher than the primary bag to infuse first if infusing by gravity. If secondary bags are hanging with a primary bag and infusing with an infusion pump, it is important to check the instruction manual.

■ Volume-controlled burettes are used for exact measurements of IV medications and fluids. These are especially important if infusion pumps are not available and small volumes of fluids must be infused precisely.

■ Intermittent peripheral infusion devices, also called saline locks or ports, are used to infuse IV medications or fluids on an intermittent basis when a continuous IV is not necessary.

■ Intermittent peripheral infusion devices are usually flushed with sterile saline. Heparin flush solutions, not exceeding 10–100 units per mL, may be used in select instances to flush an intermittent peripheral infusion device.

■ Infusion pumps are electronic devices that infuse fluids into a vein under pressure and control infusion rates.

■ Syringe pumps are used to infuse medications that cannot be mixed with other fluids or medications.

■ Patient-controlled analgesia (PCA) devices allow a patient to self-administer pain medication.

■ In IV fluid abbreviations, D identifies dextrose, W identifies water, NS identifies normal saline, LR or RL identify Lactated Ringer's or Ringer's lactate solution, and numbers identify percentage (%) strengths.

Summary Self-Test

You are to assist with some IV procedures. Answer the situational questions concerning these procedures.

1. A patient is admitted and an IV of 1,000 mL $D_5\frac{1}{2}$ NS is started at 100 mL/hour.
   What is the meaning of the term $D_5\frac{1}{2}$ NS?   _____
   What type of IV line is being started?   _____

2. All roller clamps on the IV tubing are closed before connection to the solution bag. Why?   _____

3. The IV is started in the back of the patient's left hand.
   This site indicates it is what type of IV?   _____

4. You are asked to adjust the flow rate. You will use what type of clamp to do this?   _____

5. An IV antibiotic is ordered for the patient. This is sent from the pharmacy already prepared in a small-volume IV solution bag. The setup used to infuse this medication is referred to as what?   _____

6. How is the setup in question 5 abbreviated?   _____

7. If the IV antibiotic is infusing by gravity, how will
   you set it up so that the antibiotic infuses first?   _____

8. A patient's IV fluids are to be discontinued, but the patient is to
   continue to receive IV antibiotics. How can you ensure that
   there is an IV site without continuous fluids infusing?   _____

9. A patient had a PCA pump in use for 1 day.
   What do these initials mean?   _____
   What does this device control?   _____

**Fill in the blanks to complete the following statements and answer questions as
briefly as possible.**

10. A small-volume IV medication is to be diluted in 20 mL and infused. If no infusion
    pump is available, this can be most accurately infused using a _____

11. The device mentioned in number 10 is calibrated in _____ increments.

12. When an IV medication is injected directly into the vein via a port, it is
    called an IV _____.

13. If an intravenous port is to be flushed with heparin, what dosage strengths
    would be used? _____

14. Ports may be flushed with _____ mL of _____ to prevent
    blockage every _____ hours.

15. In IV fluid abbreviations, D_5NS identifies what IV fluid? _____

Answers to Summary Self-Test

1. 5% dextrose in 0.45% saline (NaCl); primary
2. To prevent air from entering the tubing
3. peripheral
4. roller clamp
5. an IV piggyback
6. IVPB
7. The piggyback (the antibiotic) will be hung higher than the primary bag.
8. Convert the continuous IV to an intermittent
   peripheral infusion device or saline lock.
9. patient-controlled analgesia; administration of pain medication
10. calibrated burette
11. 1 mL
12. push
13. 10 units/mL or 100 units/mL
14. 1–2; normal saline; 6–8
15. 5% dextrose in normal saline or 5% dextrose in 0.9% NaCl

IV Flow Rate Calculation

Objectives

The learner will:

1. identify the calibrations in gtt/mL on IV administration sets.

2. calculate drops/minute using the method of your choice.

3. calculate mL/hour.

4. recalculate flow rates to correct off-schedule infusions.

Intravenous therapy is ordered by the physician according to the patient's needs. It is critical to administer IV fluids and medications as they are ordered. Intravenous fluids and medications can be infused by an infusion pump or by gravity. When they are infused by an infusion pump, the pump will be programmed with mL per hour. When they are infused by gravity, a calculation of drops per minute (gtt/min) will be needed in order to monitor the IV. When an infusion pump is not being used, gtt/minute will be calculated based on the available tubing and the rate ordered by the physician. In order to calculate gtt/min we will need to know the drop factor of the tubing. This will be identified as drops per mL and will be specified on the tubing packaging or the tubing itself. This chapter presents two ways to calculate IV flow rates: dimensional analysis and a formula method.

Clinical Relevance: Intravenous fluids that are ordered as continuous infusions may be ordered with a flow rate in mL per hour, for example, D_5W at 100 mL/hour. Or they may be ordered as a total volume of fluids over a total number of hours, such as 1,000 mL D_5W over 10 hours. It will be your responsibility to accurately infuse the IV at the ordered rate, whether it is by infusion pump or by gravity. If you are infusing the IV by infusion pump, you will need to program the pump accurately if the rate is already provided. However, you may also need to calculate mL/hour from the order before you program the pump. IVs that are infusing by gravity will require an additional calculation to provide a way to monitor the IV at any time we check the infusion. It will be necessary to calculate drops per minute. This will allow us to count the drops per minute at any time and get a sense of whether the IV is infusing as ordered at that point in time. We will also use these same calculations with IVs ordered on an intermittent basis, such as IV medications and fluid boluses. A fluid bolus is a rapid infusion of fluids over a short period of time and can be ordered for such conditions as hypotension or low blood pressure. Boluses, just like any IV fluid, may or may not be infused by infusion pump. A bolus of medication may be administered IV push prior to beginning an infusion of the medication.

IV Tubing Calibration

Let's look first at determining the drop factor of tubing. The size of IV drops is regulated by the type of IV set being used, which is calibrated in number of gtt/mL. Unfortunately, not all sets (or their drop size) are the same. Each clinical facility uses at least two sizes of infusion sets, a macrodrip and a microdrip. A standard **macrodrip** set calibrated at 10, 15, or 20 gtt/mL is used for routine adult IV administrations. The tubing calibrated at 20 gtt/mL is used for most infusion pump tubing. A **microdrip** set calibrated at 60 gtt/mL is used when more exact measurements are needed. Microdrip tubing may be used to infuse medications, as well as in critical care and pediatric infusions. The term *minidrip* may be used interchangeably with microdrip. Refer to Figure 19-1 for a graphic representation of the various drop sizes.

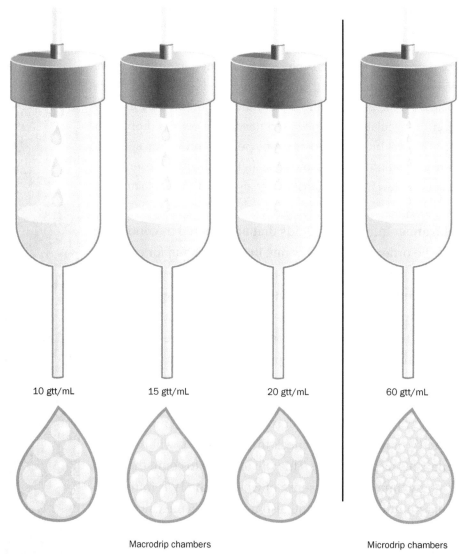

| 10 gtt/mL | 15 gtt/mL | 20 gtt/mL | 60 gtt/mL |

Macrodrip chambers   Microdrip chambers

▲ **Figure 19-1** Comparative IV drop sizes.

Keypoint: IV administration sets are calibrated in gtt/mL This is known as the drop factor and is specific for the tubing you are using. This drop factor indicates how many drops from that tubing will equal 1 mL.

The gtt/mL calibration of each IV infusion set is clearly printed on each package, and the first step in calculating flow rates is to identify the gtt/mL calibration of the set to be used for an infusion.

Problems 19.1

Identify the calibration in gtt/mL for each IV infusion set.

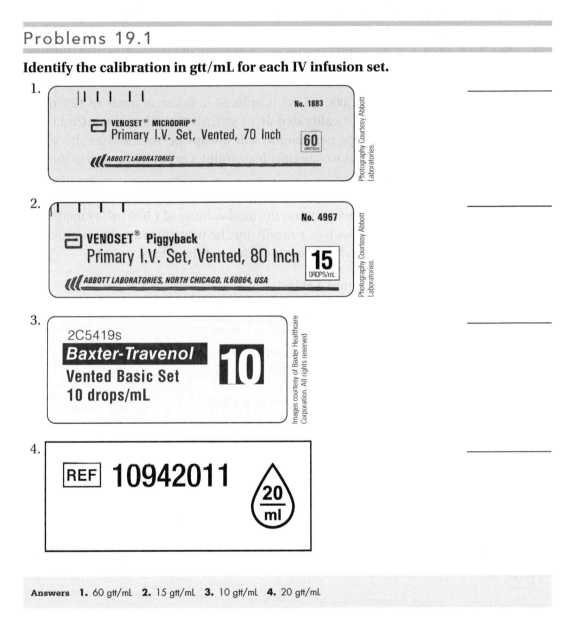

Calculating Drops Per Minute (gtt/min)

The flow rate in gtt/min is calculated from the gtt/mL calibration of the IV set being used, either 10, 15, 20, or 60 gtt/mL, and the rate per time ordered. This may be mL/hr, total mL/total hours, or mL/total minutes, which may be used with medications. To calculate this, we can use dimensional analysis or the formula method.

The formula that we use to calculate drops per minute will be slightly different from the formula we used to calculate medication dosages. For the formula method, we will use the following formula to calculate drops per minute:

$$\text{Flow rate (gtt/min)} = \frac{\text{mL} \times \text{drop factor (gtt/mL)}}{\text{time in minutes}}$$

In this formula, the mL and time must be related. For example, 125 mL/hour would be 125 mL in 60 minutes and 100 mL in 2 hours would be 100 mL in 120 minutes. The order for infusion may already be written in minutes; for example, 100 mL in 45 minutes. The mL ordered and the mL in the drop factor will cancel out, leaving drops per minute.

Let's look at a few examples using dimensional analysis, and this formula method.

Example 1 ■ An IV of 1,000 mL NS is ordered to infuse at a rate of 125 mL/hr using a set calibrated at 10 gtt/mL. Calculate the gtt/min flow rate. Drops per minute will always be rounded to the whole number, as we are unable to count a portion of a drip in the drip chamber.

You are calculating gtt/min. You will not use the total volume of 1,000 mL as there must be a time frame associated with it. You will only be using the rate that is provided of 125 mL per hour—a volume and time are included in this order.

Dimensional Analysis

$$\frac{\text{gtt}}{\text{min}} = \frac{10 \text{ gtt}}{1 \text{ mL}} \times \frac{125 \text{ mL}}{1 \text{ hr}} \times \frac{1 \text{ hr}}{60 \text{ min}}$$

$$\frac{\text{gtt}}{\text{min}} = \frac{10 \text{ gtt}}{1 \text{ mL}} \times \frac{125 \text{ mL}}{1 \text{ hr}} \times \frac{1 \text{ hr}}{60 \text{ min}}$$

$$\frac{\text{gtt}}{\text{min}} = \frac{1,250}{60} = 20.8 = 21 \text{ gtt/min}$$

Formula Method

$$\text{gtt/min} = \frac{125 \text{ mL} \times 10 \text{ gtt/mL}}{60 \text{ minutes}}$$

$$\text{gtt/min} = \frac{1,250 \text{ gtt}}{60 \text{ min}} = 20.8 = 21 \text{ gtt/min}$$

To infuse an IV at 125 mL/hr using a set with a drop factor of 10 gtt/mL, set the rate at 21 gtt/min.

 Keypoint: Flow rates are routinely rounded to the nearest whole gtt.

Example 2 ■ An IV of 150 mL is to infuse over 2 hours using a set with a drop factor of 15 gtt/mL. Calculate the flow rate in gtt/min.

Dimensional Analysis

$$\frac{\text{gtt}}{\text{min}} = \frac{15 \text{ gtt}}{1 \text{ mL}} \times \frac{150 \text{ mL}}{2 \text{ hr}} \times \frac{1 \text{ hr}}{60 \text{ min}}$$

$$\frac{\text{gtt}}{\text{min}} = \frac{15 \text{ gtt}}{1 \text{ mL}} \times \frac{150 \text{ mL}}{2 \text{ hr}} \times \frac{1 \text{ hr}}{60 \text{ min}}$$

$$\frac{\text{gtt}}{\text{min}} = \frac{2,250}{120} = 18.7 = 19 \text{ gtt/min}$$

Formula Method

$$\text{gtt/min} = \frac{150 \text{ mL} \times 15 \text{ gtt/mL}}{120 \text{ minutes}}$$

$$\text{gtt/min} = \frac{2,250 \text{ gtt}}{120 \text{ min}} = 18.7 = 19 \text{ gtt/min}$$

To infuse 150 mL in 2 hr using a set calibrated at 15 gtt/mL, set the rate at 19 gtt/min.

Example 3 ▣   The doctor orders an IV medication to be dissolved in 100 mL NS and to be infused over 45 minutes. The drop factor is 20 gtt/mL. You will be infusing this by gravity. Calculate the gtt/min.

Dimensional Analysis

$$\frac{\text{gtt}}{\text{min}} = \frac{20 \text{ gtt}}{1 \text{ mL}} \times \frac{100 \text{ mL}}{45 \text{ min}}$$

$$\frac{\text{gtt}}{\text{min}} = \frac{20 \text{ gtt}}{1 \text{ mL}} \times \frac{100 \text{ mL}}{45 \text{ min}}$$

$$\frac{\text{gtt}}{\text{min}} = \frac{2,000}{45} = 44.4 = 44 \text{ gtt/min}$$

Formula Method

$$\text{gtt/min} = \frac{100 \text{ mL} \times 20 \text{ gtt/mL}}{45 \text{ minutes}}$$

$$\text{gtt/min} = \frac{2,000 \text{ gtt}}{45 \text{ minutes}} = 44.4 = 44 \text{ gtt/min}$$

In this example, the time is already in minutes. Therefore, we do not need to convert the time to minutes. To infuse 100 mL in 45 minutes using a set with a drop factor of 20 gtt/mL, set the rate at 44 gtt/min.

Example 4 ▣   The doctor orders an IV to infuse at a KVO (keep vein open) rate. The KVO rate at your facility is defined as 20 mL/hr. You choose to use a microdrip tubing and you know this tubing drop factor is 60 gtt/mL. You will infuse this by gravity, so you calculate the drops/minute.

Dimensional Analysis

$$\frac{\text{gtt}}{\text{min}} = \frac{60 \text{ gtt}}{1 \text{ mL}} \times \frac{20 \text{ mL}}{1 \text{ hr}} \times \frac{1 \text{ hr}}{60 \text{ min}}$$

$$\frac{\text{gtt}}{\text{min}} = \frac{60 \text{ gtt}}{1 \text{ mL}} \times \frac{20 \text{ mL}}{1 \text{ hr}} \times \frac{1 \text{ hr}}{60 \text{ min}}$$

$$\frac{\text{gtt}}{\text{min}} = \frac{1,200}{60} = 20 \text{ gtt/min}$$

With a microdrip tubing, you will notice the drops per minute will be the same number as the mL per hour.

Formula Method

$$\text{gtt/min} = \frac{20 \text{ mL} \times 60 \text{ gtt/mL}}{60 \text{ minutes}}$$

$$\text{gtt/min} = \frac{1{,}200 \text{ gtt}}{60 \text{ min}} = 20 \text{ gtt/min}$$

To infuse 20 mL in 1 hour using a microdrip set, set the rate at 20 gtt/min.

Keypoint: When a 60 gtt/mL microdrip set is used, the flow rate in gtt/min is identical to the volume in mL/hr to be infused.

When using the formula method and the rate ordered is per hour, reduce numbers to easily divide the hourly rate by a number that is related to the drop factor calibration. Consider the following examples.

Example 5 ■   The physician orders an IV at 125 mL/hr. You will use a tubing with a drop factor of 10 gtt/mL. Calculate the drops per minute to infuse this by gravity by using the formula method.

$$\text{gtt/min} = \frac{125 \text{ mL} \times 10 \text{ gtt/mL}}{60 \text{ minutes}}$$

$$\text{gtt/min} = \frac{125 \times \cancel{10}^{\,1}}{\cancel{60}^{\,6}} = \frac{125}{6}$$

(Reduce 10 in the numerator and 60 in the denominator by dividing both by 10.)

$$\text{gtt/min} = 20.8 = 21 \text{ gtt/min}$$

Example 6 ■   Infuse an IV by gravity at 100 mL/hr. You will use a macrodrop tubing with a drop factor of 20 gtt/mL. Calculate the drops per minute using the formula method.

$$\text{gtt/min} = \frac{100 \text{ mL} \times 20 \text{ gtt/mL}}{60 \text{ minutes}}$$

$$\text{gtt/min} = \frac{100 \times \cancel{20}^{\,1}}{\cancel{60}^{\,3}} = \frac{100}{3}$$

(Reduce 20 in the numerator and 60 in the denominator by dividing both by 20.)

$$\text{gtt/min} = 33.3 = 33 \text{ gtt/min}$$

With these two examples, notice that if the IV is ordered as a rate per hour, we can reduce the drop factor and the 60 in the denominator. This results in a small number for quick math, even at the bedside, to calculate drops per minute. A key factor to remember, however, is the rate must be ordered as mL per 1 hour. We can quickly memorize these division factors to easily calculate drops per minute if we know the infusion rate in mL/hour.

Review the following table:

Drop Factor	Division Factor
10 gtt/mL	6
15 gtt/mL	4
20 gtt/mL	3
60 gtt/mL (microdrip tubing)	1

Example 7 ◼   The doctor orders that an IV should infuse at 120 mL per hour. You will be using tubing with a drop factor of 15. Remembering this shortcut method, you calculate as follows:

$$\frac{120}{4} = 30 \text{ gtt/min}$$ Take the mL per hour and divide by the factor of 4 to calculate the drops per minute.

Example 8 ◼   The IV is ordered to infuse at 30 mL/hr. You are using a microdrip tubing. Calculate the drops per minute by using the division factor. Recall that a microdrip tubing has a drop factor of 60 gtt/mL; therefore, the division factor will be 1. The calculation will be completed as follows:

$$\frac{30}{1} = 30 \text{ gtt/min}$$ Take the mL per hour and divide by the division factor of 1 to calculate the drops per minute.

This method can *only* be used if the rate is expressed in mL/hr (60 min). Looking at the completed equation, you will notice that because the time is restricted to 60 min, all set calibrations can be divided into the 60 to obtain a constant number for that specific tubing.

Keypoint: The division factor can be obtained for any IV set by dividing 60 by the calibration of the set. Once the division factor is known, the gtt/min rate can be calculated in one step by dividing the mL/hr rate by the division factor.

The flow rate in drops per minute is very important for any IV infusing by gravity. IVs infusing by gravity are regulated by counting the number of drops falling in the drip chamber. Use your watch or time-keeping device and count the number of drops falling in one minute. Regulate it until the number you count in one minute is the same as the number calculated for drops per minute. You will adjust this rate using the roller clamp. Knowing the drops per minute gives you a way to monitor the IV at any time you are assessing the patient and is a critical component for caring for anyone receiving IV fluids or medications by gravity.

Problems 19.2

Calculate gtt/min flow rates using the method of your choice. Round to the nearest whole gtt.

1. An IV total volume of 2,000 mL is to infuse in 12 hr using a 10 gtt/mL set.   _____

2. A total volume of 3,500 mL is ordered to infuse in 24 hr using a set calibrated at 20 gtt/mL.   _____

3. Infuse 500 mL in 3 hr using a 15 gtt/mL set.   _____

4. Infuse 150 mL in 2 hr using a 60 gtt/mL set.   _____

5. Administer an IV at 110 mL/hr using 20 gtt/mL set.   _____

6. Infuse a volume of 80 mL over 20 min using a 10 gtt/mL set.   _____

7. Infuse 125 mL over 2 hr using a microdrip set.   _____

8. A volume of 500 mL is to infuse over 4 hr on a 15 gtt/mL set.   _____

9. Infuse 750 mL over 5 hr using a calibrated 10 gtt/mL set.   _____

10. A set is calibrated at 15 gtt/mL. Infuse at 130 mL/hr.   _____

11. Infuse 200 mL over 4 hr using a microdrip set.   _____

12. 100 mL/hr is infusing on a 60 gtt/mL set.   _____

13. A set calibrated at 15 gtt/mL is used to infuse at 45 mL/hr.   _____

14. Infuse a volume of 100 mL over 30 min using a 20 gtt/mL set.   _____

15. Infuse a 50 mL IV bag of an antibiotic over 45 min using a 20 gtt/mL set.   _____

Answers 1. 28 gtt/min **2.** 49 gtt/min **3.** 42 gtt/min **4.** 75 gtt/min **5.** 37 gtt/min **6.** 40 gtt/min **7.** 63 gtt/min **8.** 31 gtt/min **9.** 25 gtt/min **10.** 33 gtt/min **11.** 50 gtt/min **12.** 100 gtt/min **13.** 11 gtt/min **14.** 67 gtt/min **15.** 22 gtt/min

Calculating Milliliter/Hour (mL/hr)

Infusion pumps are used for most IV infusions in the clinical setting. If an IV is on a pump, the pump will be programmed with the milliliter per hour rate. You will not be regulating IVs on a pump using drops per minute. Instead, if the order does not give the rate per hour, you will need to know how to calculate milliliters per hour. It is important for you to know what make and model of pump you are using. Some pumps will only allow programming to the whole number, whereas other pumps will allow programming to the tenth of a milliliter. Review the following order:

Infuse 500 mL NS over 8 hours.

This IV will be infused using an infusion pump. You will notice that the order does not give the hourly rate; therefore, you will need to calculate the hourly rate in order to program the pump. The hourly rate can be calculated with a simple formula:

$$\frac{\text{Volume in mL}}{\text{Time in hours}} = \text{mL/hr}$$

Example 1 ■   Infuse 500 mL NS over 8 hours on an infusion pump. This pump requires programming in whole numbers, therefore round to the whole number.

$$\frac{500 \text{ mL}}{8 \text{ hours}} = 62.5 \text{ mL/hr} = 63 \text{ mL/hr}$$

To infuse this IV as ordered, you will program the pump for 63 mL/hour.

Example 2 ■   Infuse 1,000 mL D$_5$NS over 12 hours. The pump you are using allows programming to the tenth, therefore round your answer to the tenth.

$$\frac{1,000 \text{ mL}}{12 \text{ hours}} = 83.33 \text{ mL/hr} = 83.3 \text{ mL/hr}$$

To infuse this IV as ordered on this pump, you will program the pump for 83.3 mL/hr.

These examples referred to IV fluids to be administered over several hours. Many times, when medications are infused on an infusion pump, they will be infused over time frames in minutes. For example, ampicillin 500 mg in 100 mL of NS IVPB over 45 minutes. To initiate this order, the vial of ampicillin would be reconstituted according to directions on the vial and then further diluted in 100 mL of NS to be administered IVPB. But, if it is being administered on an infusion pump, we will need to calculate the mL/hour to program into the pump. This can be accomplished by modifying the formula slightly. To calculate mL/hour when an IV is to infuse over several minutes, use the following formula:

$$\frac{\text{Volume in mL}}{\text{Time in minutes}} \times \frac{60 \text{ minutes}}{1 \text{ hour}} = \text{mL/hour}$$

This formula is very similar to the concepts presented in dimensional analysis. You will need to change the minutes to a portion of an hour by converting with the conversion factor of 60 minutes = 1 hour. Minutes in the numerator and denominator will cancel, and you will be left with mL/hr. Remember, it is important to multiply the numbers in the numerator first and then divide that product by the denominator. Let's look at a couple examples of how this will be applied.

Example 3 ■   Infuse ampicillin 500 mg in 100 mL NS IVPB over 45 minutes. This medication will be infused on a pump that can be programmed to the tenth. Since we are calculating mL per hour, we are only concerned with the volume and time in this order. For purposes of programming the pump, we do not need to use 500 mg anywhere in our formula.

$$\frac{100 \text{ mL}}{45 \text{ minutes}} = \frac{60 \text{ minutes}}{1 \text{ hour}} = 133.33 = 133.3 \text{ mL/hr}$$

Now you can infuse this IVPB on an infusion pump. By programming the pump for 133.3 mL/hr you will infuse this medication, as ordered, in 45 minutes.

Example 4 ■   Infuse cefuroxime 1.5 g in 100 mL D5W IVPB over 30 minutes via an infusion pump. To infuse via an infusion pump, we will need to calculate mL/hr so that the pump can be programmed.

$$\frac{100 \text{ mL}}{30 \text{ minutes}} \times \frac{60 \text{ minutes}}{1 \text{ hour}} = 200 \text{ mL/hr}$$

This order can be carried out on an infusion pump by programming it for 200 mL/hour. By doing this, the IVPB of 100 mL will infuse in 30 minutes as ordered.

 Keypoint: When an IV is ordered to infuse on an infusion pump over a time frame in minutes, the time must be converted to a portion of an hour. This is completed by using the conversion factor of 60 minutes per 1 hour.

Problems 19.3

Calculate the mL per hour in the following questions using the formula of your choice. Read the labels very carefully to locate the volume.

1. Refer to Figure 19-2 and infuse over 2 hr.   _____

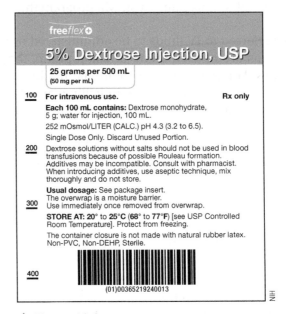

▲ **Figure 19-2**

2. Refer to Figure 19-3 and infuse over 1 hr.   _____

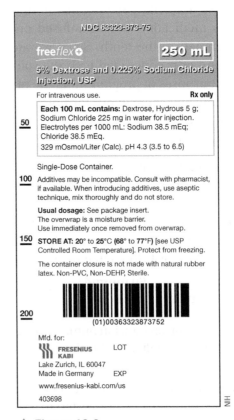

▲ **Figure 19-3**

3. Refer to Figure 19-4 and infuse over 8 hr.   _____

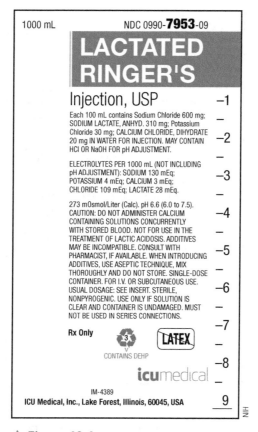

▲ **Figure 19-4**

4. Refer to Figure 19-5 and infuse over 2 hr.   _____

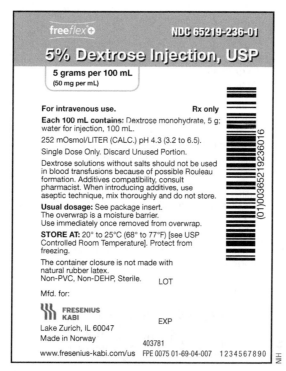

▲ **Figure 19-5**

5. Refer to Figure 19-6 and infuse over 30 min.   _____

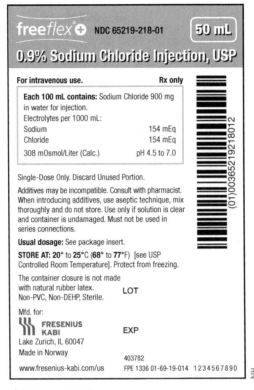

▲ **Figure 19-6**

6. Refer to Figure 19-7 and infuse over 12 hr. You are using
    an IV infusion pump that programs to the tenth mL.   _____

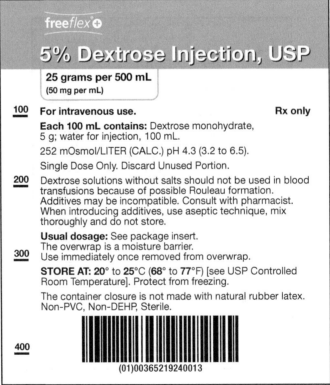

▲ **Figure 19-7**

7. Refer to Figure 19-8 and infuse the antibiotic, ciprofloxacin, over 1.5 hr. You are using an IV pump that programs to the 10th mL.

_____

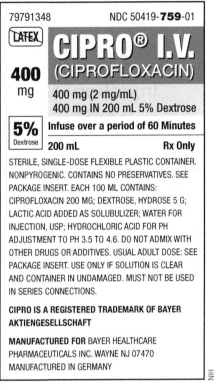

▲ **Figure 19-8**

8. See Figure 19-9 and infuse the potassium chloride IV bag over 2 hr.

_____

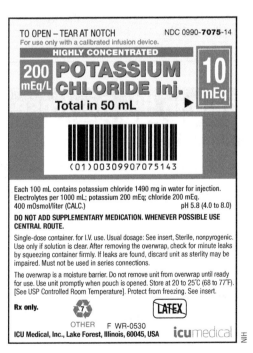

▲ **Figure 19-9**

9. Refer to Figure 19-10 and infuse the IV bag over 3 hr. You are using an IV infusion pump that does not program to the tenth.   _____

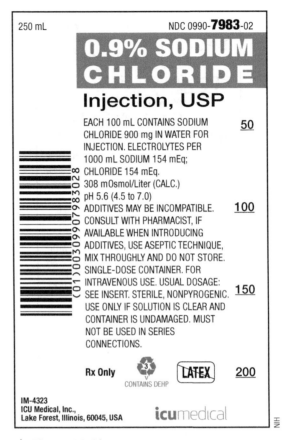

▲ **Figure 19-10**

10. Refer to Figure 19-11 and read the label for infusing the IV bag. Determine the mL/hr.   _____

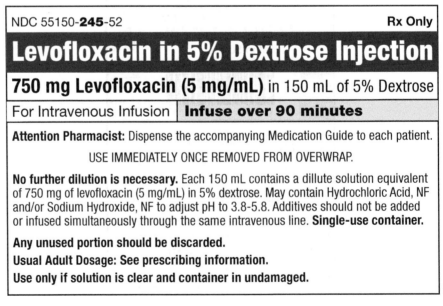

▲ **Figure 19-11**

Correcting Off-Schedule Rates

Because positional changes can alter the rate slightly, IVs occasionally infuse ahead of or behind schedule. When this occurs, the procedure in some clinical settings is to recalculate the flow rate using the volume and time remaining and to adjust the rate accordingly. However, each situation must be individually evaluated, especially if the discrepancy is large. If too much fluid has infused, immediately assess the individual's response to the increased intake and take appropriate action. If too little fluid has infused, it will be necessary to assess the individual's ability to tolerate an increased rate because many medications and fluids have restrictions on the rate of administration. These factors must be considered before rates can be increased to "catch up." In addition, most clinical facilities will have specific policies to cover over infusion or under infusion due to altered flow rates, and you will be responsible for knowing these. It is also especially critical to take the patient's age and condition into consideration. We need to be very careful with adjustment of rates for children and for the elderly.

The following are some examples of how the rate can be recalculated. Because IVs are usually checked hourly, the focus will first be on recalculation using exact hours. Some recalculations have also been included using fractions of hours rounded to the nearest quarter hour: 15 min = 0.25 hr, 30 min = 0.5 hr, and 45 min = 0.75 hr. These equivalents are close enough for uncomplicated infusions because the exact time of completion is not totally predictable. IVs needing exact infusion would be monitored by electronic infusion devices.

Example 1 ■ An IV of 1,000 mL was ordered to infuse over 10 hr. The drop factor is 15 gtt/mL and you calculated a rate of 25 gtt/min. After 5 hr, a total of 650 mL have infused instead of the 500 mL ordered. Recalculate the new gtt/min flow rate to complete the infusion on schedule.

Time remaining   10 hr − 5 hr = 5 hr

Volume remaining   1,000 mL − 650 mL = 350 mL

350 mL ÷ 5 hr = 70 mL/hr (This will be the new hourly rate required to complete the physician's order.)

Set calibration is 15 gtt/mL.

Calculate the new flow rate in drops per minute. Since this is an hourly rate, we can use the division factor to calculate our new flow rate.

70 mL/hr ÷ 4 (division factor) = 17.5 = 18 gtt/min

Slow the rate from 25 gtt/min to 18 gtt/min.

Example 2 ■ An IV of 800 mL was to infuse over 8 hr. The set calibration is 10 gtt/mL and you calculated a flow rate of 17 gtt/min. After 4 hr and 15 min only 300 mL have infused. Recalculate the gtt/min rate to complete on schedule.

Time remaining   8 hr − 4.25 hr = 3.75 hr

Volume remaining   800 mL − 300 mL = 500 mL

500 mL ÷ 3.75 hr = 133.3 = 133 mL/hr

Set calibration is 10 gtt/mL.

133 ÷ 6 (division factor) = 22.1 = 22 gtt/min

Increase the rate to 22 gtt/min.

Example 3 ■   An IV of 500 mL is infusing at 28 gtt/min. It was to complete in 3 hr, but after 1½ hr, only 175 mL have infused. Recalculate the gtt/min rate to complete the infusion on schedule. Set calibration is 10 gtt/mL.

Time remaining   3 hr − 1.5 hr = 1.5 hr

Volume remaining   500 mL − 175 mL = 325 mL

325 mL ÷ 1.5 hr = 216.6 = 217 mL/hr

Set calibration is 10 gtt/mL.

217 ÷ 6 (division factor) = 36.1 = 36 gtt/min

Increase the rate to 36 gtt/min.

Example 4 ■   A volume of 250 mL was to infuse in 1½ hr using a set calibrated at 20 gtt/mL. You calculate a flow rate of 56 gtt/min. After 30 min, 175 mL has infused. Recalculate the flow rate.

Time remaining   1.5 hr − 30 min = 1 hr

Volume remaining   250 mL − 175 mL = 75 mL

Set calibration is 20 gtt/mL.

75 ÷ 3 (division factor) = 25 gtt/min

Decrease the rate to 25 gtt/min.

Keypoint: When correcting infusion rates that are ahead or behind schedule, you must use critical thinking to determine if the change in rate that you calculate is acceptable for your patient. Take into consideration the facility policy, as well as the age and condition of the patient. Do not alter flow rates without thoughtful consideration.

Problems 19.4

Recalculate flow rates for infusions to complete on schedule.

1. An IV of 500 mL was ordered to infuse in 3 hr using a 15 gtt/mL set. With 1½ hr remaining, you discover that only 150 mL is left in the bag. At what rate will you need to reset the flow?   _____

2. An IV of 1,000 mL was scheduled to run in 12 hr. After 4 hr, only 220 mL have infused. The set calibration is 20 gtt/mL. Recalculate the rate for the remaining solution.   _____

3. An IV of 800 mL was started at 9 am to infuse in 4 hr. At 10 am, 150 mL have infused. The set is calibrated at 15 gtt/mL. Recalculate the flow rate in gtt/min.   _____

4. An IV of 600 mL was to infuse in 5 hr. After 2 hr, 400 mL have infused. Recalculate the gtt/min rate to complete on time. A 20 gtt/mL set is being used.   _____

5. A volume of 250 mL was to infuse in 2 hr. With 1 hr left, 60 mL has infused. Calculate a new gtt/min rate to complete on time using a 10 gtt/mL set.   _____

6. An infiltrated IV is restarted with a volume of 180 mL to complete in 3 hr. Calculate the gtt/min rate using a microdrip IV tubing.   _____

7. After 1 hr 30 min, 350 mL of a 1,000 mL IV has infused. It was ordered to complete in 4 hr using a set calibrated at 15 gtt/mL. Calculate the gtt/min rate to complete on time.   _____

8. A total of 400 mL of an ordered 1,000 mL in 10 hr infusion has completed in 4.5 hr. The set calibration is 20 gtt/mL. What gtt/min rate is necessary to complete on time?   _____

Answers 1. 25 gtt/min **2.** 33 gtt/min **3.** 54 gtt/min **4.** 22 gtt/min **5.** 32 gtt/min **6.** 60 gtt/min **7.** 65 gtt/min **8.** 36 gtt/min

Summary

 This concludes the chapter on IV flow rate calculation and monitoring. The important points to remember from this chapter are:

▪ IVs are ordered to infuse in measures of volume per time. This may mean the order is for mL/hr; total mL over total hours, or mL over a number of minutes.

▪ Flow rates of intravenous solutions infusing by gravity are calculated in gtt/min.

▪ IV tubings are calibrated in gtt/mL. This is called the drop factor.

▪ Macrodrip IV sets have a calibration of 10, 15, or 20 gtt/mL. Infusion pump tubings usually have a drop factor of 20 gtt/mL.

▪ Microdrip sets have a calibration of 60 gtt/mL.

▪ The formula for calculating flow rates is:

Flow rate (gtt/min) $= \frac{\text{mL} \times \text{drop factor (gtt/mL)}}{\text{time in minutes}}$

▪ The division factor method can be used to calculate flow rates only if the volume to be administered is specified in mL/hr (60 min).

▪ The division factor is obtained by dividing 60 by the set calibration.

- Flow rate by the division factor method is determined by dividing the mL/hr to be administered by the division factor.

- Because microdrip sets have a calibration of 60 gtt/mL, their division factor is 1, and the flow rate in gtt/min is the same as the mL/hr ordered.

- If an IV runs ahead of schedule or behind schedule, a possible procedure is to use the time and mL remaining to calculate a new flow rate.

- If an IV is determined to have infused ahead of schedule, immediate assessment of the individual's tolerance to the excess fluid is required and appropriate action should be taken.

- If a rate must be increased to compensate for running behind schedule, the type of fluid being infused and the individual's ability to tolerate an increased rate must be assessed.

- Before adjusting any flow rate, you must consider the age and condition of the patient, as well as the policy of the facility.

Summary Self-Test

Answer the following questions as they relate to IV administration sets.

1. Determine the division factor for the following IV sets.
   a. 60 gtt/mL   _____
   b. 15 gtt/mL   _____
   c. 20 gtt/mL   _____
   d. 10 gtt/mL   _____

2. How is the flow rate determined in the division factor method?   _____

3. You are administering an IV piggyback with a microdrip tubing. What is the relationship between gtt/min and mL/hr with the microdrip tubing?   _____

Calculate the flow rates of the following:

4. An infusion of 2,000 mL has been ordered to run 16 hr.

   Calculate the mL/hr.   _____

   Calculate the gtt/min using a 10 gtt/mL calibrated set.   _____

5. The order is for 500 mL in 8 hr. Calculate the mL/hr (round to the whole number).   _____

6. Administer 150 mL in 3 hr. A microdrip is used. Calculate gtt/min for this IV.   _____

7. An IV medication of 30 mL is to be administered in 30 min using a 15 gtt/mL set. Calculate gtt/min for this IV.   _____

8. Administer 100 mL in 1 hr using a 15 gtt/mL set. Calculate gtt/min for this IV.   _____

9. Infuse 500 mL in 6 hr. Set calibration is 10 gtt/mL. Calculate gtt/min for this IV.   _____

10. The order is to infuse a liter in 10 hr. At the end of 8 hr, you notice that there are 500 mL left. What would the new flow rate need to be to finish on schedule if the set calibration is 10 gtt/mL? _____

11. A 50 mL IV is to infuse in 15 min. The set calibration is 15 gtt/mL. After 5 min, the IV contains 40 mL. Calculate the flow rate in gtt/min to deliver the volume on time. _____

12. An infusion of 800 mL has been ordered to run in 5 hr. Set calibration is 10 gtt/mL. Calculate the gtt/min for this IV. _____

13. Administer a total volume of 1,200 mL in 8 hr, and calculate the mL/hr. _____

14. Administer 300 mL at 75 mL/hr. Determine the gtt/min with a microdrip tubing. _____

15. An IV of 1,000 mL was ordered to run in 8 hr. After 4 hr, only 250 mL have infused. The set calibration is 20 gtt/mL. Recalculate the rate in gtt/min for the remaining solution to complete on time. _____

16. The order is to infuse 50 mL in 2 hr. The set calibration is a microdrip. Calculate gtt/min for this IV. _____

17. An IV of 500 mL is to infuse in 6 hr using a set calibrated at 10 gtt/mL. Calculate gtt/min for this IV. _____

18. Infuse 120 mL in 5 hr. Use a microdrip tubing and calculate gtt/min for this IV. _____

19. Administer 12 mL in 22 min using a microdrip set. Calculate gtt/min. _____

20. A client is to receive a total of 3,000 mL in 22 hr. The infusion pump is programmed to the tenth mL. _____

21. Infuse 1 liter of sodium chloride in 5 hr using a set calibration of 15 gtt/mL. Calculate gtt/min for this IV. _____

22. A total of 1,180 mL is to infuse in 12 hr using a set calibrated at 20 gtt/mL. Calculate gtt/min for this IV. _____

23. A volume of 150 mL is to infuse in 30 min. At the end of 20 min, you discover that 100 mL have infused. The set calibration is 10 gtt/mL. What was the initial flow rate in gtt/min? _____

    Should the flow rate be adjusted? If so, what is the new rate? _____

24. The order is for 1,000 mL in 5 hr. The set calibration is 20 gtt/mL. Calculate gtt/min for this IV. _____

25. Infuse 15 mL in 14 min using a 20 gtt/mL set. Calculate gtt/min for this IV. _____

26. The order is for 1,000 mL in 18 hr to be infused on an IV pump. The IV infusion pump can be programmed to the tenth mL. _____

27. A microdrip is used to administer 12 mL in 17 min. Calculate gtt/min for this IV. _____

28. Infuse a total of 2,750 mL in 20 hr using a 10 gtt/mL set. Calculate gtt/min for this IV.   _____

29. A total IV volume of 1,800 mL is to infuse in 15 hr using a 15 gtt/mL set. Calculate gtt/min for this IV.   _____

30. Infuse 600 mL in 6 hr with a 10 gtt/mL set. Calculate gtt/min for this IV.   _____

31. Administer 22 mL in 20 min using a microdrip set. Calculate gtt/min for this IV.   _____

32. A total volume of 1,800 mL is to infuse in 15 hr. An IV infusion pump will be used. Calculate mL/hr.   _____

33. Infuse 8 mL in 9 min using a microdrip tubing. Calculate gtt/min for this IV.   _____

34. Infuse a total volume of 4,000 mL in 20 hr. A 20 gtt/mL set is used. Calculate gtt/min for this IV.   _____

35. An IV of 500 mL that was to infuse in 2 hr is discovered to have only 150 mL left after 30 min. Recalculate the flow rate in gtt/min. Set calibration is 15 gtt/mL.   _____

Answers to Summary Self-Test

1. a. 1 b. 4 c. 3 d. 6	5. 63 mL/hr	14. 75 gtt/min	23. 50 gtt/min; No, 50 gtt/min	28. 23 gtt/min
2. mL/hr ÷ division factor	6. 50 gtt/min	15. 63 gtt/min	is correct and no adjustment	29. 30 gtt/min
	7. 15 gtt/min	16. 25 gtt/min	is needed	30. 17 gtt/min
3. Flow rate will	8. 25 gtt/min	17. 14 gtt/min		31. 66 gtt/min
be the same	9. 14 gtt/min	18. 24 gtt/min	24. 67 gtt/min	32. 120 mL/hr
as mL/hr	10. 42 gtt/min	19. 33 gtt/min	25. 21 gtt/min	33. 53 gtt/min
4. 125 mL/hr, 21 gtt/min	11. 60 gtt/min	20. 136.4 mL/hr	26. 55.6 mL/hr	34. 67 gtt/min
	12. 27 gtt/min	21. 50 gtt/min	27. 42 gtt/min	35. 25 gtt/min
	13. 150 mL/hr	22. 33 gtt/min		

Calculating IV Infusion and Completion Times

There are a number of reasons for calculating IV infusion and completion times: to know when an IV solution will complete so that additional solutions ordered can be prepared in advance and ready to hang; to discontinue an IV when it has completed; and to label an IV bag with start, progress, and completion times so that the infusion can be monitored and adjusted to keep it on schedule. Knowing the infusion time is also important because laboratory studies are sometimes performed before, during, or after specified amounts of IV solutions or medications have infused. The infusion time may be calculated in hours and/or minutes, depending on the type and amount of solution ordered.

Clinical Relevance: There are many responsibilities associated with IV therapy. We have discussed the importance of consistently following the six rights of safe medication administration when administering IV fluids and medications. Accurately calculating flow rates in drops per minute or milliliters per hour is important to ensure that IV orders are carried out safely and accurately. Now we need to look at the importance of determining completion times for IVs that are prescribed for your clients. Determining completion times can help in the clinical or outpatient setting by ensuring that fluids can be ordered and prepared in advance of the IV completing so that the IV does not empty completely. It will be an important part of your ability to organize care for a group of clients. Infusion pumps have alarms and settings that alert us when there are concerns with the IV site and IV infusion. However, we must also have alternate ways of monitoring IV therapy in case infusion pumps are not available. Although many inpatient clinical settings use pumps for IV therapy, there are some inpatient settings and outpatient settings that do not have infusion pumps available. As a practitioner

Objectives

The learner will:

1. calculate infusion times.

2. calculate completion times using international/military and standard time.

3. label IV bag/bottle with start, progress, and completion times.

caring for clients in any setting, it is important to develop a comfort level with monitoring IVs that are infusing by gravity. Labels, or time-tapes, on an IV bag provide a way for continuity in monitoring IVs infusing by gravity. Knowledge of completion times is also an integral part of ensuring that IVs are administered safely and physician orders for IV therapy are implemented safely.

Calculating Infusion Time

The infusion time of any IV solution can be calculated if the flow rate in milliliters per hour or hours is known. The infusion time is calculated for each bag/bottle to be hung and infused. The largest capacity IV solution bag or bottle is 1,000 mL, but 500 mL, 250 mL, 100 mL and 50 mL bags are also commonly used. There are also times when an infusion time must be calculated for volumes of IV fluids that may be less than the standard volume in IV bags. For example, if an IV infiltrates or a site must be restarted for any reason, we must look at the volume remaining and calculate the time remaining based on the order. Infusion time for an initial IV, as well as for an IV that is stopped due to complications or other concerns, is calculated by dividing the volume being infused by the mL/hr rate ordered.

Because most IVs take several hours to infuse, the unit of time being calculated most often includes hours (hr) and minutes (min). The calculation will be performed by utilizing the following:

$$\textit{Infusion time} = \textit{Volume} \div \textit{mL/hr rate}$$

 Keypoint: IV infusion time is calculated by dividing the volume to be infused by the mL/hr flow rate.

Example 1 ■   Calculate the infusion time for an IV of 500 mL to infuse at 50 mL/hr.

Infusion time = 500 mL ÷ 50 mL/hr = 10 hr

From this calculation, we understand that the infusion time for an IV of 500 mL infusing at 50 mL/hr is 10 hr.

Example 2 ■   The order is to infuse 1,000 mL at 75 mL/hr. Calculate the infusion time.

1,000 mL ÷ 75 mL/hr = 13.33 hr

In this example, the infusion time is not a whole number in hours. We note that this IV will infuse 13 hours plus 0.33 of an hour. When we have infusion times that include a fraction of an hour, we will round our answer to the hundredth of the hour. From there we can calculate the additional minutes of infusion time. We will do this by using the conversion factor of 60 minutes per hour. After converting, we will then round the minutes to the whole number.

 Keypoint: Fractional hours are converted to minutes by multiplying 60 minutes by the fraction obtained.

In this example, we will calculate minutes by multiplying 60 min by the fractional 0.33 hr.

$$60 \text{ min/hr} \times 0.33 \text{ hr} = 19.8 = 20 \text{ min}$$

We have calculated the infusion time of this IV of 1,000 mL to be 13 hr 20 min.

Example 3 ▦ An IV of 1,000 mL is to infuse at 90 mL/hr. Calculate the infusion time.

$$1,000 \text{ mL} \div 90 \text{ mL/hr} = 11.11 \text{ hr}$$

We recognize this IV will infuse 11 hours plus 0.11 of an hour. We will convert this to minutes by multiplying 60 min by 0.11.

$$60 \text{ min/hr} \times 0.11 \text{ hr} = 6.6 = 7 \text{ min}$$

The infusion time for this IV will be 11 hr 7 min.

Example 4 ▦ Calculate the infusion time for 750 mL at a rate of 80 mL/hr.

$$750 \text{ mL} \div 80 \text{ mL/hr} = 9.38 \text{ hr}$$

$$60 \text{ min/hr} \times 0.38 \text{ hr} = 22.8 = 23 \text{ min}$$

The infusion time is 9 hr 23 min.

Example 5 ▦ A rate of 75 mL/hr is ordered for a volume of 500 mL. Calculate the infusion time.

$$500 \text{ mL} \div 75 \text{ mL/hr} = 6.67 \text{ hr}$$

$$60 \text{ min/hr} \times 0.67 \text{ hr} = 40.2 = 40 \text{ min}$$

The infusion time is 6 hr 40 min.

The calculation of infusion times gives you an estimate of when the IV infusion should be completed. This applies to IVs on infusion pumps or infusing by gravity. When the infusion time is something like 9 hours and 23 minutes, we realize that we would not allow the IV to run exactly that long; instead, it gives us an idea of when we need to change the IV bag so it does not go dry. If an IV bag goes dry, air can get into the tubing and blood can back up from the IV site and clot in the tubing. This will result in the need to change the tubing, and possibly change the IV site, due to occlusion from a blood clot. Knowing infusion time can also help us to plan to discontinue the IV solutions in situations where the IV is intermittent and the IPID needs flushed to maintain patency.

Problems 20.1

Calculate the infusion times. Remember to round fractions of an hour to the hundredth and then multiply that number by 60 min/hr to arrive at the minutes.

1. An IV of 900 mL to infuse at 80 mL/hr   _____
2. A volume of 250 mL to infuse at 30 mL/hr   _____
3. An infusion of 180 mL to run at 25 mL/hr   _____
4. A volume of 1,000 mL ordered at 60 mL/hr   _____
5. An IV of 150 mL to infuse at 80 mL/hr   _____

6. An infusion of 1,000 mL at 125 mL/hr   _____

7. A rate of 120 mL/hr for 500 mL   _____

8. A volume of 800 mL at 60 mL/hr   _____

9. An IV of 250 mL at 80 mL/hr   _____

10. A rate of 135 mL/hr for 750 mL   _____

Answers 1. 11 hr 15 min **2.** 8 hr 20 min **3.** 7 hr 12 min **4.** 16 hr 40 min **5.** 1 hr 53 min **6.** 8 hr **7.** 4 hr 10 min **8.** 13 hr 20 min **9.** 3 hr 8 min **10.** 5 hr 34 min

Determining Infusion Completion Times

The completion time is the actual hour and/or minute an infusion bag or bottle will complete or empty. Completion times are calculated in either international/military time using the 24-hour clock or standard time, depending on individual clinical facility policy.

 Keypoint: The completion time is calculated by adding the infusion time to the time the IV was started.

Facility policy will determine if international/military time or if standard time is used. A chart on the inside front cover shows the conversion of times. A facility will not use both systems of time; the facility will use one or the other system to designate time.

 Keypoint: To convert standard time to international/military time, add 12 hours to each hour beginning with 1:00 pm standard time. Minutes will be written after the hour. For example, 1620 is equivalent to 4:20 pm.

Let's look at a few examples of completion times written in international/military time. For learning purposes, we will put the standard time in parentheses so you can become comfortable with conversions between the two systems of time.

Example 1 ■   An IV started at 0400 is to be completed in 2 hr 30 min. Calculate the completion time.

Add the 2 hr 30 min infusion time to the 0400 start time.

$$\begin{array}{r} 0400 \\ + \underline{230} \\ 0630 \end{array}$$

The completion time is 0630. (This is equivalent to 6:30 am in standard time.)

Example 2 ■   An IV started at 0750 is to be completed in 5 hr 10 min. Calculate the completion time.

Add the 5 hr 10 min infusion time to the 0750 start time.

$$\begin{array}{r} 0750 \\ + \underline{510} \\ 1260 \end{array}$$

Change the 60 min to 1 hr and add to 1200 = 1300.

The completion time is 1300. (This is equivalent to 1:00 pm in standard time)

Example 3 ■   An IV started at 2250 is to be completed in 4 hr 20 min. Calculate the completion time.

Add the infusion time to the start time.

$$
\begin{array}{r}
2250 \\
+\ 420 \\
\hline
2670
\end{array}
$$

With a completion time of 2670, we note two things: we are beyond the 24 hours on the international/military clock and 70 minutes is beyond 60 minutes. We must convert the 70 minutes to an hour and a portion of an hour.

First, we will convert the 70 minutes.

Change the 70 min to 1 hr 10 min = 2710.

Now, we need to change 2710 to a time on the 24-hour clock. We will do this by subtracting 2400 from 2710.

$$2710 - 2400 = 0310$$

The completion time is 0310. (This is equivalent to 3:10 am in standard time.) If we begin this IV at 2250 in the evening, it will be completed at 0310 in the morning.

Now, review a few examples of completion times using standard time. For learning purposes, we will put the international/military time in parentheses so you can become comfortable with conversions between the two systems of time.

Keypoint: To convert international/military time to standard time, subtract 12 hours from each hour beginning with 1300, add a colon, and indicate am or pm. For example, 2330 is equivalent to 11:30 pm.

Example 4 ■   An IV medication will infuse in 20 minutes. It is now 6:14 pm. When will it be complete?

Add the 20 minutes infusion time to the 6:14 pm start time.

6:14 pm + 20 min = 6:34 pm

The completion time will be at 6:34 pm. (This is equivalent to 1834 in international/military time)

Example 5 ■   An IV is to infuse in 2 hr 33 min. It is now 4:43 pm. When will it be complete?

Add the 2 hr 33 min infusion time to the 4:43 start time.

$$
\begin{array}{r}
4:43\ \text{pm} \\
+\ 2:33 \\
\hline
6:76
\end{array}
$$

Notice that 76 minutes is more than 1 hour. Subtract 60 minutes from 76 minutes. Change the 76 min to 1 hr 16 minutes. This will be added to the 6 full hours, as follows:

6 hours + 1 hour 16 minutes = 7:16.

We have determined the completion time is 7:16 pm. (This is equivalent to 1916 in international/military time.)

Example 6 ▦   An IV infusion time is 13 hr 20 min. What is its completion time if it was started at 10:45 am?

Add the 13 hr 20 min infusion time to the 10:45 am start time.

$$
\begin{array}{r}
10:45 \text{ am} \\
+\ 13:20 \\
\hline
23:65
\end{array}
$$

Since 65 minutes is more than an hour, we must change the 65 min to 1 hr 5 min. We then need to add 1 hr 5 min to the 23 hours. This will equal 24:05. 24:05 is beyond the 24 hours in a day, so we recognize the completion time will be 5 minutes after midnight. This will be written as 12:05 am.

The completion time will be 12:05 am. (This is equivalent to 0005 in international/military time.)

Example 7 ▦   An IV with an infusion time of 10 hr 7 min is started at 9:42 am. When will it be complete?

Add the 10 hr 7 min infusion time to the 9:42 am start time.

$$
\begin{array}{r}
9:42 \text{ am} \\
+\ 10:07 \\
\hline
19:49
\end{array}
$$

Since we are working with standard time, we must remember to subtract 12 hours to determine completion time. Standard time is based on am and pm designations. Therefore, we must subtract 12 hr to make the completion time 7:49 pm.

The completion time will be 7:49 pm. (This is equivalent to 1949 in international/military time.)

Example 8 ▦   An IV with an infusion time of 12 hr 30 min is started at 2:10 am. When will it complete?

Add the 12 hr 30 min infusion time to the 2:10 am start time.

$$
\begin{array}{r}
2:10 \text{ am} \\
+\ 12:30 \\
\hline
14:40
\end{array}
$$

Since we are working with standard time, we must remember to subtract 12 hours to determine completion time. Standard time is based on am and pm designations. Therefore, we must subtract 12 hr to make the completion time 2:40 pm.

The completion time will be 2:40 pm. (This is equivalent to 1440 in international/military time.)

Problems 20.2

Calculate the international/military completion times.

1. An IV started at 0415 to infuse in 1 hr 30 min.   _____
2. An infusion started at 1735 to complete in 2 hr 40 min.   _____
3. An IV started at 1605 to complete in 3 hr 30 min.   _____
4. An IV started at 2300 to complete in 3 hr 40 min.   _____
5. An infusion time of 6 hr 20 min for an infusion started at 0325.   _____

6. An IV started at 1430 to complete in 4 hr.   _____

7. A medication infusion started at 0740 to complete in 90 min.   _____

8. An IV medication started at 1247 to complete in 45 min.   _____

Calculate IV completion using standard time.

9. An IV started at 4:40 am that has an infusion time of
   9 hr 42 min.   _____

10. An IV medication started at 7:30 am that has an infusion
    time of 45 min.   _____

11. An IV started at 2:43 pm to infuse in 40 min.   _____

12. An IV with an infusion time of 3 hr 30 min was started
    at 11:49 pm.   _____

13. An IV medication started at 10:15 am to complete in 90 min.   _____

14. An infusion started at 7:05 pm to complete in 8 hr.   _____

15. An IV started at 4:20 am to complete in 12 hr.   _____

Answers 1. 0545 **2.** 2015 **3.** 1935 **4.** 0240 **5.** 0945 **6.** 1830 **7.** 0910 **8.** 1332 **9.** 2:22 pm
10. 8:15 am **11.** 3:23 pm **12.** 3:19 am **13.** 11:45 am **14.** 3:05 am **15.** 4:20 pm

Labeling Solution Bags with Infusion and Completion Times

IV bags/bottles are calibrated so that the amount of fluid remaining can be checked at any time. When infusion pumps are used, cross check the volume that has infused from the bag with the volume infused that is showing on the pump. This provides a way to monitor the progress of the intravenous infusions that are being administered via a pump. However, if the IV is infusing by gravity, no device tracks the volume infused. In this case, it is important to label the IV bag, or place a time-tape on it, as a way to monitor the progress of the IV infusion. This provides a visual reference of the status of the infusion. Commercially prepared labels or time-tapes are available for this purpose, but you can also prepare one yourself with a strip of tape.

Figure 20-1 shows the calibrations on a 1,000 mL bag, starting at 0. Notice that each 50 mL is calibrated, but only the 100 mL calibrations are numbered: 1, 2, 3 (for 100, 200, 300), etc. Also, notice that the calibrations on the IV bag are not all the same width. They are somewhat wider at the bottom because gravity and the pressure of the solution force more fluid to the bottom of the bag.

The tape on the IV solution bag in Figure 20-1 is for an 8 hr infusion, from 9 am to 5 pm. The 9A on the strip of tape represents the start time of 9 am, and the 5P at the bottom of the strip of tape represents the completion time of 5 pm. An 8 hr infusion time for 1,000 mL means that 125 mL are to be infused per hour (1,000 mL ÷ 8 hr = 125 mL/hr). Each 125 mL is labeled on the calibrated scale along with the hour the IV should be at this level. This tape allows for constant visual monitoring of the IV. It is important to have a tape such as this on any IV infusing by gravity. Otherwise, it is very difficult to monitor and ensure the IV is infusing as ordered. Checking the label on the bag every hour to ensure the IV is infusing as ordered will help to prevent over infusion or under infusion of the IV solution. Regardless of your clinical responsibility, develop the habit of reading infusion time labeling, particularly if you have been giving personal care that involves moving or repositioning of the patient.

Figure 20-2 shows time-tape on an IV solution bag with a starting level at 1, indicating 100 mL. Unlike the bag shown in Figure 20-1, this bag does not have a 0 and you

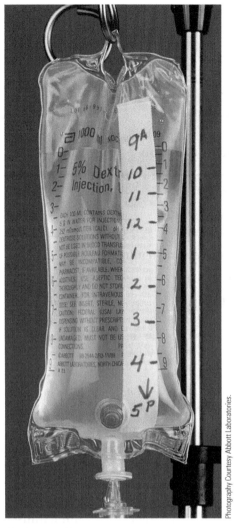

Photography Courtesy Abbott Laboratories.

▲ Figure 20-1

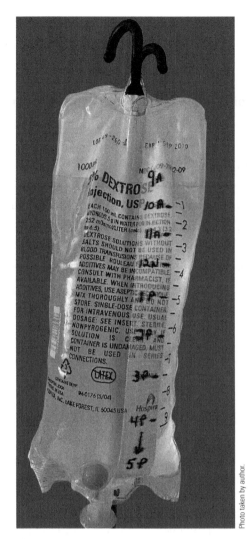

Photo taken by author.

▲ Figure 20-2

must understand that when the level of fluid is at the 1 on this bag, 100 mL has infused already. The labeling will need to take this into account, and you will find the starting time somewhere above the 1.

Let's look at an example of how you could label an IV that is just being started. You may want to use the **time-tape worksheet** in the back of the chapter and mark it as directed in the following examples. Make copies of the blank worksheet to continue to practice time-taping. The worksheet provides an opportunity to practice time-taping on an IV bag beginning with zero (left side of worksheet), and an IV bag beginning with one (right side of worksheet). When using the practice time-tape worksheet, it will not matter which side you use. The volume remains the same.

Example 1 ▪   An IV of 1,000 mL has been ordered to run at 150 mL/hr. It was started at 1:40 pm. Tape the bag with start, progress, and completion times. Before labeling the bag, calculate the infusion and completion times.

From the previous sections we know that the calculation will be as follows:

$$1,000 \text{ mL} \div 150 \text{ mL/hr} = 6.67 \text{ hours}$$

$$0.67 \text{ hr} \times 60 \text{ min/hr} = 40 \text{ minutes}$$

So, the IV should infuse for about 6 hours and 40 minutes. Determining completion time, we see that the IV should finish around 8:20 pm. To label the bag we will do the following:

Add the tape to the bag/bottle so that it is near but does not cover the calibrations. Enter the start time as 1:40 pm at the 1,000 mL level. Next, mark each 150 mL from top to bottom with the successive hours the IV will run.

$$1,000 \text{ mL} - 150 \text{ mL} = 850 \text{ mL} \qquad \text{Label } 850 \text{ mL for } 2{:}40 \text{ pm}$$
$$850 \text{ mL} - 150 \text{ mL} = 700 \text{ mL} \qquad \text{Label } 700 \text{ mL for } 3{:}40 \text{ pm}$$
$$700 \text{ mL} - 150 \text{ mL} = 550 \text{ mL} \qquad \text{Label } 550 \text{ mL for } 4{:}40 \text{ pm}$$
$$550 \text{ mL} - 150 \text{ mL} = 400 \text{ mL} \qquad \text{Label } 400 \text{ mL for } 5{:}40 \text{ pm}$$
$$400 \text{ mL} - 150 \text{ mL} = 250 \text{ mL} \qquad \text{Label } 250 \text{ mL for } 6{:}40 \text{ pm}$$
$$250 \text{ mL} - 150 \text{ mL} = 100 \text{ mL} \qquad \text{Label } 100 \text{ mL for } 7{:}40 \text{ pm}$$

This bag will not be completely empty; the bag still has 100 mL volume remaining. Recall we calculated a completion time of 8:20 pm. We do not want an IV to run dry, so most likely we would want to change this IV solution before it runs out completely. This label would give us a rough estimate of when the infusion would be complete.

Example 2 ▪   An infiltrated IV with 625 mL remaining is restarted at 5:30 pm to run at 150 mL/hr. Relabel the bag with the new start, progress, and completion times. When we are restarting a partially full IV bag, our starting time will be placed at the level of the IV solution.

Before we label the bag, we will calculate the infusion and completion times. From the previous sections we know that the calculation will be as follows:

$$625 \text{ mL} \div 150 \text{ mL/hr} = 4.17 \text{ hours}$$

$$0.17 \text{ hr} \times 60 \text{ min/hr} = 10 \text{ minutes}$$

So, we realize the IV should infuse for about 4 hours and 10 minutes. Determining completion time, we see that the IV should finish around 9:40 pm. To label the bag, we will do the following:

Label the 625 mL level with the 5:30 pm restart time.

$$625 \text{ mL} - 150 \text{ mL} = 475 \text{ mL} \qquad \text{Label } 475 \text{ mL for } 6{:}30 \text{ pm}$$
$$475 \text{ mL} - 150 \text{ mL} = 325 \text{ mL} \qquad \text{Label } 325 \text{ mL for } 7{:}30 \text{ pm}$$
$$325 \text{ mL} - 150 \text{ mL} = 175 \text{ mL} \qquad \text{Label } 175 \text{ mL for } 8{:}30 \text{ pm}$$
$$175 \text{ mL} - 150 \text{ mL} = 25 \text{ mL} \qquad \text{Label } 25 \text{ mL for } 9{:}30 \text{ pm}$$

Again, for practical purposes we estimate that this IV will be completed around 9:30 pm. With only 25 mL remaining, we would change this IV bag at that time so the IV does not empty completely.

Example 3 ▪   An infiltrated IV with 340 mL remaining is restarted at 4:15 am to run at 70 mL/hr. Relabel the bag with the new start, progress, and completion times. As we are working with a partially full IV bag, we will label our starting time at the current level of the solution.

Before we label the bag, we will calculate the infusion and completion times. From the previous sections we know that the calculation will be as follows:

$$340 \text{ mL} \div 70 \text{ mL/hr} = 4.86 \text{ hours}$$

$$0.86 \text{ hr} \times 60 \text{ min/hr} = 52 \text{ minutes}$$

So, we realize the IV should infuse for about 4 hours and 52 minutes. Determining completion time, we see that the IV should finish around 9:07 am. To label the bag, we will do the following:

Label the 340 mL level with the 4:15 am restart time.

340 mL − 70 mL = 270 mL	Label 270 mL for 5:15 am
270 mL − 70 mL = 200 mL	Label 200 mL for 6:15 am
200 mL − 70 mL = 130 mL	Label 130 mL for 7:15 am
130 mL − 70 mL = 60 mL	Label 60 mL for 8:15 am

We recognize that there will be approximately 60 mL left at 8:15 am. Remember that we calculated a completion time of 9:07 am. Although this is almost another full hour, we realize that we need to change this IV bag.

Problems 20.3

Calculate the infusion time. Label the IV bags provided with start, progress, and completion times. Have your instructor check your labeling.

1. The IV in Figure 20-3 of 1,000 mL was started at 0710 to run at 75 mL/hr.

Infusion time _____   Completion time _____

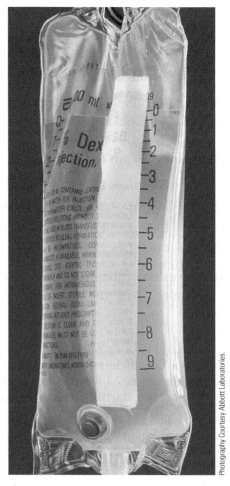

▲ **Figure 20-3**

Photography Courtesy Abbott Laboratories.

2. The 1,000 mL IV in Figure 20-4 has an ordered rate of 125 mL/hr. It was started at 6:30 pm.

    Infusion time _____   Completion time _____

3. The IV in Figure 20-5 of 1,000 mL has an ordered rate of 80 mL/hr. It was started at 5:40 am.

    Infusion time _____   Completion time _____

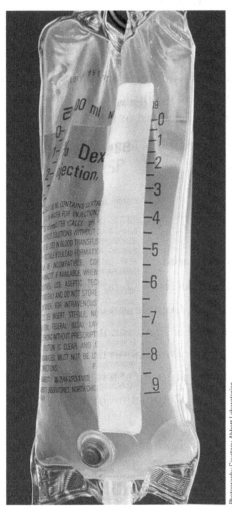

▲ Figure 20-4

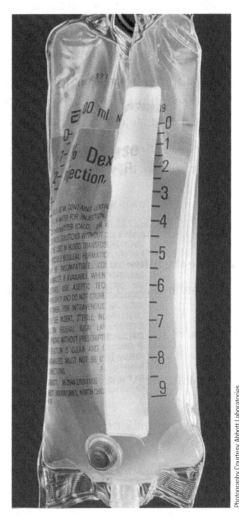

▲ Figure 20-5

Answers   **1.** 13 hr 20 min; 2030   **2.** 8 hr; 2:30 am   **3.** 12 hr 30 min; 6:10 pm

---

Summary

This concludes the chapter on calculation of infusion and completion times and labeling of IV bags/bottles with start, progress, and completion times. The important points to remember from this chapter are:

- The infusion time is the time required for an IV to infuse completely.

- The infusion time is calculated by dividing the total volume to infuse by the mL/hr rate ordered.

■ The completion time is calculated by adding the infusion time to the start time.

■ When the minutes calculated are 60 or more, an additional hr is added to the completion time and 60 min are subtracted from the total min.

■ Calculating completion times provides an opportunity to plan ahead and have the next solution ordered ready to hang. If an IV is an intermittent infusion, it also helps us plan when to discontinue the IV solution.

■ Most clinical facilities label IV solution bags/bottles that are infusing by gravity with start, progress, and finish times to provide a visual record of the infusion status.

■ Labels, or time-tapes, provide a good estimate of when the IV will need changed or discontinued. When a time-tape is present, we can check an IV at any time and recognize if it is infusing on schedule, or if it is ahead or behind schedule.

■ A label or time-tape on an IV infusing by gravity helps us identify infusion concerns before they are a significant problem.

Summary Self-Test

Calculate the infusion and completion times as indicated.

1. The order is for 50 mL to infuse at 50 mL/hr. The infusion was started at 10:10 am.
    Infusion time _____   Completion time _____

2. A total of 280 mL remains in an IV bag. The flow rate is 70 mL/hr. It is now 11:03 am.
    Infusion time _____   Completion time _____

3. An infiltrated IV with 850 mL remaining is restarted at 10 am at a rate of 150 mL/hr.
    Infusion time _____   Completion time _____

4. At 4:04 am, an IV of 500 mL is started at a rate of 50 mL/hr.
    Infusion time _____   Completion time _____

5. It is 12:00 pm, and an IV of 900 mL is to infuse at a rate of 100 mL/hr.
    Infusion time _____   Completion time _____

6. An IV of 1,000 mL is started at 0550 to infuse at 130 mL/hr.
    Infusion time _____   Completion time _____

7. An infusion of 250 mL is started at 11:20 am to infuse at a rate of 20 mL/hr.
    Infusion time _____   Completion time _____

8. The flow rate ordered for 1 L is 80 mL/hr. It was started at 8:07 pm.
    Infusion time _____   Completion time _____

9. A 250 mL volume is started at 3:40 pm to be infused at 90 mL/hr.
    Infusion time _____   Completion time _____

10. At 11:00 pm, 200 mL remain in an IV. The rate is 120 mL/hr.
    Infusion time _____   ompletion time _____

11. An IV of 425 mL is restarted at 0814 to infuse at 90 mL/hr.
    Infusion time _____   Completion time _____

12. At 1400, 500 mL is started to run at a rate of 60 mL/hr.

           Infusion time _____   Completion time _____

13. An infusion of 250 mL is started at 3:04 am to run at 100 mL/hr.

           Infusion time _____   Completion time _____

14. A liter is started at 8:42 am at a rate of 120 mL/hr.

           Infusion time _____   Completion time _____

15. An infusion of 1,000 mL is to run at 200 mL/hr. It is started at 6:40 pm.

           Infusion time _____   Completion time _____

16. An IV medication of 100 mL is started at 7:50 am to run at 150 mL/hr.

           Infusion time _____   Completion time _____

17. A volume of 500 mL is started at 4:04 pm at a rate of 75 mL/hr.

           Infusion time _____   Completion time _____

18. An IV of 950 mL is restarted at 2:10 am at 100 mL/hr.

           Infusion time _____   Completion time _____

19. An IV medication of 30 mL is started at 0915 at a rate of 60 mL/hr.

           Infusion time _____   Completion time _____

20. A medication volume of 90 mL was started at 6:15 am to be infused at 90 mL/hr.

           Infusion time _____   Completion time _____

Label the time-tape on the following solution bags for the times and rates indicated. Have your instructor check your labeling.

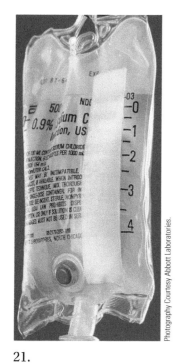 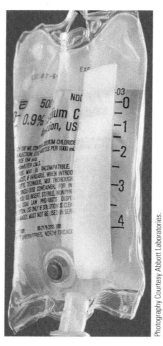 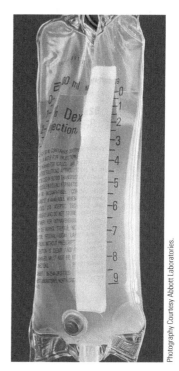

21.
Started: 10:47 am
Rate: 80 mL/hr

22.
Started: 0744
Rate: 125 mL/hr

23.
Started: 0440
Rate: 75 mL/hr

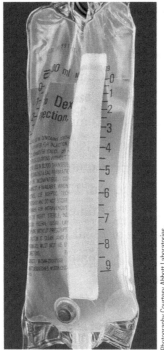

Photography Courtesy Abbott Laboratories.

Photography Courtesy Abbott Laboratories.

24.

Started: 0730

Rate: 50 mL/hr

25.

Started: 6:20 pm

Rate: 25 mL/hr

Answers to Summary Self-Test

1. 1 hr; 11:10 am **2.** 4 hr; 3:03 pm **3.** 5 hr 40 min; 3:40 pm **4.** 10 hr; 2:04 pm **5.** 9 hr; 9 pm **6.** 7 hr 41 min; 1331
7. 12 hr 30 min; 11:50 pm **8.** 12 hr 30 min; 8:37 am **9.** 2 hr 46 min; 6:26 pm **10.** 1 hr 40 min; 12:40 am
11. 4 hr 43 min; 1257 **12.** 8 hr 20 min; 2220 **13.** 2 hr 30 min; 5:34 am **14.** 8 hr 20 min; 5:02 pm **15.** 5 hr; 11:40 pm
16. 40 min; 8:30 am **17.** 6 hr 40 min; 10:44 pm **18.** 9 hr 30 min; 11:40 am **19.** 30 min; 0945 **20.** 1 hr; 7:15 am
21–25. Verify your answers with your instructor.

IV BAG – PRACTICE TIME-TAPING WORKSHEET

IV BAG STARTING   **1000 mL**   **IV BAG STARTING**

WITH 0 (zero)   **WITH 1 (one)**

WITH 0 (zero)	WITH 1 (one)
0--	
--	
1--	1--
--	--
2--	2--
--	--
3--	3--
--	--
4--	4--
--	--
5--	5--
--	--
6--	6--
--	--
7--	7--
--	--
8--	8--
--	--
9--	9--

IV BAG – PRACTICE TIME-TAPING WORKSHEET

IV BAG STARTING   **1000 mL**   **IV BAG STARTING**

WITH 0 (zero)   **WITH 1 (one)**

IV BAG STARTING WITH 0 (zero)	IV BAG STARTING WITH 1 (one)
0--	
--	
1--	1--
--	--
2--	2--
--	--
3--	3--
--	--
4--	4--
--	--
5--	5--
--	--
6--	6--
--	--
7--	7--
--	--
8--	8--
--	--
9--	9--

IV Medication Drips and Titration Calculations

Many IV drugs are used in critical and life-threatening situations to alter or maintain vital physiologic functions, such as heart rate, cardiac output, blood pressure, and respiration. In general, these drugs have a very rapid action and short duration. They are diluted in a volume of IV solution specified by the physician order or your drug reference. Some of these medications will be premixed by the manufacturer; others will be mixed by the nurse or pharmacist. The drug manufacturer will clearly label any premixed solutions with the amount of medication in the IV bag. If the nurse or pharmacist is mixing a bag, it will be extremely important to label the IV bag with the following information: the name and amount of medication (mg or mcg of the medication) placed in the IV solution, the date and time, patient name and room number, and initials of the person preparing the drip.

Intravenous medications may be ordered by dosage (mcg, mg, or units per min or hr) or based on body weight (mcg, mg, or units per kg per min or hr). They may also be ordered to infuse within a specific dosage range, such as 1–3 mcg/min, to elicit a measurable physiologic response. For example, this would be a parameter for a blood pressure medication to maintain a systolic BP above 100 mm Hg. This adjustment of rate is called titration, and dosage increments are made within the ordered range until the desired response has been established.

IV drugs require close and continuous monitoring, and an electronic infusion device, such as an infusion pump or a syringe pump, is used for their administration. If an electronic infusion device is not used, a microdrip set calibrated at 60 gtt/mL or a dosage controlled calibrated burette may be used. If a calibrated burette is used, it may be necessary to determine the minimal dilution for medications given to children or older adults, so there is no chance of administering too much fluid. The policy of facilities will vary, but some facilities will require that the volume

Objectives

The learner will:

1. calculate flow rates to infuse ordered dosages.

2. calculate flow rates based on dosages per kg of body weight.

3. calculate flow rate ranges for titrated medications.

of medication be considered in the dilution of the medicated drip, if given by calibrated burette. Due to considerable differences in facility policies and the more common use of infusion pumps and syringe pumps, the information in this chapter will focus on using an infusion or syringe pump, or microdrip tubing. As microdrip tubing has a drop factor of 60 gtt/mL, recall that mL per hour and drops per minute will be the same number.

Calculations in this chapter will include converting ordered dosages to the flow rates necessary for administration. Body weight is often a critical factor in IV dosages, and its use in calculations will also be covered. Although several electronic infusion devices provide the ability to program several medications at mcg, mg, or units per minute or hour; it is vital that you understand how to perform these calculations in the event an infusion device is not available.

IV drugs that alter a basic physiologic function generally have narrow margins of safety, and accuracy is imperative in their calculation. Triple-checking of math should be routine, but in instances where critical care medications are being administered, it is mandatory in order to prevent life-threatening errors. Due to the critical nature of these medications, dosages will be calculated to the nearest tenth and flow rates will be rounded to the nearest tenth of a mL. If infusing by gravity, the drip will be calculated to the nearest drop. Although we will calculate mL per hour to the tenth, if a device cannot be programmed to the tenth, round to the whole number for mL.

> **Key**point: All calculations assume the use of an electronic infusion device that can be programmed to the tenth. If a microdrip infusion set must be used, the flow rate will be rounded to the whole number and the mL/hr and gtt/min would be the same number.

Clinical Relevance: Some medicated drips are ordered by concentration or dosage weight, and time—for example, a medicated drip may be ordered as 20 mg per hour. This type of IV cannot be administered or monitored until it has been converted into volume per time. Use the concentration of the IV to determine volume per time based on the physician order, and calculate as you have done with other medication orders. Calculate using your preferred method: Ratio and Proportion, Dimensional Analysis, or the Formula Method. These calculations will allow us to change the weight per time order to volume per time, and we will be able to monitor the flow.

Most of these medicated drips will be on infusion pumps or will use microdrip tubing or calibrated burettes. Some of the medicated drips will be titrated based on the patient response to the medication and the doses will be individualized to the patient. When administering critical medications to children and older adults, it is important to remember that these populations may not be able to tolerate large amounts of fluid. Therefore, it is important to use critical thinking and your medication references to determine safe dilution of these medications.

Medications that are ordered as intravenous drips are usually cardiac medications, blood pressure medications, pain medications, insulin, and heparin. Heparin and insulin drips will be addressed in Chapter 22.

Flow Rates to Infuse Dosages Ordered by mg, mcg, or unit Per Time

A common calculation is to determine the mL/hr flow rate for a specific drug dosage ordered. We can calculate this using one of the three methods of calculation: Ratio and Proportion, Dimensional Analysis, or the Formula Method.

Example 1 ▣   An IV with the concentration of 125 mg/100 mL is to infuse at a rate of 20 mg/hr. Calculate the mL/hr flow rate using your preferred method. You will use the 125 mg/100 mL solution strength to calculate the mL/hr rate for 20 mg/hr.

Method 1: Ratio and Proportion

$$\frac{125 \text{ mg}}{100 \text{ mL}} = \frac{20 \text{ mg}}{x \text{ mL}} \qquad or \qquad 125 \text{ mg} : 100 \text{ mL} = 20 \text{ mg} : x \text{ mL}$$

$$125x = 100 \times 20 \qquad\qquad\qquad 125x = 100 \times 20$$

$$x = 16 \text{ mL/hr} \qquad\qquad\qquad\quad x = 16 \text{ mL/hr}$$

To infuse 20 mg/hr, set the flow rate at 16 mL/hr.

Method 2: Dimensional Analysis

To calculate mL/hr from the 20 mg per hour that is ordered, use dimensional analysis as follows:

$$\frac{\text{mL}}{\text{hr}} = \frac{100 \text{ mL}}{125 \text{ mg}} \times \frac{20 \text{ mg}}{1 \text{ hr}}$$

$$= \frac{100 \text{ mL}}{125 \text{ mg}} \times \frac{20 \text{ mg}}{1 \text{ hr}}$$

$$= 16 \text{ mL/hr}$$

Method 3: Formula Method

When using the formula method, use the prescriber's order of 20 mg per hour as the desire. This does not change; the desire is the doctor's order for the dose per time. The have and the quantity will come from the IV solution. Consider the IV solution to be the supply, or equivalent to a "vial." The setup using the formula method will be as follows:

$$\frac{20 \text{ mg/hr (D)} \times 100 \text{ mL(Q)}}{125 \text{ mg (H)}} = x \text{ mL/hr}$$

$$\frac{2,000}{125} = 16 \text{ mL/hr}$$

Any of the three methods of calculation will give you the flow rate of 16 mL/hr. If placed on an infusion pump, the rate would be set at 16 mL/hr. If this medication drip is infused by gravity, microdrip tubing would be used and the drops per minute would be 16 gtt/min.

Example 2 ◼   A maintenance dose of 2 mcg/min has been ordered using an 8 mg dose in 250 mL solution. Calculate the mL/hr flow rate.

When an order is written as a unit of weight per minute, the easiest approach is to convert the rate to an hourly rate. To convert 2 mcg per minute to an hourly rate, we will multiply 2 mcg/min by the conversion of 60 minutes in 1 hour. We will calculate the following:

$$2 \text{ mcg/min} \times 60 \text{ min/hr} = 120 \text{ mcg/hr}$$

The next thing we notice with this medication order is that the supply is in mg and the order is in mcg. One of these will need to be converted so that both the order and the supply are in the same system and same unit of measure. It might be easiest to convert so that you are not using decimals, so convert mg to mcg, using the conversion of 1,000 mcg = 1 mg.

$$8 \text{ m\!g} \times 1,000 \text{ mcg/m\!g} = 8,000 \text{ mcg}$$

Our supply is equivalent to 8,000 mcg in 250 mL. Now we can apply either of the three methods of calculation.

Method 1: Ratio and Proportion

$$\frac{8,000 \text{ mcg}}{250 \text{ mL}} = \frac{120 \text{ mcg}}{x \text{ mL}} \qquad or \qquad 8,000 \text{ mcg} : 250 \text{ mL} = 120 \text{ mcg} : x \text{ mL}$$

$$8,000x = 30,000 \qquad\qquad\qquad\qquad 8,000x = 30,000$$

$$x = 3.75 = 3.8 \text{ mL/hr} \qquad\qquad\qquad x = 3.75 = 3.8 \text{ mL/hr}$$

Most likely, a medicated drip would be placed on an infusion pump that can be programmed to the tenth. Therefore, we would calculate this to the hundredth and round to the tenth. If infusing by gravity or on a pump that can only be programmed in whole numbers, we would infuse this drip at 4 mL/hr or 4 gtt/min.

Method 2: Dimensional Analysis

We will use the hourly dosage that we calculated to complete the calculation using dimensional analysis. We will complete the conversion from mg to mcg within the dimensional analysis equation.

$$\frac{\text{mL}}{\text{hr}} = \frac{250 \text{ mL}}{8 \text{ m\!g}} \times \frac{1 \text{ m\!g}}{1,000 \text{ m\!c\!g}} \times \frac{120 \text{ m\!c\!g}}{1 \text{ hr}}$$

$$\frac{\text{mL}}{\text{hr}} = \frac{30,000}{8,000}$$

$$\frac{\text{mL}}{\text{hr}} = 3.75 = 3.8 \text{ mL/hr}$$

Method 3: Formula Method

The desire will be 120 mcg per hour. The have and quantity will be the concentration of the solution. We will use 8,000 mcg in 250 mL. Calculation using the formula method will be as follows:

$$\frac{120 \text{ m\!c\!g/hr (D)} \times 250 \text{ mL (Q)}}{8,000 \text{ m\!c\!g (H)}} = x \text{ mL/hr}$$

$$\frac{30,000}{8,000} = 3.75 = 3.8 \text{ mL/hr}$$

All three methods of calculation arrive at the same answer. We will program an electronic pump at 3.8 mL/hr if it can be programmed to the tenth. If not, we will round the rate to 4 mL/hr. If we are infusing this medication by gravity, we will use microdrip tubing and regulate it at 4 gtt/min.

> **Key**point: Metric conversions may be made in either direction: solution strength to dosage ordered or dosage ordered to solution strength. Sometimes it is easier to convert so that you do not have to calculate with decimals.

Example 3 ■   Refer to Figure 21-1 for the medication for this order. A nitroglycerin drip of 50 mg in 250 mL is prepared and a dosage of 200 mcg/min is ordered.

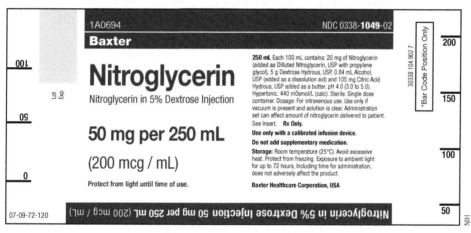

▲ **Figure 21-1**

We need to calculate the flow rate in mL/hr. Our first step will be to calculate the hourly rate.

200 mcg/min × 60 min/hr = 12,000 mcg/hr

Our next step will be to ensure the dosage and the supply are in the same system and unit of measure. We will convert mcg to mg – this will make the number smaller, and we will not have any decimals.

12,000 mcg = 12 mg

We have converted the ordered dosage to 12 mg/hr. Now we can apply any of the three methods of calculation to calculate the rate of infusion.

Method 1: Ratio and Proportion

$$\frac{50 \text{ mg}}{250 \text{ mL}} \times \frac{12 \text{ mg}}{x \text{ mL}} \qquad or \qquad 50 \text{ mg} : 250 \text{ mL} = 12 \text{ mg} : x \text{ mL}$$

$$50x = 3{,}000 \qquad\qquad\qquad\qquad 50x = 3{,}000$$

$$x = 60 \text{ mL/hr} \qquad\qquad\qquad\qquad x = 60 \text{ mL/hr}$$

Method 2: Dimensional Analysis

In this example, we will use the conversions we have already completed—the dosage ordered is 12 mg/hr.

$$\frac{mL}{hr} = \frac{250 \text{ mL}}{50 \text{ mg}} \times \frac{12 \text{ mg}}{1 \text{ hr}}$$

$$\frac{mL}{hr} = \frac{3{,}000}{50}$$

$$\frac{mL}{hr} = 60 \text{ mL/hr}$$

Method 3: Formula Method

We will use the conversions we have already completed. The desire will be 12 mg per hour and the supply will be the nitroglycerin solution of 50 mg in 250 mL.

$$\frac{12 \text{ mg/hr (D)} \times 250 \text{ mL (Q)}}{50 \text{ mg (H)}} = x \text{ mL/hr}$$

$$\frac{3{,}000}{50} = 60 \text{ mL/hr}$$

To infuse 200 mcg/min of this nitroglycerin drip, set the flow rate at 60 mL/hr. If it is infusing by gravity, use a microdrip tubing and infuse at 60 gtt/min.

Problems 21.1

Calculate and round these mL/hr flow rates to the tenth.

1. A physician has ordered IV furosemide to infuse at 9.5 mg/hr.
   See Figure 21-2 to calculate the mL/hr.   _____

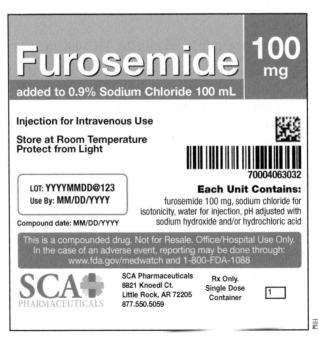

Furosemide 100 mg
added to 0.9% Sodium Chloride 100 mL

Injection for Intravenous Use

Store at Room Temperature
Protect from Light

LOT: YYYYMMDD@123
Use By: MM/DD/YYYY

Compound date: MM/DD/YYYY

70004063032
Each Unit Contains:
furosemide 100 mg, sodium chloride for
isotonicity, water for injection, pH adjusted with
sodium hydroxide and/or hydrochloric acid

This is a compounded drug. Not for Resale. Office/Hospital Use Only.
In the case of an adverse event, reporting may be done through:
www.fda.gov/medwatch and 1-800-FDA-1088

SCA✚
PHARMACEUTICALS

SCA Pharmaceuticals
8821 Knoedl Ct.
Little Rock, AR 72205
877.550.5059

Rx Only.
Single Dose
Container   1

▲ **Figure 21-2**

2. An IV medication is ordered at the rate of 3 mcg/min. The solution strength is 8 mg in 250 mL.   _____

3. A solution strength of 2 g in 500 mL is used to administer a dosage of 2 mg/min.   _____

4. A rate of 2 mcg/min is ordered. The solution strength is 1 mg/250 mL.   _____

5. A client has been ordered an IV infusion of amiodarone at a rate of 500 mcg/min. Refer to Figure 21-3 to calculate the mL/hr.   _____

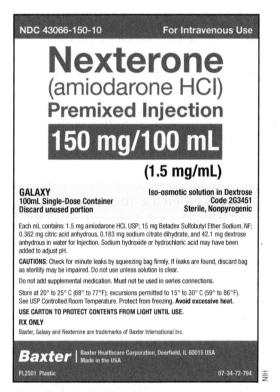

▲ **Figure 21-3**

6. A patient with angina pectoris has been ordered a nicardipine IV infusion at 1.2 mg/hr. Refer to Figure 21-4 for the dosage strength of solution. Determine the flow rate in mL/hr.   _____

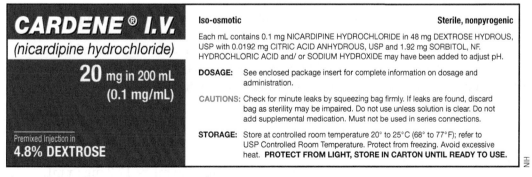

▲ **Figure 21-4**

7. A solution strength of 75 mg/250 mL is to infuse at 10 mg/hr.   _____

8. A 1 g/500 mL solution is to infuse at 1 mg/min.   _____

9. A 100 mg/250 mL solution is to infuse at 8 mg/hr.   _____

10. A 1 g/150 mL solution is to infuse at 175 mg/hr.   _____

Flow Rates to Infuse Dosages per Time Based on Body Weight

Many drug dosages per time are calculated based on body weight—for example, 5 mg/kg/hr. Body weight, to the nearest tenth kg, is used for these calculations. A preliminary step of calculating dosage based on weight is necessary before the flow rate can be calculated. Fractional dosage answers are expressed to the nearest tenth and mL/hr rates should be expressed to the nearest tenth of a mL. Again, it is important to recognize that if an infusion pump cannot be programmed to the tenth, we would round the mL/hr to the nearest whole number. This will also be important if we are infusing the medication by gravity.

Example 1 ■   A drug is ordered at the rate of 3 mcg/kg/min for a body weight of 95.9 kg. The solution strength is 400 mg in 250 mL. Calculate the mL/hr flow rate.

Our first step will be to calculate the dosage per minute for this individual who weighs 95.9 kg.

3 mcg/kg/min × 95.9 kg = 287.7 mcg/min

Now we must convert the rate per minute to the rate per hour. We will do this by multiplying the rate per minute by 60 minutes in one hour.

287.7 mcg/min × 60 min/hr = 17,262 mcg/hr

Our solution is mixed with milligrams per mL; therefore we must convert either milligrams to micrograms, or micrograms to milligrams. We will choose to convert micrograms to milligrams. This will make the number smaller and easier to work with. Convert 17,262 mcg to mg by applying the conversion of 1,000 mcg in 1 mg.

17,262 mcg/hr ÷ 1,000 mcg/mg = 17.26 = 17.3 mg/hr

Remember to round the mg/hr to the tenth instead of the whole number for greater accuracy. Now that we have completed our conversions, we can apply any of the three methods of calculation to this order to calculate the flow rate.

Method 1: Ratio and Proportion

$$\frac{400\text{ mg}}{250\text{ mL}} = \frac{17.3\text{ mg}}{x\text{ mL}}$$

$$400x = 250 \times 17.3$$

$$x = 10.81 = 10.8\text{ mL/hr}$$

or   400 mg : 250 mL = 17.3 mg : x mL

$$400x = 250 \times 17.3$$

$$x = 10.81 = 10.8\text{ mL/hr}$$

Method 2: Dimensional Analysis

$$\frac{mL}{hr} = \frac{250 \text{ mL}}{400 \text{ mg}} \times \frac{17.3 \text{ mg}}{1 \text{ hr}}$$

$$\frac{mL}{hr} = \frac{4{,}325}{400}$$

$$\frac{mL}{hr} = 10.81 = 10.8 \text{ mL/hr}$$

Method 3: Formula Method

$$\frac{17.3 \text{ mg/hr (D)} \times 250 \text{ mL (Q)}}{400 \text{ mg (H)}} = x \text{ mL/hr}$$

$$\frac{4{,}325}{400} = 10.81 = 10.8 \text{ mL/hr}$$

To infuse this IV at 3 mcg/kg/min for this patient, we will set the flow rate at 10.8 mL/hr. If the infusion pump cannot be programmed to the tenth, we would round to the whole number of 11 mL/hr. If we must infuse it by gravity, we would select a microdrip tubing and infuse it at 11 gtt/min.

Example 2 ■   A 2.5 g in 250 mL solution is ordered at a rate of 100 mcg/kg/min for a body weight of 104.6 kg.

Calculate the mL/hr flow rate using the following steps:

    Step 1   Calculate the dosage per min for 104.6 kg.

        100 mcg/kg/min $\times$ 104.6 kg = 10,460 mcg/min

    Step 2   Convert 10,460 mcg to mg and 2.5 g to mg so that both the order and the supply are in the same unit of measure.

        10,460 mcg/min $\div$ 1,000 mcg/mg = 10.46 = 10.5 mg/min

        2.5 g $\times$ 1,000 mg/g = 2,500 mg

        There are 2,500 mg of medication in the 250 mL IV bag.

    Step 3   Now we need to convert 10.5 mg/min to mg/hr.

        10.5 mg/min $\times$ 60 min/hr = 630 mg/hr

Finally, we can calculate the flow rate using any of the three methods of calculation.

Method 1: Ratio and Proportion

$$\frac{2{,}500 \text{ mg}}{250 \text{ mL}} = \frac{630 \text{ mg}}{x \text{ mL}} \qquad or \qquad 2{,}500 \text{ mg} : 250 \text{ mL} = 630 \text{ mg} : x \text{ mL}$$

$$2{,}500x = 250 \times 630 \qquad\qquad\qquad 2{,}500x = 250 \times 630$$

$$x = \frac{250 \times 630}{2{,}500} \qquad\qquad\qquad x = \frac{250 \times 630}{2{,}500}$$

$$x = 63 \text{ mL/hr} \qquad\qquad\qquad\qquad x = 63 \text{ mL/hr}$$

Method 2: Dimensional Analysis

$$\frac{mL}{hr} = \frac{250 \text{ mL}}{2,500 \text{ mg}} \times \frac{630 \text{ mg}}{1 \text{ hr}}$$

$$\frac{mL}{hr} = \frac{157,500}{2,500}$$

$$\frac{mL}{hr} = 63 \text{ mL/hr}$$

Method 3: Formula Method

$$\frac{630 \text{ mg/hr (D)} \times 250 \text{ mL (Q)}}{2,500 \text{ mg (H)}} = x \text{ mL/hr}$$

$$\frac{157,500}{2,500} = 63 \text{ mL/hr}$$

To infuse 100 mcg/kg/min for this patient, set the rate at 63 mL/hr on an infusion device. If it is infusing by gravity, set the drops per minute at 63 gtt/min using a microdrip tubing.

Example 3 ■   An IV medication has been ordered at 4 mcg/kg/min using a solution of 50 mg in 250 mL. The body weight is 107.3 kg.

Calculate the mL/hr flow rate using the following steps:

Step 1   Calculate the dosage per min for the patient weighing 107.3 kg.

4 mcg/kg/min $\times$ 107.3 kg = 429.2 mcg/min

Step 2   Convert mcg/min to mcg/hr.

429.2 mcg/min $\times$ 60 min/hr = 25,752 mcg/hr

Step 3   Convert mcg to mg so the order and the supply unit of measurement are the same.

25,752 mcg/hr $\div$ 1,000 mcg/mg = 25.75 = 25.8 mg/hr

Now we can calculate the flow rate using any of the methods of calculation.

Method 1: Ratio and Proportion

$$\frac{50 \text{ mg}}{250 \text{ mL}} = \frac{25.8 \text{ mg}}{x \text{ mL}} \qquad or \qquad 50 \text{ mg} : 250 \text{ mL} = 25.8 \text{ mg} : x \text{ mL}$$

$$50x = 6,450 \qquad\qquad\qquad 50x = 250 \times 25.8 = 6,450$$

$$x = 129 \text{ mL/hr} \qquad\qquad\qquad x = 129 \text{ mL/hr}$$

Method 2: Dimensional Analysis

$$\frac{mL}{hr} = \frac{250 \text{ mL}}{50 \text{ mg}} \times \frac{25.8 \text{ mg}}{1 \text{ hr}}$$

$$\frac{mL}{hr} = \frac{6,450}{50}$$

$$\frac{mL}{hr} = 129 \text{ mL/hr}$$

Method 3: Formula Method

$$\frac{25.8 \text{ mg/hr (D)} \times 250 \text{ mL (Q)}}{50 \text{ mg (H)}} = x \text{ mL/hr}$$

$$\frac{6{,}450}{50} = 129 \text{ mL/hr}$$

To infuse 4 mcg/kg/min to this patient who weighs 107.3 kg, set the rate at 129 mL/hr.

Problems 21.2

Calculate and round the dosage per min to the tenth, and the mL/hr flow rates to the tenth.

	mcg/min	mL/hr

1. A dosage of 50 mcg/kg/min of esmolol has been ordered for an 87.4 kg adult. Refer to Figure 21-5 for the solution strength.   _____   _____

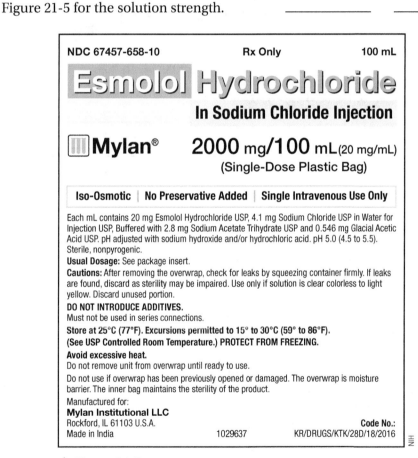

NDC 67457-658-10   Rx Only   100 mL

Esmolol Hydrochloride

In Sodium Chloride Injection

Mylan®   **2000 mg/100 mL** (20 mg/mL)
(Single-Dose Plastic Bag)

| Iso-Osmotic | No Preservative Added | Single Intravenous Use Only |

Each mL contains 20 mg Esmolol Hydrochloride USP, 4.1 mg Sodium Chloride USP in Water for Injection USP, Buffered with 2.8 mg Sodium Acetate Trihydrate USP and 0.546 mg Glacial Acetic Acid USP. pH adjusted with sodium hydroxide and/or hydrochloric acid. pH 5.0 (4.5 to 5.5). Sterile, nonpyrogenic.

Usual Dosage: See package insert.

Cautions: After removing the overwrap, check for leaks by squeezing container firmly. If leaks are found, discard as sterility may be impaired. Use only if solution is clear colorless to light yellow. Discard unused portion.

DO NOT INTRODUCE ADDITIVES.

Must not be used in series connections.

Store at 25°C (77°F). Excursions permitted to 15° to 30°C (59° to 86°F).

(See USP Controlled Room Temperature.) PROTECT FROM FREEZING.

Avoid excessive heat.

Do not remove unit from overwrap until ready to use.

Do not use if overwrap has been previously opened or damaged. The overwrap is moisture barrier. The inner bag maintains the sterility of the product.

Manufactured for:

Mylan Institutional LLC

Rockford, IL 61103 U.S.A.

Made in India   1029637   **Code No.:**
KR/DRUGS/KTK/28D/18/2016

▲ **Figure 21-5**

2. A dosage has been ordered at 4 mcg/kg/min using a 400 mg/250 mL solution. The body weight is 92.4 kg.   _____   _____

3. A dosage of 2.5 mcg/kg/min has been ordered. The solution is 0.5 g/250 mL. The body weight is 80.7 kg.   _____   _____

4. A dosage of 150 mcg/kg/min has been ordered for a body weight of 92.1 kg. The solution strength is 2.5 g/250 mL.   _____   _____

5. A 5 mcg/kg/min infusion is ordered for a body weight of 80.3 kg. The solution strength is 1 g/500 mL.   _____   _____

6. A milrinone dosage of 0.5 mcg/kg/min has been ordered for an adult weighing 78.2 kg. Refer to Figure 21-6 for solution information.   _____   _____

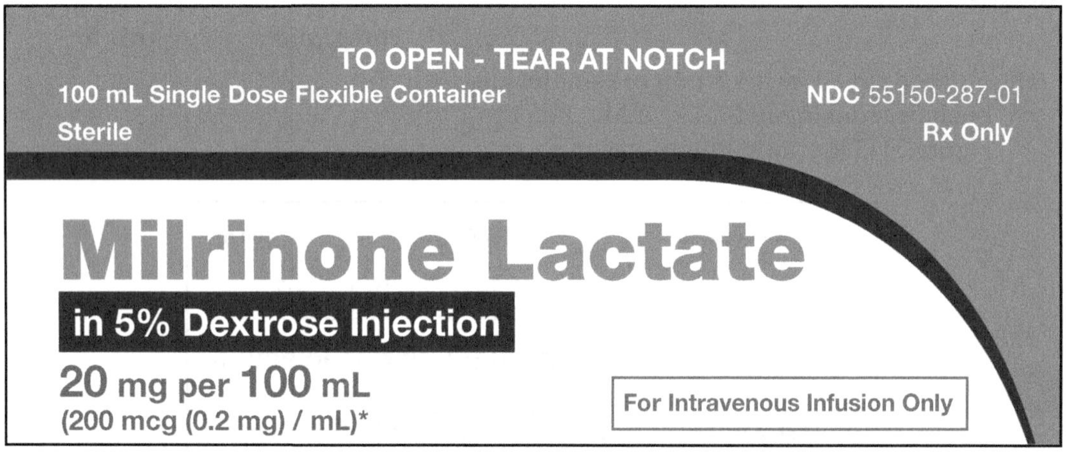

TO OPEN - TEAR AT NOTCH

100 mL Single Dose Flexible Container   NDC 55150-287-01

Sterile   Rx Only

Milrinone Lactate

in 5% Dextrose Injection

20 mg per 100 mL
(200 mcg (0.2 mg) / mL)*

For Intravenous Infusion Only

▲ Figure 21-6

7. A dosage of 6 mcg/kg/min has been ordered for an adult weighing 88.7 kg. A solution strength of 100 mg/500 mL is to be infused.   _____   _____

8. The body weight is 91.2 kg and a 1.5 mcg/kg/min rate is ordered using a 0.3 g/250 mL solution.   _____   _____

9. A 2 mcg/kg/min infusion is ordered for a 90.3 kg adult. The solution to be used has a strength of 0.5 g/250 mL.   _____   _____

10. A 0.4 mcg/kg/min dosage of phenylephrine is ordered for a body weight of 65 kg. Refer to Figure 21-7 for solution strength.   _____   _____

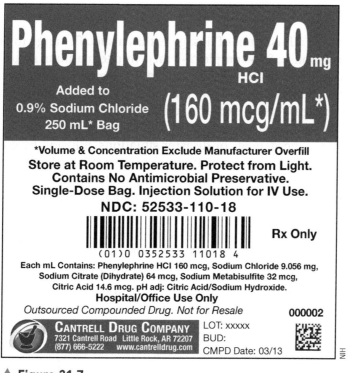

▲ **Figure 21-7**

11. A 2 mcg/kg/min dosage has been ordered for an adult weighing 79.9 kg. The solution strength available is 50 mg/250 mL.

    _____   _____

12. A dosage of 3 mcg/kg/min has been ordered using a 350 mg/250 mL solution strength. The body weight is 86.9 kg.

    _____   _____

13. An adult weighing 84.3 kg has a dosage of 3 mcg/kg/min ordered. The solution to be used is 0.75 g/300 mL.

    _____   _____

14. A 6 mcg/kg/min dosage is ordered for an adult weighing 85.8 kg. The solution strength is 800 mg/500 mL.

    _____   _____

15. An adult weighing 91.4 kg has a dosage of 4 mcg/kg/min ordered. The solution to be used is 700 mg/500 mL.

    _____   _____

Answers **1.** 4,370 mcg/min; 13.1 mL/hr **2.** 369.6 mcg/min; 13.9 mL/hr **3.** 201.8 mcg/min; 6.1 mL/hr **4.** 13,815 mcg/min; 82.9 mL/hr **5.** 401.5 mcg/min; 12.1 mL/hr **6.** 39.1 mcg/min; 11.5 mL/hr **7.** 532.2 mcg/min; 159.5 mL/hr **8.** 136.8 mcg/min; 6.8 mL/hr **9.** 180.6 mcg/min; 5.4 mL/hr **10.** 26 mcg/min; 9.8 mL/hr (if using mcg/mL); 10 mL/hr (if using mg/mL) **11.** 159.8 mcg/min; 48 mL/hr **12.** 260.7 mcg/min; 11.1 mL/hr **13.** 252.9 mcg/min; 6.1 mL/hr **14.** 514.8 mcg/min; 19.3 mL/hr **15.** 365.6 mcg/min; 15.6 mL/hr

Calculation of Infusion Titrations

Titration refers to the adjustment of dosage within a specific range to obtain a measurable physiologic response; for example, 2–4 mcg/min to maintain systolic BP >100. The dosage is increased or decreased within the ordered range until the desired response is obtained. The lowest dosage is set first and adjusted upward and downward as necessary. The upper dosage is never exceeded unless a new order is obtained.

Electronic infusion devices are used for administration of medications requiring titration. In extreme emergencies or disaster situations, infusion by gravity may be the only option. This would require constant monitoring until an electronic infusion device became available. Flow rates are calculated in mL/hr for the lowest and highest dosage ordered and adjusted within this range to elicit the desired physiologic response.

Example 1 ■   Norepinephrine has been ordered for your patient with severe hypotension. A dosage of 2–4 mcg/min has been ordered to maintain systolic BP > 100 mm Hg. Refer to Figure 21-8 for the label on your IV bag, notice the solution being titrated has 8 mg in 250 mL. Calculate the flow rate for the 2–4 mcg range.

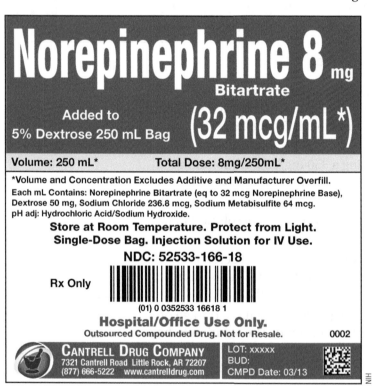

▲ Figure 21-8

First, calculate the lower 2 mcg/min flow rate.

Step 1   Convert 2 mcg/min to mcg/hr.

$$2 \text{ mcg/min} \times 60 \text{ min/hr} = 120 \text{ mcg/hr}$$

As the bag is supplied in milligrams (8 mg per 250 mL), you will need to convert mg to mcg or mcg to mg. It may be preferable to convert mg to mcg to avoid decimals.

Step 2   We will convert 8 mg to mcg.

$$8 \text{ mg} = 8,000 \text{ mcg}$$

Step 3   Now we will calculate the flow rate for 120 mcg per hour using any of the three methods of calculation.

Method 1: Ratio and Proportion

$$\frac{8{,}000 \text{ mcg}}{250 \text{ mL}} = \frac{120 \text{ mcg}}{x \text{ mL}} \qquad or \qquad 8{,}000 \text{ mcg} : 250 \text{ mL} = 120 \text{ mcg} : x \text{ mL}$$

$$8{,}000x = 30{,}000 \qquad\qquad\qquad 8{,}000x = 30{,}000$$

$$x = 3.75 = 3.8 \text{ mL/hr} \qquad\qquad x = 3.75 = 3.8 \text{ mL/hr}$$

Method 2: Dimensional Analysis

$$\frac{\text{mL}}{\text{hr}} = \frac{250 \text{ mL}}{8{,}000 \text{ meg}} \times \frac{120 \text{ meg}}{1 \text{ hr}}$$

$$\frac{\text{mL}}{\text{hr}} = \frac{30{,}000}{8{,}000}$$

$$\frac{\text{mL}}{\text{hr}} = 3.75 = 3.8 \text{ mL/hr}$$

Method 3: Formula Method

$$\frac{120 \text{ meg/hr (D)} \times 250 \text{ mL (Q)}}{8{,}000 \text{ meg (H)}} = x \text{ mL/hr}$$

$$\frac{30{,}000}{8{,}000} = 3.75 = 3.8 \text{ mL/hr}$$

From these calculations, we see that the lowest range of 2 mcg/min would be infused by setting the IV pump at 3.8 mL/hr. If we had to run this by gravity, we would choose a microdrip tubing and set the flow rate at 4 gtt/min.

In this example, the upper level of 4 mcg/min flow rate is exactly double the 2 mcg/min rate, so it can be calculated by multiplying the 3.8 mL/hr rate by 2.

$$3.8 \text{ mL/hr} \times 2 = 7.6 \text{ mL/hr}$$

The flow rate for the upper level of 4 mcg/min dosage is 7.6 mL/hr on an electronic pump. If we had to infuse this IV by gravity using a microdrip tubing, we would round to 8 and infuse it at 8 gtt/min. Therefore, the flow rate range to titrate a dosage of 2–4 mcg/min is 3.8–7.6 mL/hr.

We would monitor the patient's blood pressure and if the systolic was not above 100 mm Hg, we would slowly titrate the medicated drip within this range. We cannot go above this range without new orders from the physician.

Example 2 ▦   A drug is to be titrated between 415 and 830 mcg/min. The solution concentration is 100 mg in 40 mL. Calculate the mL/hr flow rate range.

Our first step will be to calculate the lower 415 mcg/min flow rate first.

Step 1   Convert 415 mcg/min to mcg/hr.

415 mcg/min × 60 min/hr = 24,900 mcg/hr

Notice the supply is in a different unit of measure than the order. We can convert either the order in mcg to mg, or the supply in mg to mcg.

Step 2   In this example, we will convert 24,900 mcg/hr to mg/hr.

24,900 mcg/hr ÷ 1,000 mcg/mg = 24.9 mg/hr

Step 3   Calculate the flow rate for 24.9 mg/hr using the three methods of calculation.

Method 1: Ratio and Proportion

$$\frac{100 \text{ mg}}{40 \text{ mL}} = \frac{24.9 \text{ mg}}{x \text{ mL}} \qquad or \qquad 100 \text{ mg} : 40 \text{ mL} = 24.9 \text{ mg} : x \text{ mL}$$

$$100x = 40 \times 24.9 \qquad\qquad\qquad 100x = 40 \times 24.9$$

$$x = 9.96 = 10 \text{ mL/hr} \qquad\qquad x = 9.96 = 10 \text{ mL/hr}$$

Method 2: Dimensional Analysis

$$\frac{\text{mL}}{\text{hr}} = \frac{40 \text{ mL}}{100 \text{ mg}} \times \frac{24.9 \text{ mg}}{1 \text{ hr}}$$

$$\frac{\text{mL}}{\text{hr}} = \frac{996}{100}$$

$$\frac{\text{mL}}{\text{hr}} = 9.96 = 10 \text{ mL/hr}$$

Method 3: Formula Method

$$\frac{24.9 \text{ mg/hr (D)} \times 40 \text{ mL (Q)}}{100 \text{ mg (H)}} = x \text{ mL/hr}$$

$$\frac{996}{100} = 9.96 = 10 \text{ mL/hr}$$

In this example, the upper level of 830 mcg/min dosage is exactly double the 415 mcg/min dosage. It can be calculated by multiplying the 10 mL/hr rate by 2.

$$10 \text{ mL/hr} \times 2 = 20 \text{ mL/hr}$$

The flow rate for the upper level of 830 mcg/min dosage is 20 mL/hr on an electronic pump. If we had to infuse this IV by gravity using a microdrip tubing, we would infuse it at 20 gtt/min. Therefore, the flow rate range to titrate a dosage of 415–830 mcg/min is 10–20 mL/hr.

Example 3 ■   A dose is ordered by weight. An adult weighing 103.1 kg has orders for a titration between 0.3 and 3 mcg/kg/min. The solution concentration is 50 mg in 250 mL.

First, calculate the lower and upper dosage ranges for the patient weighing 103.1 kg.

Step 1   Calculate the lower end of the titration range of 0.3 mcg/kg per min.

0.3 mcg/kg/min × 103.1 kg = 30.93 = 30.9 mcg/min

Step 2   Calculate the upper end of the titration range of 3 mcg/kg per min.

3 mcg/kg/min × 103.1 kg = 309.3 mcg/min

The dosage range for the patient weighing 103.1 kg is 30.9 to 309.3 mcg/min. Next, calculate the flow rate for the lower 30.9 mcg/min dosage.

Step 3	Convert 30.9 mcg/min to mcg/hr.

$$30.9 \text{ mcg/min} \times 60 \text{ min/hr} = 1{,}854 \text{ mcg/hr}$$

Step 4	Since the dosage is ordered in mcg per hour, and the supply is in milligrams, we must convert so they are both in the same unit of measure. We will convert 1,854 mcg/hr to mg/hr.

$$1{,}854 \text{ mcg/hr} \div 1{,}000 \text{ mcg/mg} = 1.85 = 1.9 \text{ mg/hr}$$

Step 5	Calculate the flow rate for 1.9 mg/hr using the three methods of calculation.

Method 1: Ratio and Proportion

$$\frac{50 \text{ mg}}{250 \text{ mL}} = \frac{1.9 \text{ mg}}{x \text{ mL}} \quad or \quad 50 \text{ mg} : 250 \text{ mL} = 1.9 \text{ mg} : x \text{ mL}$$

$$50x = 250 \times 1.9 \qquad\qquad 50x = 250 \times 1.9$$

$$x = 9.5 \text{ mL/hr} \qquad\qquad x = 9.5 \text{ mL/hr}$$

Method 2: Dimensional Analysis

$$\frac{\text{mL}}{\text{hr}} = \frac{250 \text{ mL}}{50 \text{ mg}} \times \frac{1.9 \text{ mg}}{1 \text{ hr}}$$

$$\frac{\text{mL}}{\text{hr}} = \frac{475}{50}$$

$$\frac{\text{mL}}{\text{hr}} = 9.5 \text{ mL/hr}$$

Method 3: Formula Method

$$\frac{1.9 \text{ mg/hr (D)} \times 250 \text{ mL (Q)}}{50 \text{ mg (H)}} = x \text{ mL/hr}$$

$$\frac{475}{50} = 9.5 \text{ mL/hr}$$

The upper level of the titration range is 309.3 mcg/min. Next, calculate the flow rate for this upper end of the range.

Step 6	Convert 309.3 mcg/min to mcg/hr.

$$309.3 \text{ mcg/min} \times 60 \text{ min/hr} = 18{,}558 \text{ mcg/hr}$$

Step 7	Since the dosage is ordered in mcg per hour, and the supply is in milligrams, we must convert so they are both in the same unit of measure. We will convert 18,558 mcg/hr to mg/hr.

$$18{,}558 \text{ mcg/hr} \div 1{,}000 \text{ mcg/mg} = 18.55 = 18.6 \text{ mg/hr}$$

Step 8	Calculate the flow rate for 18.6 mg/hr using the three methods of calculation.

Method 1: Ratio and Proportion

$$\frac{50 \text{ mg}}{250 \text{ mL}} = \frac{18.6 \text{ mg}}{x \text{ mL}} \qquad or \qquad 50 \text{ mg} : 250 \text{ mL} = 18.6 \text{ mg} : x \text{ mL}$$

$$50x = 250 \times 18.6 \qquad\qquad\qquad 50x = 250 \times 18.6$$

$$x = 93 \text{ mL/hr} \qquad\qquad\qquad x = 93 \text{ mL/hr}$$

Method 2: Dimensional Analysis

$$\frac{\text{mL}}{\text{hr}} = \frac{250 \text{ mL}}{50 \text{ mg}} \times \frac{18.6 \text{ mg}}{1 \text{ hr}}$$

$$\frac{\text{mL}}{\text{hr}} = \frac{4{,}650}{50}$$

$$\frac{\text{mL}}{\text{hr}} = 93 \text{ mL/hr}$$

Method 3: Formula Method

$$\frac{18.6 \text{ mg/hr (D)} \times 250 \text{ mL (Q)}}{50 \text{ mg (H)}} = x \text{ mL/hr}$$

$$\frac{4{,}650}{50} = 93 \text{ mL/hr}$$

The flow rate for the upper level of the titration range is 93 mL/hr. Therefore, this medication can be titrated between a low flow rate of 9.5 mL/hr to a high flow rate of 93 mL/hr for the patient who weighs 103.1 kg.

Problems 21.3

Calculate these mL/hr flow rate ranges. Express answers to the nearest tenth.

1. A physician has ordered IV procainamide for a patient with arrhythmias. The solution is to titrate at 1–4 mg/min. Refer to Figure 21-9 for supply strength.   _____

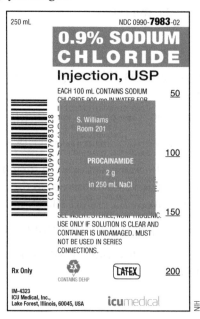

250 mL   NDC 0990-**7983**-02

0.9% SODIUM CHLORIDE
Injection, USP

EACH 100 mL CONTAINS SODIUM   50
CHLORIDE 900 mg IN WATER FOR

S. Williams
Room 201

100

PROCAINAMIDE
2 g
in 250 mL NaCl

150

USE ONLY IF SOLUTION IS CLEAR AND
CONTAINER IS UNDAMAGED. MUST
NOT BE USED IN SERIES
CONNECTIONS.

Rx Only   CONTAINS DEHP   [LATEX]   200

IM-4323
ICU Medical, Inc.,
Lake Forest, Illinois, 60045, USA   icumedical

▲ **Figure 21-9**

2. A drug is ordered to titrate between 1 and 3 mcg/min. The
   solution strength is 1 mg per 250 mL.   _____

3. Dopamine IV has been ordered to titrate at 1–5 mcg/kg/min.
   The adult weighs 103.7 kg. Refer to Figure 21-10 for the solution strength.   _____

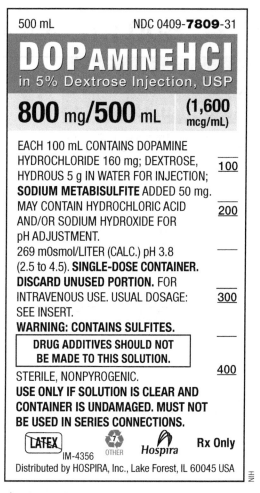

500 mL   NDC 0409-**7809**-31

DOPAMINEHCl
in 5% Dextrose Injection, USP
800 mg/**500** mL   (1,600 mcg/mL)

EACH 100 mL CONTAINS DOPAMINE
HYDROCHLORIDE 160 mg; DEXTROSE,   ‾‾ 100
HYDROUS 5 g IN WATER FOR INJECTION;
SODIUM METABISULFITE ADDED 50 mg.
MAY CONTAIN HYDROCHLORIC ACID   ‾‾ 200
AND/OR SODIUM HYDROXIDE FOR
pH ADJUSTMENT.
269 mOsmol/LITER (CALC.) pH 3.8   ‾‾
(2.5 to 4.5). **SINGLE-DOSE CONTAINER.**
DISCARD UNUSED PORTION. FOR
INTRAVENOUS USE. USUAL DOSAGE: ‾‾ 300
SEE INSERT.
WARNING: CONTAINS SULFITES.
  ┌─────────────────────────────┐   ‾‾
  │ **DRUG ADDITIVES SHOULD NOT** │
  │ **BE MADE TO THIS SOLUTION.** │   ‾‾ 400
  └─────────────────────────────┘
STERILE, NONPYROGENIC.
USE ONLY IF SOLUTION IS CLEAR AND
CONTAINER IS UNDAMAGED. MUST NOT
BE USED IN SERIES CONNECTIONS.
[LATEX]   ⟳   Hospira   **Rx Only**
       IM-4356   OTHER
Distributed by HOSPIRA, Inc., Lake Forest, IL 60045 USA

▲ **Figure 21-10**

4. A drug is to titrate between 50 and 100 mcg/kg/min. The
   adult weighs 78.7 kg, and the solution strength is 2,500 mg in
   250 mL.   _____

5. An adult weighing 73.2 kg has a solution of 500 mg in 250 mL
   ordered to titrate between 3 and 10 mcg/kg/min.   _____

6. A dosage of 4–6 mg/min has been ordered using a solution
   strength of 2.5 g/400 mL.   _____

7. A dosage of 2–4 mcg/min has been ordered using a solution
   strength of 2 mg/250 mL.   _____

8. A male patient with ventricular tachycardia has been ordered
   a lidocaine IV drip titrated at 20–50 mcg/kg/min. The patient
   weighs 99.5 kg. Refer to Figure 21-11 for the supply strength. _____

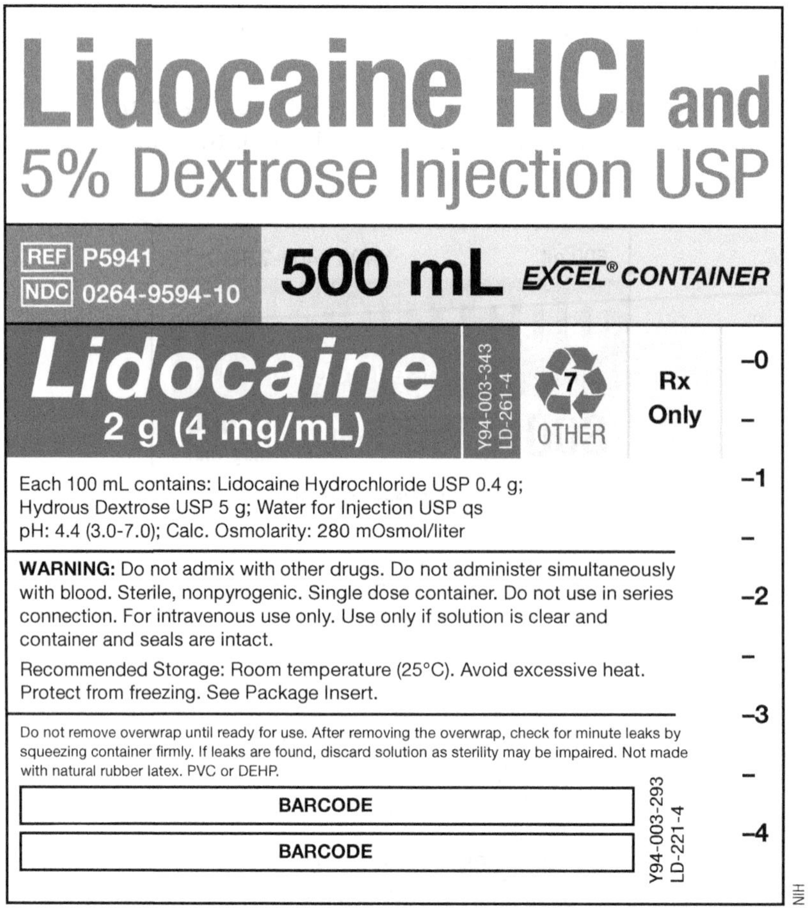

Lidocaine HCl and 5% Dextrose Injection USP

| REF P5941 | **500 mL** *EXCEL® CONTAINER* |
| NDC 0264-9594-10 | |

Lidocaine 2 g (4 mg/mL)

Y94-003-343 LD-261-4

7 OTHER

Rx Only

–0
–
–1
–
–2
–
–3
–
–4

Each 100 mL contains: Lidocaine Hydrochloride USP 0.4 g; Hydrous Dextrose USP 5 g; Water for Injection USP qs pH: 4.4 (3.0-7.0); Calc. Osmolarity: 280 mOsmol/liter

WARNING: Do not admix with other drugs. Do not administer simultaneously with blood. Sterile, nonpyrogenic. Single dose container. Do not use in series connection. For intravenous use only. Use only if solution is clear and container and seals are intact.

Recommended Storage: Room temperature (25°C). Avoid excessive heat. Protect from freezing. See Package Insert.

Do not remove overwrap until ready for use. After removing the overwrap, check for minute leaks by squeezing container firmly. If leaks are found, discard solution as sterility may be impaired. Not made with natural rubber latex. PVC or DEHP.

| BARCODE |
| BARCODE |

Y94-003-293 LD-221-4

▲ **Figure 21-11**

9. A range of 30–70 mcg/kg/min infusion is ordered for an 84.3 kg adult. The solution to be used has a strength of 2 g/250 mL. _____

10. A 75–125 mcg/kg/min dosage is ordered for a body weight of 81.2 kg. The solution available is 2.5 g/250 mL. _____

11. An adult weighing 101.6 kg has a dosage of 4–7 mcg/kg/min ordered. The solution to be used is 75 mg/50 mL. _____

12. A 30–70 mcg/kg/min dosage is ordered for an 80.4 kg adult. The solution strength is 3 g/250 mL. _____

13. A 4–8 mcg/kg/min dosage is ordered for an adult weighing 72.1 kg. The solution strength is 400 mg/250 mL. _____

14. An IV infusion of amiodarone is initiated on a patient with arrythmias. The medication is to be titrated at 1–2 mcg/kg/min. The patient weighs 74.2 kg. Refer to Figure 21-12 for the solution strength. _____

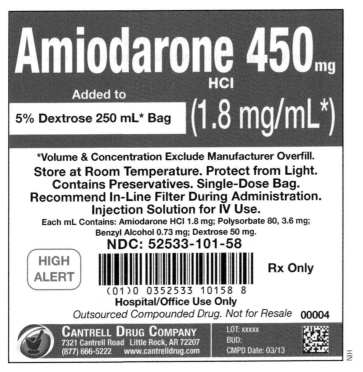

Amiodarone 450mg
HCl
Added to
5% Dextrose 250 mL* Bag   (1.8 mg/mL*)

*Volume & Concentration Exclude Manufacturer Overfill.
**Store at Room Temperature. Protect from Light.
Contains Preservatives. Single-Dose Bag.
Recommend In-Line Filter During Administration.
Injection Solution for IV Use.**
Each mL Contains: Amiodarone HCl 1.8 mg; Polysorbate 80, 3.6 mg;
Benzyl Alcohol 0.73 mg; Dextrose 50 mg.
NDC: 52533-101-58

HIGH
ALERT   Rx Only

(01)0 0352533 10158 8
Hospital/Office Use Only
Outsourced Compounded Drug. Not for Resale **00004**

CANTRELL DRUG COMPANY   LOT: xxxxx
7321 Cantrell Road Little Rock, AR 72207   BUD:
(877) 666-5222   www.cantrelldrug.com   CMPD Date: 03/13

▲ **Figure 21-12**

15. A titration at 150–200 mcg/kg/min has been ordered for a patient
who weighs 83.3 kg. The solution strength is 3.5 g in 250 mL.   _____

Answers 1. 7.5–30 mL/hr **2.** 15-45 mL/hr **3.** 3.9–19.4 mL/hr **4.** 23.6–47.2 mL/hr **5.** 6.6–22 mL/hr **6.** 38.4–
57.6 mL/hr **7.** 15–30 mL/hr **8.** 29.9–74.6 mL/hr **9.** 19–44.3 mL/hr **10.** 36.5–60.9 mL/hr **11.** 16.3–28.5 mL/hr
12. 12.1–28.1 mL/hr **13.** 10.8–21.6 mL/hr **14.** 2.5–4.9 mL/hr **15.** 53.6–71.4 mL/hr

---

Summary

This concludes the chapter on titration of IV medications. The important points to
remember about these medications are:

▪ They have a rapid action.

▪ They have a narrow margin of safety, and continuous monitoring is required in
their use.

▪ They are frequently titrated within a specific dosage or flow rate to elicit a measurable physiologic response.

▪ When titrated, they are initiated at the lowest dosage ordered and increased or
decreased slowly to obtain the desired response.

▪ They are infused using an electronic infusion device, or, in an emergency, a 60
gtt/mL microdrip set. Sometimes with children or elderly, a calibrated burette
may be used if an electronic pump or syringe pump is not available.

▪ The mL/hr flow rate for infusion pumps and the gtt/min for gravity drips using
microdrip tubing are identical.

When IV drips are prepared by the nurse or the pharmacy, they must be labeled with the name and amount of medication (mg, mcg of medication) placed in the IV solution, the date and time, patient name and room number, and initials of the person preparing the drip.

Summary Self-Test

Calculate dosages and flow rates to the nearest tenth using the calculation method of your choice. All IV infusions will be administered using an IV infusion device that programs to the tenth.

1. Dobutamine 6 mcg/kg/min dosage is ordered for an adult weighing 75.4 kg. Refer to Figure 21-13 for the available solution strength.

   mcg/min dosage _____   mL/hr flow rate _____

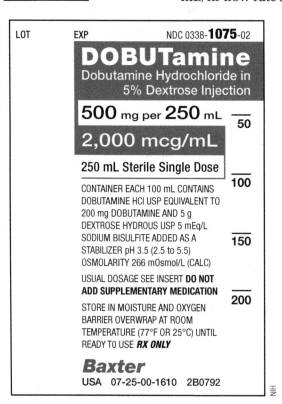

▲ **Figure 21-13**

2. The order is to infuse a solution of 30 mg in 250 mL at 0.6 mcg/kg/min. Calculate the dosage and flow rate for a 62.7 kg adult.

   mcg/min dosage _____   mL/hr flow rate _____

3. A solution of 275 mg in 500 mL is to infuse between 0.5 and 0.7 mg/kg/hr. The adult weighs 82.4 kg.

   mg/hr dosage range _____   mL/hr flow rate range _____

4. A client is ordered nitroprusside IV to treat a hypertensive crisis. The client weighs 68.5 kg. The medication is ordered at 0.3 mcg/kg/min. Refer to Figure 21-14 for supply strength.

mcg/min dosage _____   mL/hr flow rate _____

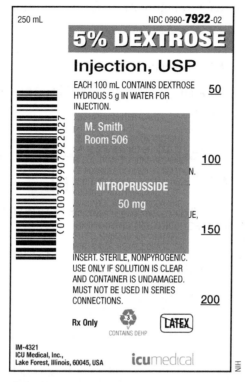

▲ Figure 21-14

5. A 1–6 mg/min dosage is ordered. The solution strength is 2 g/500 mL.

mL/hr flow rate range _____

6. A client weighs 62.8 kg and is ordered a dopamine IV infusion to control and sta-
bilize the blood pressure. The order is to titrate the infusion at 5–15 mcg/kg/min.
Refer to Figure 21-15 for the solution strength.

mL/hr flow rate range _____

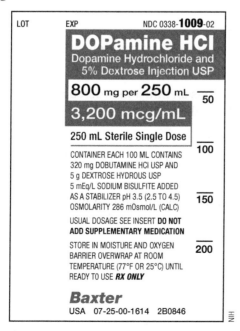

▲ Figure 21-15

7. A patient weighs 52.2 kg and is ordered a potassium chloride IV infusion to titrate at 0.3–0.5 mEq/kg/hr. Refer to Figure 21-16 for the solution strength.

   mL/hr flow rate range _____

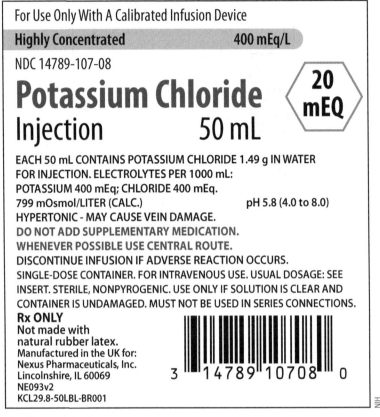

For Use Only With A Calibrated Infusion Device

Highly Concentrated   **400 mEq/L**

NDC 14789-107-08

Potassium Chloride

〈 **20 mEQ** 〉

Injection   50 mL

EACH 50 mL CONTAINS POTASSIUM CHLORIDE 1.49 g IN WATER
FOR INJECTION. ELECTROLYTES PER 1000 mL:
POTASSIUM 400 mEq; CHLORIDE 400 mEq.
799 mOsmol/LITER (CALC.)   pH 5.8 (4.0 to 8.0)
HYPERTONIC - MAY CAUSE VEIN DAMAGE.
DO NOT ADD SUPPLEMENTARY MEDICATION.
WHENEVER POSSIBLE USE CENTRAL ROUTE.
DISCONTINUE INFUSION IF ADVERSE REACTION OCCURS.
SINGLE-DOSE CONTAINER. FOR INTRAVENOUS USE. USUAL DOSAGE: SEE
INSERT. STERILE, NONPYROGENIC. USE ONLY IF SOLUTION IS CLEAR AND
CONTAINER IS UNDAMAGED. MUST NOT BE USED IN SERIES CONNECTIONS.
Rx ONLY
Not made with
natural rubber latex.
Manufactured in the UK for:
Nexus Pharmaceuticals, Inc.
Lincolnshire, IL 60069
NE093v2
KCL29.8-50LBL-BR001

3 14789 10708 0

▲ **Figure 21-16**

8. A solution of 100 mg in 40 mL is ordered to infuse at 5 mcg/kg/min for an adult weighing 77.1 kg.

   mL/hr flow rate _____

9. A drug is ordered at 5 mcg/min. The solution available is 1 mg in 250 mL.

   mL/hr flow rate _____

10. An adult weighing 80 kg has an infusion ordered at 8 mcg/kg/min. The solution strength is 800 mg in 500 mL.

    mcg/min dosage _____   mL/hr flow rate _____

11. A 10 mcg/min dosage is ordered using an 8 mg/250 mL solution.

    mL/hr flow rate _____

12. A client has been ordered an IV infusion of Brevibloc to be titrated at 50–200 mcg/kg/min. The client weighs 72.4 kg. Refer to Figure 21-17 for the solution strength.

mL/hr flow rate range _____

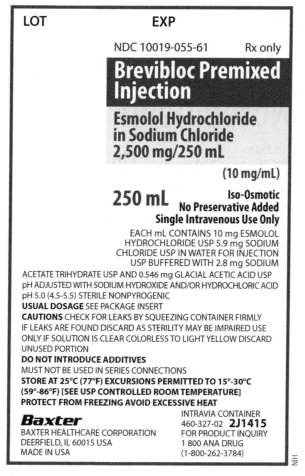

▲ **Figure 21-17**

13. An adult weighing 77.9 kg is to receive 80 mcg/kg/min. The solution strength is 2.5 g in 250 mL.

    mcg/min dosage _____   mL/hr flow rate _____

14. A dosage of 4 mcg/min has been ordered using an 8 mg in 250 mL solution.

    mL/hr flow rate _____

15. An adult who weighs 81.7 kg has orders for 8–10 mcg/kg/min. The solution strength is 400 mg in 250 mL.

    mcg/min dosage range _____   mL/hr flow rate _____

16. A 6 mcg/kg/min dosage has been ordered for a 90.7 kg adult. The solution strength is 50 mg in 250 mL.

    mcg/min dosage _____   mL/hr flow rate _____

17. A dosage of 5 mcg/kg/min is ordered. The solution available is 400 mg in 250 mL. The adult weighs 70.7 kg.

    mcg/min dosage _____   mL/hr flow rate _____

18. A 3 mg/min dosage is ordered. The solution strength is 2 g in 500 mL.

    mL/hr flow rate _____

19. A norepinephrine IV is ordered to titrate 2–4 mcg/min. Refer to Figure 21-18 for the solution strength.

    mcg/hr dosage range _____   mL/hr flow rate range _____

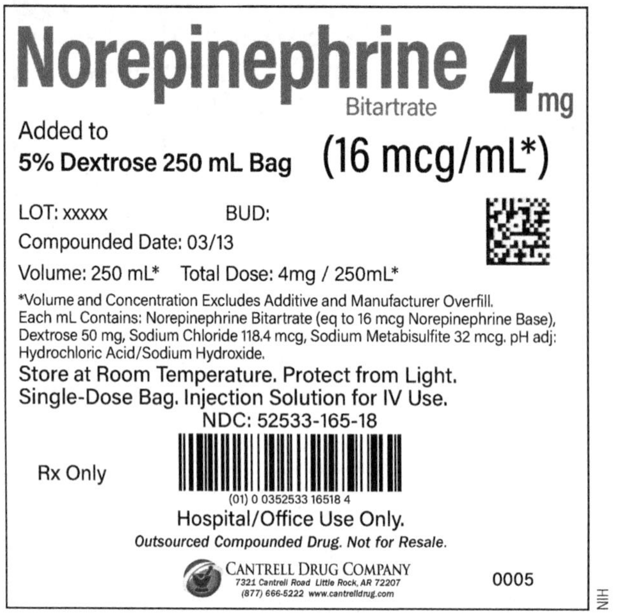

▲ **Figure 21-18**

20. A 500 mg in 250 mL solution is ordered for a 101.2 kg adult to titrate at 3–10 mcg/kg/min.

    mg/min dosage range _____   mL/hr flow rate _____

Answers to Summary Self-Test

1. 452.4 mcg/min; 13.6 mL/hr
2. 37.6 mcg/min; 19.2 mL/hr
3. 41.2–57.7 mg/hr; 74.9–104.9 mL/hr
4. 20.6 mcg/min; 6 mL/hr
5. 15–90 mL/hr
6. 5.9–17.7 mL/hr
7. 39.3–65.3 mL/hr
8. 9.2 mL/hr
9. 75 mL/hr
10. 640 mcg/min; 24 mL/hr
11. 18.8 mL/hr
12. 21.7–86.9 mL/hr
13. 6,232 mcg/min; 37.4 mL/hr
14. 7.5 mL/hr
15. 653.6–817 mcg/min; 24.5–30.6 mL/hr
16. 544.2 mcg/min; 163.5 mL/hr
17. 353.5 mcg/min; 13.3 mL/hr
18. 45 mL/hr
19. 120–240 mcg/hr; 7.5–15 mL/hr
20. 303.6–1,012 mcg/min; 9.1–30.4 mL/hr

Critical Thinking Questions

1. The physician has ordered the client, J. Smith, an isoproterenol IV infusion to titrate at 0.05–2 mcg/kg/min beginning the infusion at the lowest end of the range for the management of bradycardia. The client weighs 140 lb. The IV bag of this medication has arrived from pharmacy, and the nurse is calculating the flow rate. Refer to Figure 21-19. In the following matrix, determine if the choices are appropriate or inappropriate.

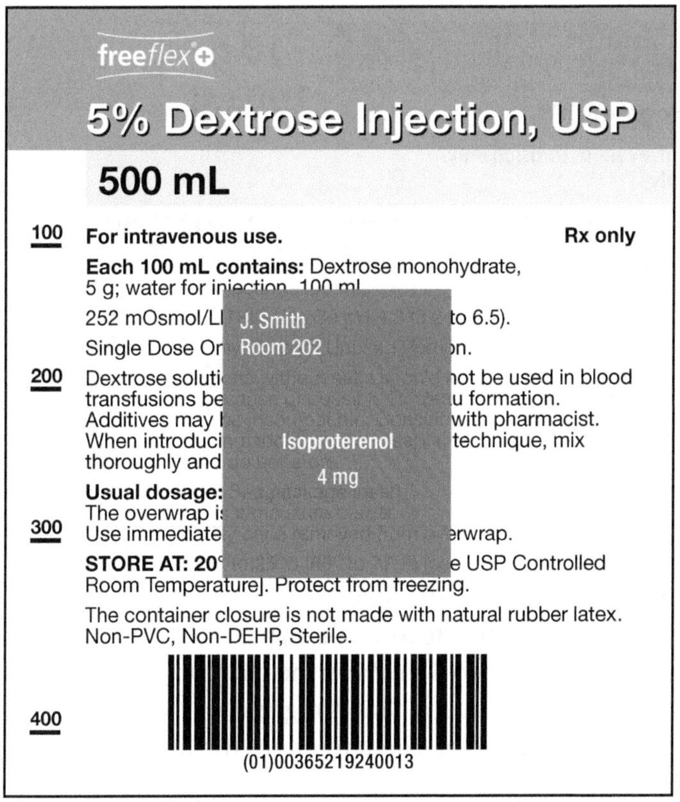

▲ Figure 21-19

Choice	Appropriate action	Inappropriate action
Calculate the mcg/min range at 3.2–12.7.		
Start the infusion at 25 mL/hr.		
Calculate the mg/hr range at 0.2–7.6.		
Determine kg weight to be 63.6 kg.		
Start the IV infusion at 127 mL/hr.		

2. A 56-year-old male client is ordered an IV Immune Globulin infusion for treatment of primary immune deficiency. The order is for 0.5 mg/kg/min, and if tolerated after an hour, increase to 0.8 mg/kg/min. The client weighs 64.3 kg. Utilize the label in Figure 21-20, and the client information, to choose the pertinent information as it relates to the calculation and administration of the IV medication. Select all that apply.

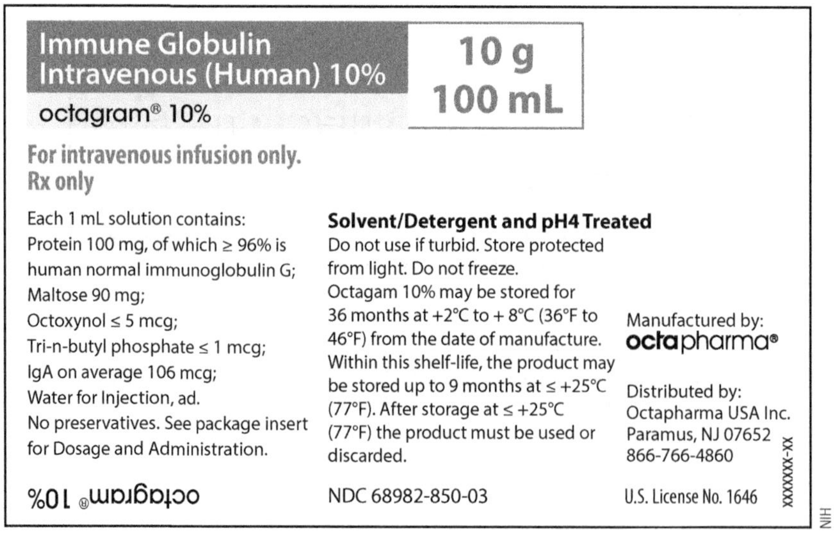

Immune Globulin
Intravenous (Human) 10%

10 g
100 mL

octagram® 10%

For intravenous infusion only.
Rx only

Each 1 mL solution contains:
Protein 100 mg, of which ≥ 96% is
human normal immunoglobulin G;
Maltose 90 mg;
Octoxynol ≤ 5 mcg;
Tri-n-butyl phosphate ≤ 1 mcg;
IgA on average 106 mcg;
Water for Injection, ad.
No preservatives. See package insert
for Dosage and Administration.

Solvent/Detergent and pH4 Treated
Do not use if turbid. Store protected
from light. Do not freeze.
Octagam 10% may be stored for
36 months at +2°C to + 8°C (36°F to
46°F) from the date of manufacture.
Within this shelf-life, the product may
be stored up to 9 months at ≤ +25°C
(77°F). After storage at ≤ +25°C
(77°F) the product must be used or
discarded.

Manufactured by:
octapharma®

Distributed by:
Octapharma USA Inc.
Paramus, NJ 07652
866-766-4860

octagram® 10%

NDC 68982-850-03

U.S. License No. 1646

▲ **Figure 21-20**

a. Calculate 32.2 mg/hr for the first dose.

b. Calculate the first flow rate to 19.3 mL/hr.

c. Increase the flow rate by 5 mL/hr if the client tolerates the first dose.

d. Calculate the second dose at 3,084 mg/hr.

e. Double the flow rate if the client tolerates the first dose.

Answers to Critical Thinking Questions

1.

Choice	Appropriate Action	Inappropriate Action
Calculate the mcg/min range at 3.2–12.7.		X
Start the infusion at 25 mL/hr.	X	
Calculate the mg/hr range at 0.2–7.6.	X	
Determine kg weight to be 63.6 kg.	X	
Start the IV infusion at 127 mL/hr.		X

Rationale:
The mcg/min range is not appropriate. Calculate the correct range at 3.2–127.2 mcg/min.
This is an appropriate answer. Start the infusion at 25 mL/hr. (Using 0.2 mg/hr as the desired)
The mg/hr range of 0.2–7.6 is appropriate.
The kg weight of 63.6 is appropriate.
The infusion flow rate is not appropriate. The initial flow rate is 25 mL/hr.

2. b, d (Rationale: a is incorrect—the first dose is 1,932 mg/hr; c is incorrect—the increase would be by 11.5 mL; e is incorrect—the answer is 30.8 mL/hr.)

Heparin and Insulin Drip Calculations

Heparin is a powerful anticoagulant drug that inhibits new blood clot formation or the extension of already-existing clots. Heparin dosages are expressed in USP units and may be given subcutaneously, mixed in IV solutions, or by IV push or bolus. Heparin that is mixed in IV solutions may come from the pharmaceutical companies already premixed in solutions, and these standard mixes of IV solutions are most frequently used for heparin drips. Frequent checks of a lab test known as an activated partial thromboplastin time or aPTT during heparin therapy is essential. Heparin dosages are ordered and titrated based on aPTT and/or on an individual's body weight in kg. Subcutaneous heparin injections are given deeply at a 45–90° angle, to discourage medication leakage from the injection site, and subsequent bruising. Heparin should never be given intramuscularly, as it can cause bleeding in the muscle and a resultant hematoma.

Recall from Chapter 14, that insulin is a hormone that is used to treat diabetes mellitus and lower blood sugar. Insulin may be given not only subcutaneously but may also be given intravenously to individuals who have rapidly changing needs for insulin to control their blood sugar. Intravenous administration may include IV push or bolus, as well as IV drips. When given intravenously, only clear insulin can be given. This is usually regular insulin. If administered as an IV drip, the solution is usually mixed by the pharmacy or the nurse administering the IV drip, using a vial of regular insulin of the concentration 100 units per mL. Insulin is usually added to NS solution for blood sugar control. The patient's blood glucose is monitored by the lab and/or bedside fingerstick blood sugars.

There is no essential difference in the calculations you have already practiced for IV medication drips and those for heparin or insulin drips. The calculations can be performed using any of the three methods of calculation. When given subcutaneously, heparin dosages are measured

Objectives

The learner will:

1. calculate the volume of heparin to add to an IV bag for heparin drips.

2. calculate mL/hr flow rates for heparin drips based on an order for units/hr.

3. calculate mL/hr flow rate for heparin drips based on an order for units/kg/hr.

4. calculate mL/hr flow rates for insulin drips based on an order for units/hr.

using a 0.5 or 1 mL TB syringe. Insulin given subcutaneously is only given in an insulin syringe calibrated in units. Remember, although heparin and insulin are ordered in units, only insulin is given in the specially designed insulin syringe calibrated in units. The insulin syringe should never be used to measure or administer any other medication.

In this chapter, we will review a variety of labels of heparin and insulin and perform calculations related to intravenous administration of heparin and insulin. Both medications will be ordered as units per hour if they are ordered as IV drips.

Clinical Relevance: Heparin and insulin are common medications used for subcutaneous injections, as well as IV bolus injections. They are given as IV drips and are titrated based on the patient's physiological response. These medications are both **high-alert medications,** and they have an increased risk of causing harm to the patient if not administered correctly. Heparin is an anticoagulant. Effectiveness is based on lab results and the patient's response. Insulin is given to lower the blood sugar and is also based on lab results or fingerstick blood glucose. In addition, the patient must be assessed for symptoms of hypoglycemia and hyperglycemia.

As the person caring for patients on heparin or insulin drips, you must have a knowledge of the medications and the expected results, as well as adverse reactions that might occur from overdosage or underdosage of these medications. Both medicated IV drips will be infused on an electronic infusion device. If there is any instance where an electronic infusion device is not available, these medicated drips would be infused by gravity with careful monitoring of the drops per minute and the patient's response. Microdrip tubing would most likely be the IV tubing of choice for infusion if an electronic pump is not available. Many facilities have a policy requiring double and triple checking of the doses of these medications, including setting up IV drips, to ensure that the chance of error is decreased significantly. Your policy may require a second health professional to be present when programming the infusion pump. All your math should be triple-checked; if you are using a calculator, triple-check your entries.

Heparin and Insulin Labels

Heparin vial dosage strengths are available in a wide variety of concentrations. There is an enormous difference between dosage strengths used for heparin flushes and dosage strengths used for treatment with heparin. Strengths for a heparin flush will be 10 units per mL or 100 units per mL. Heparin used to treat or prevent blood clots is supplied in higher concentrations—up to 40,000 units per mL. This is a significant difference in dosage strengths and may be a cause of medication error if the labels are not read very carefully. This is one of the reasons heparin is a high-alert drug and why it is policy at many clinical facilities to include double and triple checks for heparin therapy. Extreme caution with reading labels is necessary when preparing heparin flushes or heparin for treatment administration. Refer to Figure 22-1 for a label for heparin that would be a strength for flush only. Refer to Figure 22-2 for a label for a strength that would be used for treatment, not flush.

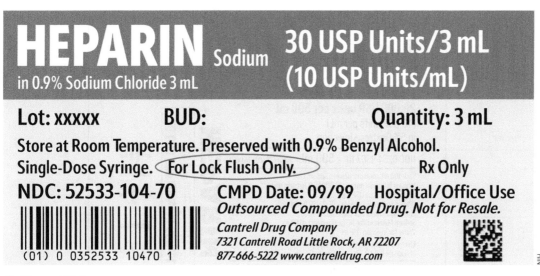

HEPARIN Sodium
in 0.9% Sodium Chloride 3 mL

30 USP Units/3 mL
(10 USP Units/mL)

Lot: xxxxx   BUD: Quantity: 3 mL

Store at Room Temperature. Preserved with 0.9% Benzyl Alcohol.
Single-Dose Syringe. For Lock Flush Only.   Rx Only

NDC: 52533-104-70   CMPD Date: 09/99   Hospital/Office Use
                           Outsourced Compounded Drug. Not for Resale.
                           Cantrell Drug Company
                           7321 Cantrell Road Little Rock, AR 72207
(01) 0 0352533 10470 1   877-666-5222 www.cantrelldrug.com

▲ Figure 22-1

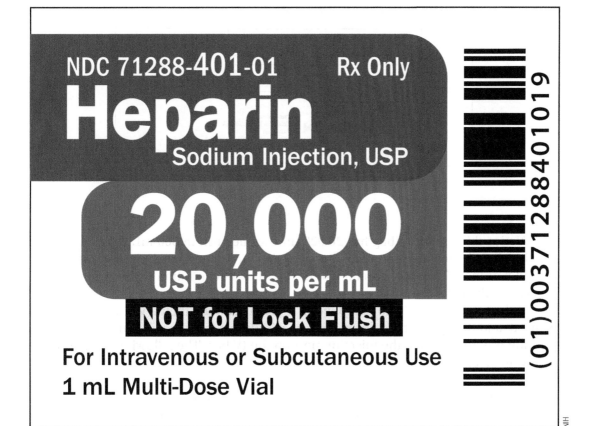

NDC 71288-401-01   Rx Only

Heparin
Sodium Injection, USP

20,000
USP units per mL
NOT for Lock Flush

For Intravenous or Subcutaneous Use
1 mL Multi-Dose Vial

(01)003712884010 19

▲ Figure 22-2

Notice the heparin with a strength of 10 units/mL is labeled with the warning that it is to be used for lock flush only. The heparin with a strength of 20,000 units/mL is clearly labeled **not** to be used for lock flush. The best safeguard on avoiding critical errors with heparin is to read the labels carefully.

Heparin used for IV drips can be supplied in a premixed bag, as shown in Figure 22-3.

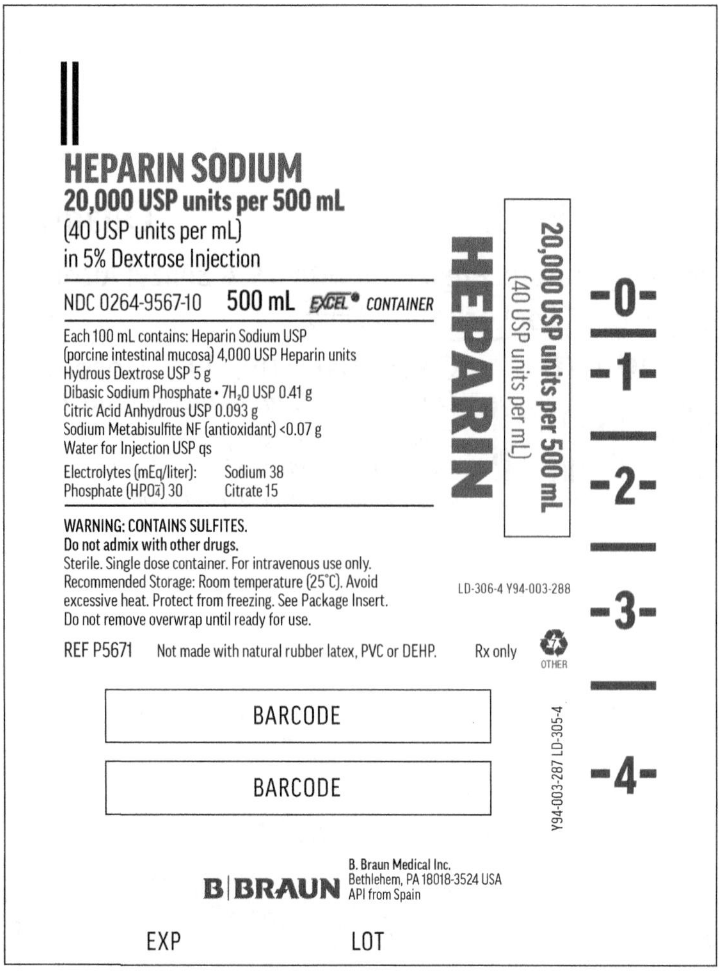

▲ Figure 22-3

Notice this premixed bag has 20,000 units of heparin in 500 mL D$_5$W. The bag is clearly labeled showing it contains heparin. Again, it is extremely important to read the label of the IV bag very carefully to ensure the concentration is the concentration ordered by the physician.

If the heparin drip is not supplied in a premixed bag, then a vial of heparin will be used, and the appropriate dosage will be withdrawn from the vial and added to the solution ordered through the injection port on the IV bag. The following is an example of how to mix a bag yourself.

Example 1 ■   The order is for 10,000 units of heparin in 250 mL D5W. How much heparin would be required from the vial shown in Figure 22-4 to mix this bag of heparin?

Use your preferred calculation method to determine the volume of heparin required from this vial to mix your IV bag. In this example, we will use the formula method. The desired will be the physician order of 10,000 units of heparin. The have and quantity will come from the vial and will be 5,000 units per mL.

$$\frac{10,000 \text{ units} \times 1 \text{ mL}}{5,000 \text{ units}} = 2 \text{ mL}$$

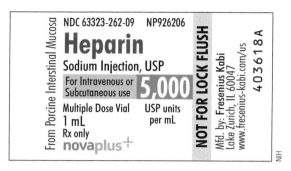

▲ **Figure 22-4**

Using the method of your choice, you should have calculated that you would need 2 mL of this strength of heparin to add to the 250 mL bag of D₅W. Depending on the total volume of heparin in the vial, you may need to use more than one vial. After adding this heparin to the IV bag, you must clearly label the IV bag with the amount of heparin added (10,000 units), the date and time, the patient's name and room number, and your initials as the person who mixed the bag.

Insulin drips will be mixed the same way. Regular insulin will be used to mix insulin drips and the IV solution will typically be NS. There is one standard concentration of regular insulin—100 units per mL. As a word of caution, there is also a highly concentrated strength of insulin that should not be used to mix an insulin drip. Insulin with a concentration of 500 units per mL is extremely concentrated and is rarely used. Refer to the labels in Figures 22-5 and 22-6.

The U-100 label in Figure 22-5 indicates the medication should be used with a U-100 syringe only and is for subcutaneous or IV use. It has 100 units per mL. The U-500 label in Figure 22-6 clearly indicates a warning that it is highly concentrated and should only be used with a U-500 syringe. It also indicates on the label that it is

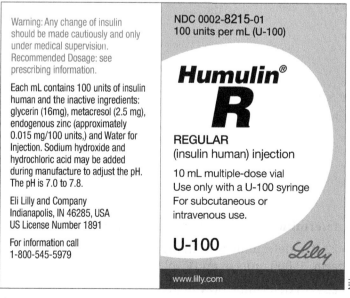

▲ **Figure 22-5**

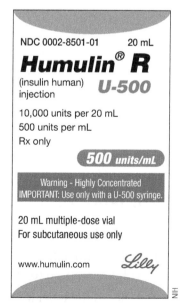

▲ **Figure 22-6**

for subcutaneous use only. The information on these labels must be read carefully. Incorrect selection of insulin can result in death; consequently, most facilities do not stock U-500 insulin on the nursing units. The following is an example of mixing an insulin IV drip.

Example 2 ■   The order is for 50 units regular insulin in 250 mL of NS. You obtain a vial of regular insulin U-100 and a U-100 insulin syringe and withdraw 50 units of insulin from the vial. This insulin will be injected into the 250 mL bag of NS, and a label will be placed on the bag indicating that regular insulin (50 units) was added to the bag of IV solution. Refer to Figure 22-7 for the IV bag with a label.

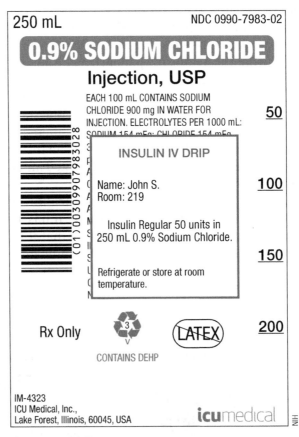

▲ **Figure 22-7**

Problems 22.1

Utilize the labels provided to determine how to prepare the solutions indicated.

1. Refer to the label in Figure 22-8 to determine how many mL will be required to add heparin 20,000 units to an IV solution.   _____

2. Refer to the label in Figure 22-9 to determine how many mL will be required to add heparin 20,000 units to an IV solution.   _____

3. Refer to the label in Figure 22-10 to determine how many mL
   of heparin will be required to add 25,000 units to an IV solution.   _____

4. Refer to the label in Figure 22-11 to determine how many mL
   will be required to add heparin 10,000 units to an IV solution.   _____

5. The physician has ordered 40 units of regular insulin to be
   added to a 250 mL IV bag. Refer to the label in Figure 22-12
   to determine how many units will be withdrawn from the vial.   _____

6. What syringe will be used in question 5? Be specific.   _____

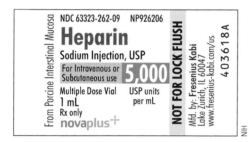

▲ **Figure 22-8**

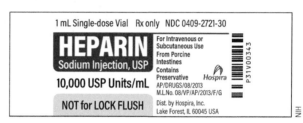

▲ **Figure 22-9**

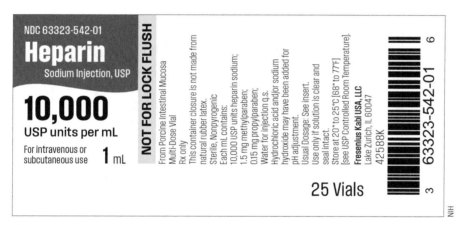

▲ **Figure 22-10**

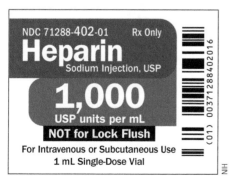

▲ **Figure 22-11**

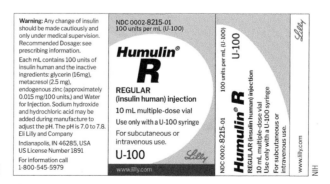

▲ **Figure 22-12**

Answers **1.** 4 mL **2.** 2 mL **3.** 2.5 mL **4.** 10 mL **5.** 40 units **6.** Insulin syringe

Heparin Drips

Intravenous heparin drips are most frequently ordered in units/hr to be administered. For example, 1,000 units/hr is ordered to infuse using an electronic infusion device. In order to place this drip on an electronic infusion device, the units/hr would have to be converted to mL/hr. Although an electronic infusion device will be the preferred method of infusion, there may be times when an electronic device is not available. In that case, microdrip tubing should be used. Recall that the mL/hr flow rate will be identical to the gtt/min for a gravity flow using a microdrip tubing. The calculations will be performed as they were in Chapter 21. The following are examples of calculations for heparin drips using the three methods of calculation.

Example 1 ▪   The order is to infuse 1,000 units per hour from the solution shown in Figure 22-13. You will infuse this on an electronic infusion device that can be programmed to the tenth.

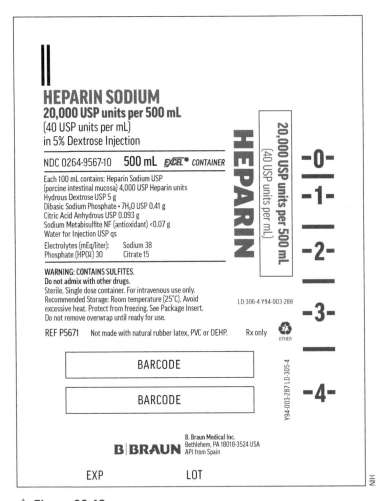

▲ **Figure 22-13**

Method 1: Ratio and Proportion

$$\frac{20{,}000 \text{ units}}{500 \text{ mL}} = \frac{1{,}000 \text{ units}}{x \text{ mL}} \quad or \quad 20{,}000 \text{ units} : 500 \text{ mL} = 1{,}000 \text{ units} : x \text{ mL}$$

$$20{,}000x = 500 \times 1{,}000 \qquad\qquad 20{,}000x = 500 \times 1{,}000$$

$$x = 25 \text{ mL/hr} \qquad\qquad\qquad x = 25 \text{ mL/hr}$$

Method 2: Dimensional Analysis

$$\frac{mL}{hr} = \frac{500\ mL}{20{,}000\ \cancel{units}} \times \frac{1{,}000\ \cancel{units}}{1\ hr}$$

$$\frac{mL}{hr} = \frac{500{,}000}{20{,}000} = 25\ mL/hr$$

Method 3: Formula Method

$$\frac{1{,}000\ \cancel{units}/hr\ (D) \times 500\ mL\ (Q)}{20{,}000\ \cancel{units}\ (H)} = x\ mL/hr$$

$$\frac{500{,}000}{20{,}000} = 25\ mL/hr$$

The flow rate to infuse 1,000 units/hr from a solution of 20,000 units in 500 mL is 25 mL/hr.

Example 2 ■   The order is to infuse heparin 1,100 units/hr from a solution of 60,000 units in 1 L of D_5W. You will infuse this on an electronic infusion device that can be programmed to the tenth. We will calculate the flow rate using the three methods of calculation.

Method 1: Ratio and Proportion

$$\frac{60{,}000\ units}{1{,}000\ mL} = \frac{1{,}100\ units}{x\ mL} \quad or \quad 60{,}000\ units : 1{,}000\ mL = 1{,}100\ units : x\ mL$$

$$60{,}000x = 1{,}000 \times 1{,}100 \qquad\qquad 60{,}000x = 1{,}000 \times 1{,}100$$

$$x = 18.33 = 18.3\ mL/hr \qquad\qquad x = 18.33 = 18.3\ mL/hr$$

Method 2: Dimensional Analysis

$$\frac{mL}{hr} = \frac{1{,}000\ mL}{60{,}000\ \cancel{units}} \times \frac{1{,}100\ \cancel{units}}{1\ hr}$$

$$\frac{mL}{hr} = \frac{1{,}100{,}000}{60{,}000} = 18.33 = 18.3\ mL/hr$$

Method 3: Formula Method

$$\frac{1{,}100\ \cancel{units}/hr\ (D) \times 1{,}000\ mL\ (Q)}{60{,}000\ \cancel{units}\ (H)} = x\ mL/hr$$

$$\frac{1{,}100{,}000}{60{,}000} = 18.33 = 18.3\ mL/hr$$

The flow rate to infuse 1,100 units/hr from a solution of 60,000 units in 1 L is 18.3 mL/hr.

Sometimes heparin drips are ordered on a protocol and the dosage is based on weight. The heparin protocols may differ from facility to facility. These protocols may order a heparin bolus to be given IV push, followed by a heparin drip ordered in units per hour. The protocol may also include titration of the heparin drip based on results of the lab test for aPTT. The protocol will also be specific regarding rounding of the heparin doses.

The following is an example of weight-based dosage of heparin for a bolus and for the initiation of a drip.

Example 3 ■   A bolus of 70 units/kg of heparin IV push is ordered for an adult weighing 60 kg. This is to be followed by an infusion of 15 units/kg/hr. The solution is premixed and has a concentration of 25,000 units of heparin in 500 mL D₅W. Calculate the bolus, using the heparin in the label in Figure 22-14. Then, calculate the infusion rate in mL/hr. It will be infused on an electronic infusion pump that can be programmed to the tenth.

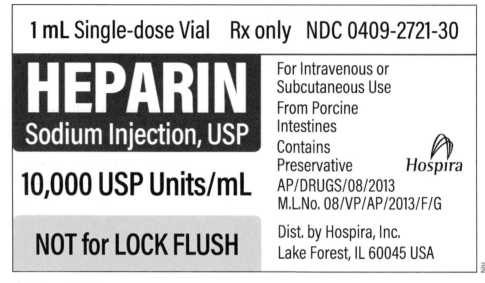

1 mL Single-dose Vial   Rx only   NDC 0409-2721-30

HEPARIN
Sodium Injection, USP

10,000 USP Units/mL

NOT for LOCK FLUSH

For Intravenous or Subcutaneous Use
From Porcine Intestines
Contains Preservative
Hospira
AP/DRUGS/08/2013
M.L.No. 08/VP/AP/2013/F/G

Dist. by Hospira, Inc.
Lake Forest, IL 60045 USA

▲ **Figure 22-14**

First, calculate the bolus. The dose will be 70 units/kg × 60 kg. The dose for the IV push bolus will be 4,200 units. Using the supply in the label in Figure 22-14, we calculate that we will administer 0.42 mL IV push. We could prepare this in a 0.5 mL or 1 mL tuberculin syringe.

Next, calculate the rate of infusion. For the rate of infusion, we will need the dose: 15 units/kg/hr. For this patient, who weighs 60 kg, the dose will be 900 units/hr. Our supply will be the premixed IV bag, which has a concentration of 25,000 units in 500 mL.

Then, calculate the flow rate using the three methods of calculation.

Method 1: Ratio and Proportion

$$\frac{25,000 \text{ units}}{500 \text{ mL}} = \frac{900 \text{ units}}{x \text{ mL}} \quad or \quad 25,000 \text{ units} : 500 \text{ mL} = 900 \text{ units} : x \text{ mL}$$

$$25,000x = 500 \times 900 \qquad\qquad 25,000x = 500 \times 900$$

$$x = 18 \text{ mL/hr} \qquad\qquad\qquad x = 18 \text{ mL/hr}$$

Method 2: Dimensional Analysis

$$\frac{\text{mL}}{\text{hr}} = \frac{500 \text{ mL}}{25,000 \text{ units}} \times \frac{900 \text{ units}}{1 \text{ hr}}$$

$$\frac{\text{mL}}{\text{hr}} = \frac{450,000}{25,000} = 18 \text{ mL/hr}$$

Method 3: Formula Method

$$\frac{900 \text{ units/hr (D)} \times 500 \text{ mL (Q)}}{25{,}000 \text{ units (H)}} = x \text{ mL/hr}$$

$$\frac{450{,}000}{25{,}000} = 18 \text{ mL/hr}$$

For this adult weighing 60 kg, we will administer an IV bolus of 0.42 mL of heparin IV push. We will follow the bolus with an infusion of heparin at a rate of 18 mL/hr using a premixed IV of 25,000 units of heparin in 500 mL D_5W. At this rate, the patient will receive 900 units per hour.

Problems 22.2

Calculate bolus doses and mL/hr flow rates as indicated using the calculation method you prefer. Use standard rounding for bolus calculations; less than 1, round to the hundredth; greater than 1, round to the tenth. Round all flow rates to the tenth.

1. The order is to infuse 1,000 units heparin per hour. Refer to Figure 22-15 for the available solution strength. _____

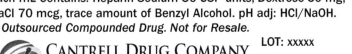

HEPARIN Sodium
25,000 USP Units

Added to 5% Dextrose 500 mL Bag

(50 USP units/mL) *Volume & Concentration Exclude Manufacturer Overfill
Store at Room Temperature. Single-Dose Bag.
Hospital/Office Use Only. Injection Solution For IV Use.

HIGH
ALERT

NDC: 52533-106-32

D5

(01) 0 0352533 10632 3

Rx Only

Each mL Contains: Heparin Sodium 50 USP units, Dextrose 50 mg, NaCl 70 mcg, trace amount of Benzyl Alcohol. pH adj: HCl/NaOH.
Outsourced Compounded Drug. Not for Resale.

00003

CANTRELL DRUG COMPANY
7321 Cantrell Road Little Rock, AR 72207
(877) 666-5222 www.cantrelldrug.com

LOT: xxxxx
BUD:
CMPD Date: 03/13

▲ **Figure 22-15**

2. A bolus of heparin 60 units/kg IV push has been ordered for a client weighing 72 kg. At the completion of the bolus, the client is ordered a heparin IV infusion at 18 units/kg/hr. The solution is premixed with a concentration of 40,000 units in 1,000 mL D$_5$W.

  A. Calculate the bolus dose to administer utilizing the vial in Figure 22-16. _____

  B. Calculate the mL/hr for the heparin infusion. _____

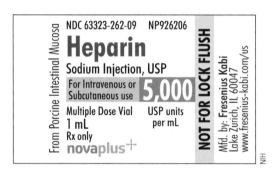

▲ Figure 22-16

3. The order is to infuse IV heparin at 350 units per hour. Refer to Figure 22-17 for the solution strength. _____

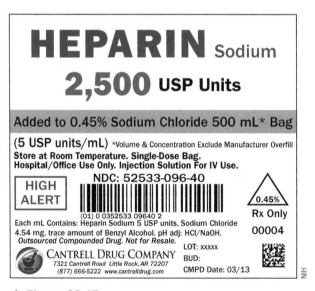

▲ Figure 22-17

4. An adult has orders for IV heparin infusion at a rate of 1,000 units per hour IV. You must administer a bolus of heparin 40 units per kg prior to the infusion. The patient weighs 74 kg.

  A. Refer to Figure 22-18 for the heparin vial to calculate the bolus. _____

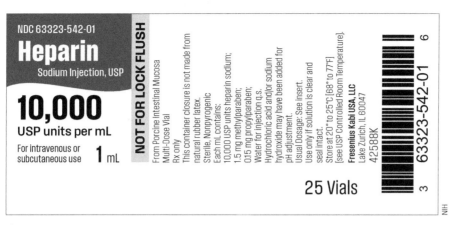

▲ **Figure 22-18**

B. Refer to Figure 22-19 to calculate the heparin infusion flow rate. _____

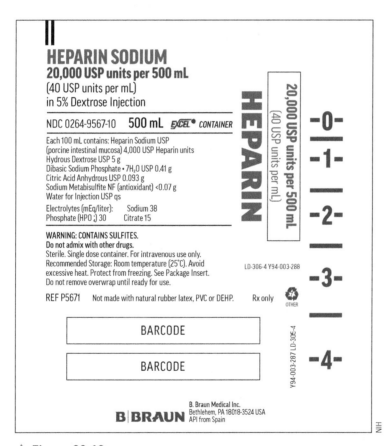

▲ **Figure 22-19**

5. Administer 1,500 units per hour of heparin from an available
    prepared IV bag. See Figure 22-20 for the solution strength. _____

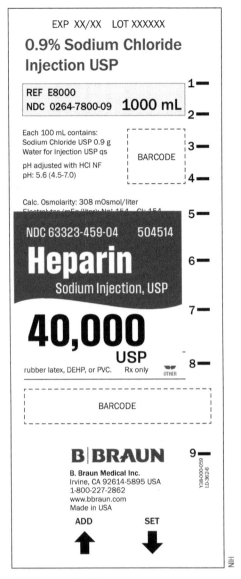

▲ **Figure 22-20**

6. Determine the heparin IV bolus for an ordered dose of 45 units/kg for a patient weighting 62 kg. Refer to Figure 22-21 to calculate the dose to be administered.

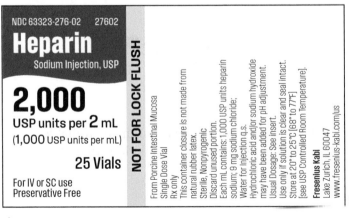

▲ **Figure 22-21**

7. A patient is ordered a heparin infusion of 34 units/kg/hr. The patient weighs 63 kg. Refer to Figure 22-22 for the solution strength to determine the mL/hr for the heparin infusion.   _____

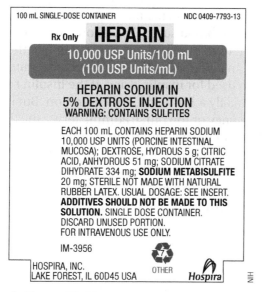

▲ **Figure 22-22**

8. The physician has ordered a patient a heparin bolus of 45 units/kg prior to a heparin infusion of 22 units/kg/hr. The patient weighs 90 kg.

   A. Utilizing a heparin vial of 2,500 units/mL, calculate the mL to be administered for the heparin IV push bolus.   _____

   B. Refer to Figure 22-23 for the solution strength to calculate the mL/hr for the heparin infusion.   _____

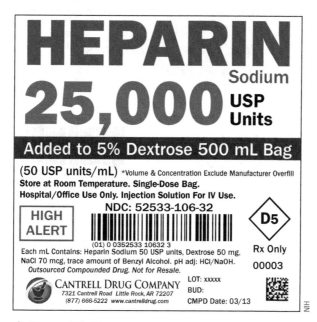

▲ **Figure 22-23**

Answers **1.** 20 mL/hr **2. A.** 0.86 mL; **B.** 32.4 mL/hr **3.** 70 mL/hr **4. A.** 0.3 mL; **B.** 25 mL/hr **5.** 37.5 mL/hr **6.** 2.8 mL **7.** 21.4 mL/hr **8. A.** 1.6 mL; **B.** 39.6 mL/hr

Insulin Drips

Intravenous insulin drips are used primarily in critical care settings where glucose levels may fluctuate significantly. Regular insulin, which has a quick onset of action and a short duration, is the type of insulin used in insulin drips. When insulin drips are administered, they are titrated according to blood sugar. This allows for better control of blood sugar in critical care settings, but it remains a high alert situation and the drip must be monitored carefully and frequently. Insulin drips are also ordered as units per hour. Regular U-100 insulin is the only insulin used for insulin drips. If the insulin infusion is a commercially prepared infusion, it is usually a 1 unit/mL concentration. But many times the IV insulin drip is mixed by the pharmacy or the nurse administering the drip. Therefore, it will be a two-step process: addition of the insulin to the IV fluid and calculation of the rate based on the ordered units/hr. Recall from Chapter 14, insulin is ordered in units, supplied in units, and measured in units; so unlike heparin, we do not need to calculate mL of insulin to add to the IV bag. We will just need to prepare the ordered amount of insulin in units in a U-100 insulin syringe and inject it into the IV bag. Usually, it is mixed in NS.

Example 1 ■   Prepare an insulin drip of 50 units regular insulin in 100 mL NS. Administer the insulin drip at 6 units/hr. As the nurse preparing this insulin drip, you will add 50 units of regular insulin to the IV bag of 100 mL NS. You will need to label this bag. Refer to Figure 22-24.

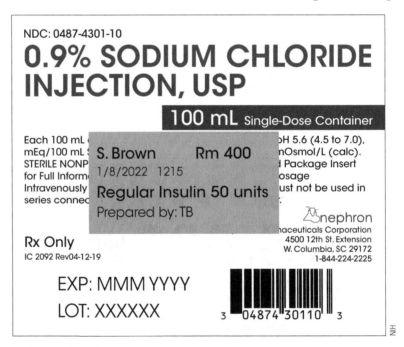

▲ **Figure 22-24**

Calculate the infusion rate for the order of 6 units/hr using the three methods of calculation.

Method 1: Ratio and Proportion

$$\frac{50 \text{ units}}{100 \text{ mL}} = \frac{6 \text{ units}}{x \text{ mL}} \quad or \quad 50 \text{ units} : 100 \text{ mL} = 6 \text{ units} : x \text{ mL}$$

$$50x = 600 \qquad\qquad 50x = 600$$

$$x = 12 \text{ mL/hr} \qquad\qquad x = 12 \text{ mL/hr}$$

Method 2: Dimensional Analysis

$$\frac{mL}{hr} = \frac{100 \text{ mL}}{50 \text{ units}} \times \frac{6 \text{ units}}{1 \text{ hr}}$$

$$\frac{mL}{hr} = \frac{600}{50} = 12 \text{ mL/hr}$$

Method 3: Formula Method

$$\frac{6 \text{ units/hr (D)} \times 100 \text{ mL (Q)}}{50 \text{ units (H)}} = x \text{ mL/hr}$$

$$\frac{600}{50} = 12 \text{ mL/hr}$$

This insulin drip will infuse at 12 mL/hr and will deliver 6 units per hour.

Problems 22.3

Use your calculation method of choice to determine the mL/hr of the following insulin IV drips. Round all flow rates to the tenth.

1. A patient has been ordered an IV infusion of regular insulin at 5 units/hr. Refer to Figure 22-25 for the solution strength. _____

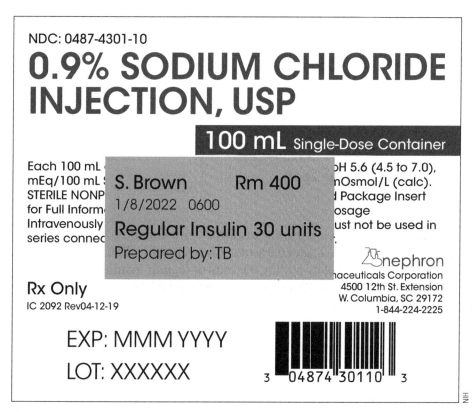

NDC: 0487-4301-10

0.9% SODIUM CHLORIDE INJECTION, USP

100 mL Single-Dose Container

Each 100 mL ... pH 5.6 (4.5 to 7.0),
mEq/100 mL ... nOsmol/L (calc).
STERILE NONP... Package Insert
for Full Inform... osage
Intravenously... ust not be used in
series connec...

S. Brown   Rm 400
1/8/2022 0600
Regular Insulin 30 units
Prepared by: TB

nephron
aceuticals Corporation
4500 12th St. Extension
W. Columbia, SC 29172
1-844-224-2225

Rx Only
IC 2092 Rev04-12-19

EXP: MMM YYYY
LOT: XXXXXX

3 04874 30110 3

▲ **Figure 22-25**

2. An IV infusion of regular insulin has been ordered at 12 units/hr. The order includes instructions to add 40 units of regular insulin to a 250 mL IV bag. Calculate the mL/hr of the insulin infusion. _____

3. You will apply a label to the IV bag in question 2. What will you include on this label? _____

4. A patient has a blood sugar of 500 and has been ordered an insulin infusion of 15 units/hr. Refer to Figure 22-26 for the solution strength. _____

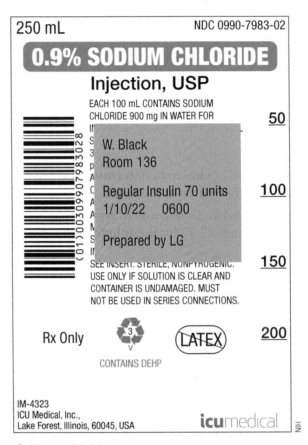

▲ Figure 22-26

5. A client has been ordered a regular insulin IV infusion to be prepared in a 250 mL IV bag of 0.9% of sodium chloride. You are to prepare the IV bag by adding 80 units of regular insulin. Refer to Figures 22-27 and 22-28 to choose which vial you will use to withdraw the 80 units. _____

A.

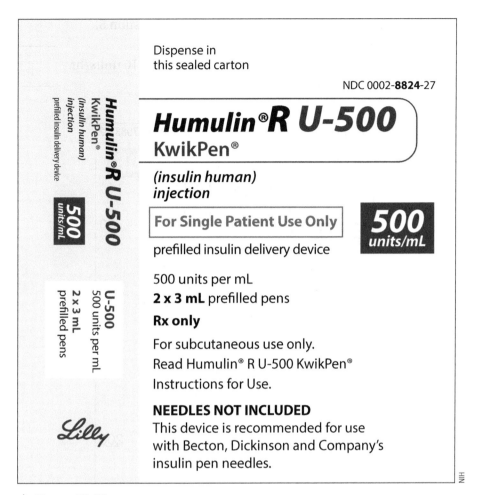

▲ **Figure 22-27**

B.

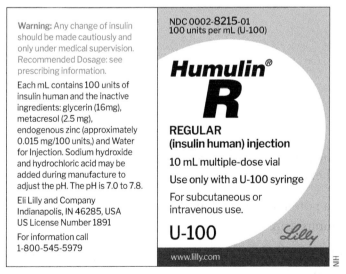

▲ **Figure 22-28**

6. After you prepare the IV regular insulin infusion in question 5, administer 6 units/hr. Calculate the mL/hr.   _____

7. A physician orders a client a regular insulin infusion at 10 units/hr. Refer to Figure 22-29. Calculate the mL/hr.   _____

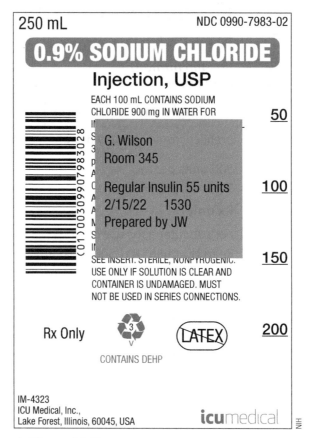

250 mL   NDC 0990-7983-02

0.9% SODIUM CHLORIDE

Injection, USP

EACH 100 mL CONTAINS SODIUM CHLORIDE 900 mg IN WATER FOR

50

G. Wilson
Room 345

Regular Insulin 55 units   100
2/15/22   1530
Prepared by JW

SEE INSERT. STERILE, NONPYROGENIC.   150
USE ONLY IF SOLUTION IS CLEAR AND
CONTAINER IS UNDAMAGED. MUST
NOT BE USED IN SERIES CONNECTIONS.

Rx Only   200

CONTAINS DEHP

IM-4323
ICU Medical, Inc.,
Lake Forest, Illinois, 60045, USA   icumedical

▲ **Figure 22-29**

Answers **1.** 16.7 mL/hr **2.** 75 mL/hr **3.** patient name, room number, medication and dose (units), date & time, your initials **4.** 53.6 mL/hr **5.** B, U-100 **6.** 18.8 mL/hr **7.** 45.5 mL/hr

Summary

This concludes the chapter on IV heparin and insulin administration. The important points to remember are:

- Heparin is a potent anticoagulant that may be added to IV solutions and infused as a continuous drip.

- Heparin therapy requires a frequent check of coagulation times to monitor and adjust dosage.

- Subcutaneous heparin injections are given deeply at a 45–90˚ angle, to discourage medication leakage from the injection site and subsequent bruising.

- IV heparin drip dosages may be ordered per kg of body weight.

- Regular insulin may be added to IV fluids, most commonly NS, and infused as a continuous drip with careful monitoring of blood sugar.

- Heparin and insulin are measured in USP units.

- IV heparin and insulin drips are usually ordered by units/hr to infuse.

- An electronic infusion device or microdrip tubing may be used for heparin and insulin infusion.

- Commercially prepared IV heparin solutions are available in several strengths.

- Additional IV heparin solution strengths may require the preparation of heparin drips from available vial strengths.

- Insulin drips are usually prepared by the pharmacy or the nurse administering the IV and use U-100 regular insulin for preparation.

- When IV drips are prepared by the nurse or the pharmacy, they must be labeled with the name and amount of medication (units for heparin and insulin) placed in the IV solution, the date and time, patient name and room number, and initials of the person preparing the drip.

Summary Self-Test

Calculate bolus doses and mL/hr flow rates as indicated using the calculation method you prefer. Use standard rounding for bolus calculations; less than 1, round to the hundredth; greater than 1, round to the tenth. Round all flow rates to the tenth.

1. An adult patient is to receive IV heparin at 1,200 units/hr. Prior to the infusion, the patient is to receive a 16 unit/kg IV push heparin bolus. The patient's weight is 92 kg. Calculate the bolus dose utilizing the label in Figure 22-30.   _____

   Refer to Figure 22-31 for the solution strength. Calculate the heparin infusion mL/hr.   _____

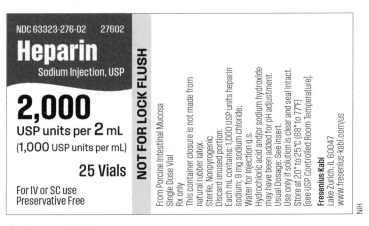

▲ **Figure 22-30**

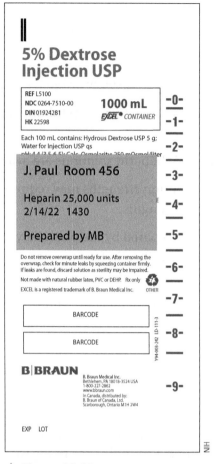

▲ Figure 22-31

2. A solution of 35,000 units heparin in 1 L D₅W is to infuse via an IV infusion pump at 15 units/kg/hr. The patient weighs 75 kg.

3. The order is for 325 units heparin per hour. Refer to Figure 22-32 for the solution strength.

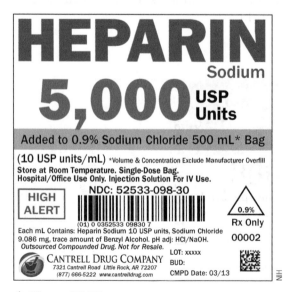

▲ Figure 22-32

4. A patient is to receive 18 units/kg/hr of IV heparin. The solution strength is 15,000 units in 500 mL D$_5$W. The patient weighs 84 kg. _____

5. A solution of 10,000 units heparin in 500 mL D$_5$W is ordered to infuse at 1,100 units/hr. The patient is to receive a bolus of 35 units/kg of heparin prior to the infusion. The patient weighs 74 kg. Calculate the bolus dose using the label in Figure 22-33. _____

Calculate the flow rate for the heparin infusion. _____

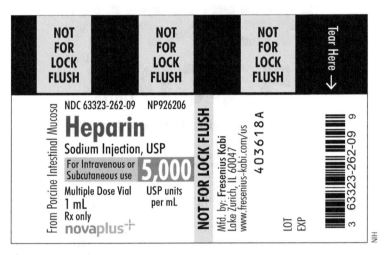

▲ **Figure 22-33**

6. An IV of 1,000 mL D$_5$W with 40,000 units heparin is to infuse at 1,200 units/hr via a pump. _____

7. Refer to Figure 22-34 to infuse a heparin drip at 1,600 units/hr. _____

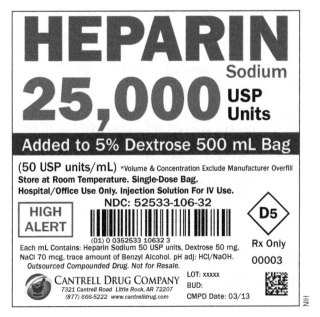

▲ **Figure 22-34**

8. A patient is ordered a heparin IV infusion at 16 units/kg/hr. The solution supply is 500 mL D_5W with 30,000 units of heparin. The patient weighs 88 kg.   _____

9. The order is to infuse 1 L D_5W with 45,000 units of heparin at 1,875 units/hr.   _____

10. A client is ordered 9 units/kg/hr of heparin IV. The client weighs 63 kg. Refer to Figure 22-35 for the supply solution to calculate the flow rate.   _____

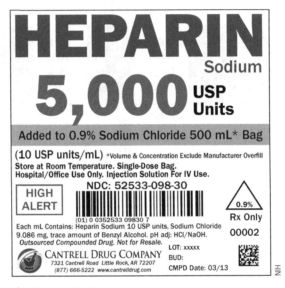

▲ **Figure 22-35**

11. A patient is ordered a regular insulin drip infusion at 6 units per hr. Refer to the supply solution in Figure 22-36 to calculate the flow rate.   _____

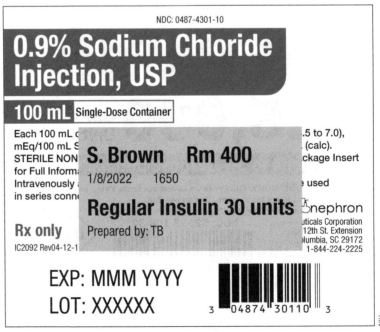

▲ **Figure 22-36**

12. You are preparing an IV insulin infusion, and you discover the following insulin label in the medication room on the clinical unit. Refer to Figure 22-37 and the chapter information. List two reasons why this medication will not be used during this preparation.

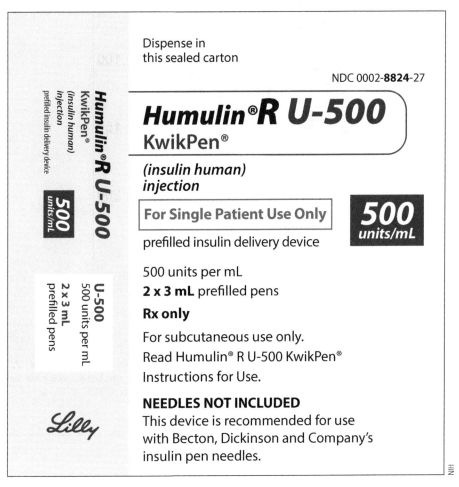

Dispense in
this sealed carton

NDC 0002-**8824**-27

Humulin®*R U-500*
KwikPen®

(insulin human)
injection

For Single Patient Use Only

500
units/mL

prefilled insulin delivery device

500 units per mL

2 x 3 mL prefilled pens

Rx only

For subcutaneous use only.
Read Humulin® R U-500 KwikPen®
Instructions for Use.

NEEDLES NOT INCLUDED
This device is recommended for use
with Becton, Dickinson and Company's
insulin pen needles.

Lilly

▲ **Figure 22-37**

13. A physician has ordered a client 4 units per hour of IV regular insulin infusion. You are to prepare the IV with 75 units of insulin in a 250 mL IV sodium chloride bag. Calculate the flow rate.

14. A patient is to receive 125 units of regular insulin in a 250 mL IV bag of 0.9% sodium chloride. The order is for 12 units per hour.

15. Refer to Figure 22-38 to determine the flow rate for an insulin drip ordered to infuse at 8 units/hr.

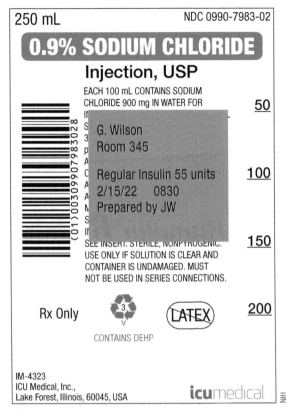

▲ Figure 22-38

Critical Thinking Questions

1. Mr. Kline, a 60-year-old male client, has been admitted with a glucose level of 450 mg/dL. The client weighs 120 kg and is scheduled to receive an insulin drip to infuse at 9 units/hr. The IV bag will be prepared by the nurse. The order is to add 35 units to a 250 mL sodium chloride IV bag. Choose the following relevant data as it relates to the preparation and administration of this IV drip. Select all that apply.

   a. Add regular insulin to the IV bag with a 1 mL syringe.
   b. Calculate the flow rate at 7.1 mL/hr.
   c. Use a 50-unit insulin syringe to prepare the IV bag.
   d. Calculate the flow rate at 64.3 mL/hr.
   e. Choose a D_5 NS IV bag for preparation.

2. A 72-year-old female client has been admitted to the hospital with a pulmonary embolus. The physician has ordered a 40 unit/kg IV push heparin bolus, followed by an IV heparin drip to infuse according to the client's weight at 25 units/kg/hr. The client's weight is 230 lb. Refer to Figure 22-39 to calculate the bolus. Refer to Figure 22-40 for the premixed heparin IV bag. Select all that apply.

a. Prepare the bolus in a 3 mL syringe.

b. Administer a 0.42 mL bolus.

c. Calculate the flow rate at 25 mL/hr.

d. Administer a 4.2-unit bolus.

e. Calculate the flow rate at 26.1 mL/hr.

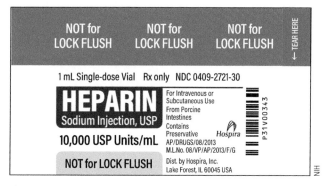

▲ **Figure 22-39**

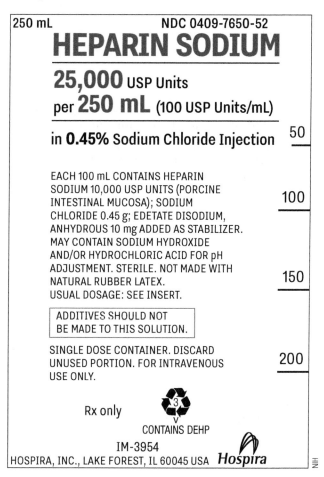

▲ **Figure 22-40**

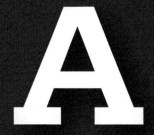

Appendix

A

Equivalents

Agencies such as The Joint Commission, Institute for Safe Medication Practices (ISMP), and the Food and Drug Administration (FDA) recommend using the metric system in prescribing and labeling medications. However, the metric system is not uniformly used in either prescribing or labeling. It is useful to know various equivalents in order to convert orders or supplies of medications.

The apothecary system is relatively inaccurate and can lead to errors based on the abbreviations and notation used. The metric system has generally replaced the apothecary system, which is basically obsolete. However, you may still see references to various measures in the apothecary system on equipment or some resources. The apothecary system, when used for prescribing and dispensing medications, includes measures for weight and volume. The most commonly used measure of weight in the apothecary system is the grain (gr). Commonly used measurements of volume in the apothecary system include measurements such as minim (min), drams (dr), and ounces (oz).

Metric measures are more commonly used in medication administration, but household measures are still seen, especially when communicating with clients. Many clients recognize household measures such as teaspoon and tablespoon more easily than metric measures. The ounce and dram measures still appear on some disposable medication cups, so it is very important to read your equipment very carefully to avoid errors in measurement.

Please see the following chart for common equivalents. All three systems (metric, apothecary, and household) are represented, but the most common in use currently is the metric system. Conversions related to the apothecary system are provided for information purposes only.

EQUIVALENTS USED FOR CONVERSIONS			
Volume		**Weight**	
1 liter	= 1,000 milliliters	1 kilogram	= 1,000 grams
1 ounce	= 30 milliliters	1 gram	= 1,000 milligrams
1 teaspoon	= 5 milliliters	1 milligram	= 1,000 micrograms
1 tablespoon	= 15 milliliters	1 kilogram	= 2.2 pounds
1 cup	= 8 ounces	1 pound	= 16 ounces
1 cup	= 240 milliliters	1 grain	= 60 milligrams (for information only)
1 dram	= 4 milliliters (for information only)	½ grain	= 30 milligrams (for information only)
		¼ grain	= 15 milligrams (for information only)

Appendix B

ISMP List of Error-Prone Abbreviations, Symbols, and Dose Designations

The abbreviations, symbols, and dose designations in the **Table** below were reported to ISMP through the ISMP National Medication Errors Reporting Program (ISMP MERP) and have been misinterpreted and involved in harmful or potentially harmful medication errors. These abbreviations, symbols, and dose designations should **NEVER** be used when communicating medical information verbally, electronically, and/or in handwritten applications. This includes internal communications; verbal, handwritten, or electronic prescriptions; handwritten and computer-generated medication labels; drug storage bin labels; medication administration records; and screens associated with pharmacy and prescriber computer order entry systems, automated dispensing cabinets, smart infusion pumps, and other medication-related technologies.

In the **Table**, error-prone abbreviations, symbols, and dose designations that are included on The Joint Commission's "**Do Not Use**" list (Information Management standard IM.02.02.01) are identified with a double asterisk (******) and must be included on an organization's "**Do Not Use**" list. Error-prone abbreviations, symbols, and dose designations that are relevant mostly in handwritten communications of medication information are highlighted with a dagger (†).

Table. Error-Prone Abbreviations, Symbols, and Dose Designations			
Error-Prone Abbreviations, Symbols, and Dose Designations	Intended Meaning	Misinterpretation	Best Practice
Abbreviations for Doses/Measurement Units			
cc	Cubic centimeters	Mistaken as u (units)	Use mL
IU**	International unit(s)	Mistaken as IV (intravenous) or the number 10	Use unit(s) (International units can be expressed as units alone.)
l **ml**	Liter Milliliter	Lowercase letter l mistaken as the number 1	Use L (UPPERCASE) for liter Use mL (lowercase m, UPPERCASE L) for milliliter
MM or M **M or K**	Million Thousand	Mistaken as thousand Mistaken as million M has been used to abbreviate both million and thousand (M is the Roman numeral for thousand)	Use million Use thousand
Ng or ng	Nanogram	Mistaken as mg Mistaken as nasogastric	Use nanogram or nanog
U or u**	Unit(s)	Mistaken as zero or the number 4, causing a 10-fold overdose or greater (e.g., 4U seen as 40 or 4u seen as 44) Mistaken as cc, leading to administering volume instead of units (e.g., 4u seen as 4cc)	Use unit(s)
μg	Microgram	Mistaken as mg	Use mcg
Abbreviations for Route of Administration			
AD, AS, AU	Right ear, left ear, each ear	Mistaken as OD, OS, OU (right eye, left eye, each eye)	Use right ear, left ear, or each ear
IN	Intranasal	Mistaken as IM or IV	Use NAS (all UPPERCASE letters) or intranasal

On The Joint Commission's "Do Not Use**" list

†Relevant mostly in handwritten medication information

List — continued on page 472

List — continued from page 471

Error-Prone Abbreviations, Symbols, and Dose Designations	Intended Meaning	Misinterpretation	Best Practice
IT	Intrathecal	Mistaken as intratracheal, intratumor, intratympanic, or inhalation therapy	Use intrathecal
OD, OS, OU	Right eye, left eye, each eye	Mistaken as AD, AS, AU (right ear, left ear, each ear)	Use right eye, left eye, or each eye
Per os	By mouth, orally	The os was mistaken as left eye (OS, oculus sinister)	Use PO, by mouth, or orally
SC, SQ, sq, or sub q	Subcutaneous(ly)	SC and sc mistaken as SL or sl (sublingual) SQ mistaken as "5 every" The q in sub q has been mistaken as "every"	Use SUBQ (all UPPER-CASE letters, without spaces or periods between letters) or subcutaneous(ly)
Abbreviations for Frequency/Instructions for Use			
HS hs	Half-strength At bedtime, hours of sleep	Mistaken as bedtime Mistaken as half-strength	Use half-strength Use HS (all UPPERCASE letters) for bedtime
o.d. or OD	Once daily	Mistaken as right eye (OD, oculus dexter), leading to oral liquid medications administered in the eye	Use daily
Q.D., QD, q.d., or qd**	Every day	Mistaken as q.i.d., especially if the period after the q or the tail of a handwritten q is misunderstood as the letter i	Use daily
Qhs	Nightly at bedtime	Mistaken as qhr (every hour)	Use nightly or HS for bedtime
Qn	Nightly or at bedtime	Mistaken as qh (every hour)	Use nightly or HS for bedtime
Q.O.D., QOD, q.o.d., or qod**	Every other day	Mistaken as qd (daily) or qid (four times daily), especially if the "o" is poorly written	Use every other day
q1d	Daily	Mistaken as qid (four times daily)	Use daily
q6PM, etc.	Every evening at 6 PM	Mistaken as every 6 hours	Use daily at 6 PM or 6 PM daily

On The Joint Commission's **"Do Not Use" list

†Relevant mostly in handwritten medication information

List — continued on page 473

List — continued from page 472

Error-Prone Abbreviations, Symbols, and Dose Designations	Intended Meaning	Misinterpretation	Best Practice
SSRI	Sliding scale regular insulin	Mistaken as selective-serotonin reuptake inhibitor	Use sliding scale (insulin)
SSI	Sliding scale insulin	Mistaken as Strong Solution of Iodine (Lugol's)	
TIW or tiw	3 times a week	Mistaken as 3 times a day or twice in a week	Use 3 times weekly
BIW or biw	2 times a week	Mistaken as 2 times a day	Use 2 times weekly
UD	As directed (ut dictum)	Mistaken as unit dose (e.g., an order for "dilTIAZem infusion UD" was mistakenly administered as a unit [bolus] dose)	Use as directed
Miscellaneous Abbreviations Associated with Medication Use			
BBA	Baby boy A (twin)	B in BBA mistaken as twin B rather than gender (boy)	When assigning identifiers to newborns, use the mother's last name, the baby's gender (boy or girl), and a distinguishing identifier for all multiples (e.g., Smith girl A, Smith girl B)
BGB	Baby girl B (twin)	B at end of BGB mistaken as gender (boy) not twin B	
D/C	Discharge or discontinue	Premature discontinuation of medications when D/C (intended to mean discharge) on a medication list was misinterpreted as discontinued	Use discharge and discontinue or stop
IJ	Injection	Mistaken as IV or intrajugular	Use injection
OJ	Orange juice	Mistaken as OD or OS (right or left eye); drugs meant to be diluted in orange juice may be given in the eye	Use orange juice
Period following abbreviations (e.g., mg., mL.)†	mg or mL	Unnecessary period mistaken as the number 1, especially if written poorly	Use mg, mL, etc., without a terminal period

On The Joint Commission's **"Do Not Use" list

†Relevant mostly in handwritten medication information

List — continued on page 474

List — continued from page 473

Error-Prone Abbreviations, Symbols, and Dose Designations	Intended Meaning	Misinterpretation	Best Practice
Drug Name Abbreviations			
To prevent confusion, avoid abbreviating drug names entirely. Exceptions may be made for multi-ingredient drug formulations, including vitamins, when there are electronic drug name field space constraints; however, drug name abbreviations should NEVER be used for any medications on the *ISMP List of High-Alert Medications* (in Acute Care Settings [www.ismp.org/node/103], Community/Ambulatory Settings [www.ismp.org/node/129], and Long-Term Care Settings [www.ismp.org/node/130]). Examples of drug name abbreviations involved in serious medication errors include:			
Antiretroviral medications (e.g., DOR, TAF, TDF)	DOR: doravirine TAF: tenofovir alafenamide TDF: tenofovir disoproxil fumarate	DOR: Dovato (dolutegravir and lami**VUD**ine) TAF: tenofovir disoproxil fumarate TDF: tenofovir alafenamide	Use complete drug names
APAP	acetaminophen	Not recognized as acetaminophen	Use complete drug name
ARA A	vidarabine	Mistaken as cytarabine ("ARA C")	Use complete drug name
AT II and AT III	AT II: angiotensin II (Giapreza) AT III: antithrombin III (Thrombate III)	AT II (angiotensin II) mistaken as AT III (antithrombin III) AT III (antithrombin III) mistaken as AT II (angiotensin II)	Use complete drug names
AZT	zidovudine (Retrovir)	Mistaken as azithromycin, aza**THIO**prine, or aztreonam	Use complete drug name
CPZ	Compazine (prochlorperazine)	Mistaken as chlorpro**MAZINE**	Use complete drug name
DTO	diluted tincture of opium or deodorized tincture of opium (Paregoric)	Mistaken as tincture of opium	Use complete drug name
HCT	hydrocortisone	Mistaken as hydro**CHLORO**thiazide	Use complete drug name
HCTZ	hydro**CHLORO**thiazide	Mistaken as hydrocortisone (e.g., seen as HCT250 mg)	Use complete drug name
MgSO4**	magnesium sulfate	Mistaken as morphine sulfate	Use complete drug name
MS, MSO4**	morphine sulfate	Mistaken as magnesium sulfate	Use complete drug name

On The Joint Commission's "Do Not Use**" list

†Relevant mostly in handwritten medication information

List — continued on page 475

List — continued from page 474

Error-Prone Abbreviations, Symbols, and Dose Designations	Intended Meaning	Misinterpretation	Best Practice
MTX	methotrexate	Mistaken as mito**XANTRONE**	Use complete drug name
Na at the beginning of a drug name (e.g., Na bicarbonate)	Sodium bicarbonate	Mistaken as no bicarbonate	Use complete drug name
NoAC	novel/new oral anticoagulant	Mistaken as no anticoagulant	Use complete drug name
OXY	oxytocin	Mistaken as oxy**CODONE**, Oxy**CONTIN**	Use complete drug name
PCA	procainamide	Mistaken as patient-controlled analgesia	Use complete drug name
PIT	Pitocin (oxytocin)	Mistaken as Pitressin, a discontinued brand of vasopressin still referred to as PIT	Use complete drug name
PNV	prenatal vitamins	Mistaken as penicillin VK	Use complete drug name
PTU	propylthiouracil	Mistaken as Purinethol (mercaptopurine)	Use complete drug name
T3	Tylenol with codeine No. 3	Mistaken as liothyronine, which is sometimes referred to as T3	Use complete drug name
TAC or tac	triamcinolone or tacrolimus	Mistaken as tetracaine, Adrenalin, and cocaine; or as Taxotere, Adriamycin, and cyclophosphamide	Use complete drug names Avoid drug regimen or protocol acronyms that may have a dual meaning or may be confused with other common acronyms, even if defined in an order set
TNK	TNKase	Mistaken as TPA	Use complete drug name
TPA or tPA	tissue plasminogen activator, Activase (alteplase)	Mistaken as TNK (TNKase, tenecteplase), TXA (tranexamic acid), or less often as another tissue plasminogen activator, Retavase (retaplase)	Use complete drug names
TXA	tranexamic acid	Mistaken as TPA (tissue plasminogen activator)	Use complete drug name
ZnSO4	zinc sulfate	Mistaken as morphine sulfate	Use complete drug name

**On The Joint Commission's "Do Not Use" list

†Relevant mostly in handwritten medication information

List — continued on page 476

List — continued from page 475

Error-Prone Abbreviations, Symbols, and Dose Designations	Intended Meaning	Misinterpretation	Best Practice
Stemmed/Coined Drug Names			
Nitro drip	nitroglycerin infusion	Mistaken as nitroprusside infusion	Use complete drug name
IV vanc	Intravenous vancomycin	Mistaken as Invanz	Use complete drug name
Levo	levofloxacin	Mistaken as Levophed (norepinephrine)	Use complete drug name
Neo	Neo-Synephrine, a well known but discontinued brand of phenylephrine	Mistaken as neostigmine	Use complete drug name
Coined names for compounded products (e.g., magic mouthwash, banana bag, GI cocktail, half and half, pink lady)	Specific ingredients compounded together	Mistaken ingredients	Use complete drug/ product names for all ingredients Coined names for compounded products should only be used if the contents are standardized and readily available for reference to prescribers, pharmacists, and nurses
Number embedded in drug name (not part of the official name) (e.g., 5-fluorouracil, 6-mercaptopurine)	fluorouracil mercaptopurine	Embedded number mistaken as the dose or number of tablets/capsules to be administered	Use complete drug names, without an embedded number if the number is not part of the official drug name
Dose Designations and Other Information			
1/2 tablet	Half tablet	1 or 2 tablets	Use text (half tablet) or reduced font-size fractions (½ tablet)
Doses expressed as Roman numerals (e.g., V)	5	Mistaken as the designated letter (e.g., the letter V) or the wrong numeral (e.g., 10 instead of 5)	Use only Arabic numerals (e.g., 1, 2, 3) to express doses
Lack of a leading zero before a decimal point (e.g., .5 mg)**	0.5 mg	Mistaken as 5 mg if the decimal point is not seen	Use a leading zero before a decimal point when the dose is less than one measurement unit
Trailing zero after a decimal point (e.g., 1.0 mg)**	1 mg	Mistaken as 10 mg if the decimal point is not seen	Do not use trailing zeros for doses expressed in whole numbers

On The Joint Commission's **"Do Not Use" list

†Relevant mostly in handwritten medication information

List — continued on page 477

List — continued from page 476

Error-Prone Abbreviations, Symbols, and Dose Designations	Intended Meaning	Misinterpretation	Best Practice
Ratio expression of a strength of a single-entity inject-able drug product (e.g., EPINEPHrine 1:1,000; 1:10,000; 1:100,000)	1:1,000: contains 1 mg/mL 1:10,000: contains 0.1 mg/mL 1:100,000: contains 0.01 mg/mL	Mistaken as the wrong strength	Express the strength in terms of quantity per total volume (e.g., **EPINEPH**rine 1 mg per 10 mL) **Exception:** combination local anesthetics (e.g., lidocaine 1% and **EPINEPH**rine 1:100,000)
Drug name and dose run together (problematic for drug names that end in the letter l [e.g., propranolol20 mg; TEGretol300 mg])	propranolol 20 mg **TEG**retol 300 mg	Mistaken as propranolol 120 mg Mistaken as **TEG**retol 1300 mg	Place adequate space between the drug name, dose, and unit of measure
Numerical dose and unit of measure run together (e.g., 10mg, 10Units)	10 mg 10 mL	The m in mg, or U in Units, has been mistaken as one or two zeros when flush against the dose (e.g., 10mg, 10Units), risking a 10- to 100-fold overdose	Place adequate space between the dose and unit of measure
Large doses with-out properly placed commas (e.g., 100000 units; 1000000 units)	100,000 units 1,000,000 units	100000 has been mistaken as 10,000 or 1,000,000 1000000 has been mis-taken as 100,000	Use commas for dosing units at or above 1,000 or use words such as 100 thousand or 1 million to improve readability **Note:** Use commas to separate digits only in the US; commas are used in place of decimal points in some other countries
Symbols			
℥ or ℳ †	Dram Minim	Symbol for dram mistaken as the number 3 Symbol for minim mis-taken as mL	Use the metric system
x1	Administer once	Administer for 1 day	Use explicit words (e.g., for 1 dose)

**On The Joint Commission's "Do Not Use" list

†Relevant mostly in handwritten medication information

List — continued on page 478

List — continued from page 477

Error-Prone Abbreviations, Symbols, and Dose Designations	Intended Meaning	Misinterpretation	Best Practice
> **and** <	More than and less than	Mistaken as opposite of intended Mistakenly have used the incorrect symbol < mistaken as the number 4 when handwritten (e.g., <10 misread as 40)	Use more than or less than
↑ **and** ↓†	Increase and decrease	Mistaken as opposite of intended Mistakenly have used the incorrect symbol ↑ mistaken as the letter T, leading to misinterpretation as the start of a drug name, or mistaken as the numbers 4 or 7	Use increase and decrease
/ (slash mark)†	Separates two doses or indicates per	Mistaken as the number 1 (e.g., 25 units/10 units misread as 25 units and 110 units)	Use per rather than a slash mark to separate doses
@†	At	Mistaken as the number 2	Use at
&†	And	Mistaken as the number 2	Use and
+†	Plus or and	Mistaken as the number 4	Use plus, and, or in addition to
°	Hour	Mistaken as a zero (e.g., q2° seen as q20)	Use hr, h, or hour
Φ **or** φ†	Zero, null sign	Mistaken as the numbers 4, 6, 8, and 9	Use 0 or zero, or describe intent using whole words
#	Pound(s)	Mistaken as a number sign	Use the metric system (kg or g) rather than pounds Use lb if referring to pounds

---

On The Joint Commission's "Do Not Use**" list

†Relevant mostly in handwritten medication information

List — continued on page 479

List — continued from page 478

Error-Prone Abbreviations, Symbols, and Dose Designations	Intended Meaning	Misinterpretation	Best Practice
Apothecary or Household Abbreviations			
Explicit apothecary or household measurements may **ONLY** be safely used to express the directions for mixing dry ingredients to prepare topical products (e.g., dissolve 2 capfuls of granules per gallon of warm water to prepare a magnesium sulfate soaking aid). Otherwise, metric system measurements should be used.			
gr	Grain(s)	Mistaken as gram	Use the metric system (e.g., mcg, g)
dr	Dram(s)	Mistaken as doctor	Use the metric system (e.g., mL)
min	Minim(s)	Mistaken as minutes	Use the metric system (e.g., mL)
oz	Ounce(s)	Mistaken as zero or 0_2	Use the metric system (e.g., mL)
tsp	Teaspoon(s)	Mistaken as tablespoon(s)	Use the metric system (e.g., mL)
tbsp or Tbsp	Tablespoon(s)	Mistaken as teaspoon(s)	Use the metric system (e.g., mL)

Common Abbreviations with Contradictory Meanings	Contradictory Meanings		Correction
For additional information and tables from Neil Davis (MedAbbrev.com) containing additional examples of abbreviations with contradictory or ambiguous meanings, please visit: www.ismp.org/ext/638.			
B	Breast, brain, or bladder		Use breast, brain, or bladder
C	Cerebral, coronary, or carotid		Use cerebral, coronary, or carotid
D or d	Day or dose (e.g., parameter-based dosing formulas using D or d [mg/kg/d] could be interpreted as either day or dose [mg/kg/day or mg/kg/dose]; or x3d could be interpreted as either 3 days or 3 doses)		Use day or dose
H	Hand or hip		Use hand or hip
I	Impaired or improvement		Use impaired or improvement
L	Liver or lung		Use liver or lung
N	No or normal		Use no or normal
P	Pancreas, prostate, preeclampsia, or psychosis		Use pancreas, prostate, preeclampsia, or psychosis

**On The Joint Commission's "Do Not Use" list

†Relevant mostly in handwritten medication information

List — continued on page 480

List — continued from page 479

Error-Prone Abbreviations, Symbols, and Dose Designations	Intended Meaning	Misinterpretation	Best Practice
S	Special or standard		Use special or standard
SS or ss	Single strength, sliding scale (insulin), signs and symptoms, or ½ (apothecary) SS has also been mistaken as the number 55		Use single strength, sliding scale, signs and symptoms, or one-half or ½

On The Joint Commission's "Do Not Use**" list

†Relevant mostly in handwritten medication information

While the abbreviations, symbols, and dose designations in the **Table** should **NEVER** be used, not allowing the use of **ANY** abbreviations is exceedingly unlikely. Therefore, the person who uses an organization-approved abbreviation must take responsibility for making sure that it is properly interpreted. If an uncommon or ambiguous abbreviation is used, and it should be defined by the writer or sender. Where uncertainty exists, clarification with the person who used the abbreviation is required.

Insulin

Chapter 14 focuses on insulin types, syringes, pens, and injection sites, and implications related to the administration of insulin. Below is an insulin table of all of the types of insulins according to their time of action.

Types of Insulin and Action Times

Insulin Combinations	Onset	Peak	Duration
Humalog 75/25® insulin lispro protamine suspension-insulin lispro injection mixtures, rDNA origin	15–30 min	2.8 hr	24 hr
Humalog 50/50® insulin lispro protamine suspension-insulin lispro injection mixtures, rDNA origin	15–30 min	2.8 hr	24 hr
Novolog 70/30® insulin aspart protamine suspension— insulin aspart injection mixtures, rDNA origin	15 min	1–4 hr	18–24 hr
Humulin/Novolin 70/30® NPH 70% Regular 30%	30 min	2–12 hr	24 hr
Rapid-acting Insulin	**Onset**	**Peak**	**Duration**
Novolog® or Fiasp® insulin aspart	Within 15 min	1–2 hr	3–4 hr
Apidra® insulin glulisine	Within 15 min	1–2 hr	3–4 hr
Humalog® Admelog® Lyumjev® insulin lispro	Within 15 min	1–2 hr	3–4 hr

(continued)

Short-acting Insulin	Onset	Peak	Duration
Afrezza® insulin, inhalation	Within 30 min	30–60 min	160 min
Humulin R® Novolin R® insulin regular (Intravenous-IV)	10–30 min	15–30 min	30–60 min
Humulin R® Novolin R® insulin regular (Subcutaneous-SUBQ)	30–60 min	2–4 hr	5–7 hr
Intermediate-acting Insulin	Onset	Peak	Duration
Humulin N® Novolin N® NPH	2–4 hr	4–10 hr	10–16 hr
Long-acting Insulin	Onset	Peak	Duration
Levemir® insulin detemir	3–4 hr	3–14 hr	6–24 hr
Lantus® Basaglar® insulin glargine – 100u/mL	3–4 hr	No Peak	24 hr
Toujeo® insulin glargine – 300u/mL	Develops over 6 hr	No Peak	24 hr
Tresiba® insulin degludec	Within 2 hr	12 hr	Up to 42 hr

Administering insulin based on a sliding scale, or coverage, during hospitalization is needed when clients are ill. Insulin needs change with infection, surgery, medications, etc. A sliding-scale chart will be included with the physician's orders. Sliding-scale orders will not be the same for every client. The client's blood sugar will be checked before meals and at bedtime, and the sliding scale will be used for insulin coverage at those times. See the following chart for an example of a sliding-scale order:

Glucose (mg/dL) (blood sugar)	Insulin Dose (Regular Insulin) Administer Subcutaneously
0–140	No coverage
141–200	2 units
201–260	4 units
261–320	6 units
321–399	8 units
400 or greater	Call the physician stat

Medication Label Index

Index